I0882099

Decision Making

Decision Making is an exciting new collection of recent research into the actual processes that people use when making decisions in their everyday lives. Rather than use the more traditional mathematical theories that seldom match real behaviour, the contributors use cognitive psychological techniques to break down the constituent processes and set them in their social context.

Containing contributions from well-respected international researchers into decision making, the book offers overviews and critical evaluations of significant recent studies. It examines the nature of the psychological processes underlying decision making, and addresses a range of important topics including the role of emotions, coping with uncertainty, time pressure and confidence in decisions. *Decision Making* first places the process approach to decision research in a historical and theoretical context and provides a critical evaluation of its principal research methods. Contributors then consider the influence of values, involvement and emotions upon decision making and issues concerning risk and uncertainty. A final section examines time pressure, the effects of past decisions, and post-decision processes. Decision making is regarded as an interaction between decision maker, problem and context and is thus placed in a social environment.

Decision Making provides an overview of current thinking in the psychology of decision making and will be a valuable resource for cognitive psychologists in applied settings, economists and managers.

Rob Ranyard is Reader in Psychology at the Bolton Institute. **Ray Crozier** is Senior Lecturer in Psychology of Education at the University of Wales, Cardiff. His previous publications include *Individual Learners: Personality Differences in Education* (1997). **Ola Svenson** is Professor of Psychology at Stockholm University. His previous publications include *Time Pressure and Stress in Human Judgement and Decision Making* (1993). All three are founder members of the European Group of Process Studies of Decision Making.

Frontiers of Cognitive Science
Series Advisor: Tim Valentine
Goldsmiths College, University of London

Cognitive Science is a new interdisciplinary area including cognitive psychology, neuroscience, computer science, linguistics and philosophy. In 'Frontiers of Cognitive Science', authors from a range of backgrounds have been encouraged to present up-to-date and comprehensive coverage of a central area of current research interest. New applied areas and emerging topics showing special promise will be included alongside the purely theoretical. The books will be particularly useful to researchers and graduate students wishing to access a new topic in this exciting field.

Forthcoming titles:

The Nature, Representation and Evolution of Concepts
Philip van Loocke

Understanding driving:
Cognitive aspects of an everyday task
John Groeger

Decision Making

Cognitive models and explanations

Edited by Rob Ranyard,
W. Ray Crozier and Ola Svenson

Routledge
Taylor & Francis Group
London and New York

First published 1997 by Routledge
2 Park Square, Milton Park, Abingdon, Oxon, OX14 4RN

Simultaneously published in the USA and Canada
by Routledge
711 Third Avenue, New York, NY 10017

Routledge is an imprint of the Taylor & Francis Group

First issued in paperback 2011

Typeset in Times by Florencetype Ltd, Stoodleigh, Devon

British Library Cataloguing in Publication Data
A catalogue record for this book is available from the British Library

Library of Congress Cataloguing in Publication Data
Decision making: cognitive models and explanations / edited by Rob Ranyard, W. Ray Crozier, and Ola Svenson.
p. cm. – (Frontiers of cognitive science)
Includes bibliographical references and index.
ISBN 0–415–15818–4 (hardcover)
1. Decision-making. 2. Cognition. I. Ranyard, Rob. II. Crozier, W. Ray, 1945– . III. Svenson, Ola. IV. Series.
BF448.D42 1997
153.8′3–DC21 97–15835
CIP

ISBN13: 978-0-415-15818-3 (hbk)
ISBN13: 978-0-415-51359-3 (pbk)

Publisher's Note
The publisher has gone to great lengths to ensure the quality of this reprint but points out that some imperfections in the original may be apparent

Contents

List of figures and tables

FIGURES

TABLES

Contributors

Wibecke Brun is a research fellow at the Research Centre for Health Promotion, University of Bergen, Norway. She received her Ph.D. degree from the University of Bergen in 1995. Her main research interests are in the areas of risk perception and subjective probability judgement. [*The Hemil Centre, University of Bergen, Christiesgt, 13, 5015 Bergen, Norway.*]

Ray Crozier is Senior Lecturer in the Psychology of Education in the University of Wales, Cardiff. His current research interests are in decision making, psychological aesthetics and shyness. [*School of Education, University of Wales, 21 Senghennydd Road, Cardiff CF2 4YG, UK.*]

Anne C. Edland is a member of the Risk Analysis and Decision Group at the University of Stockholm, Sweden. She has completed her doctorate and published several academic papers on time pressure. [*Department of Psychology, University of Stockholm, S-106 91 Stockholm, Sweden.*]

Tommy Gärling is Professor of Psychology at Göteborg University, Sweden. His primary research area is judgement and decision making including applications to travel demand modelling and environmentally friendly consumption. [*Department of Psychology, Göteborg University, Haraldsgatan 1, S-413 14 Göteborg, Sweden.*]

Johanna M. Harte is a Research Psychologist at the Pieter Baan Centre, Utrecht. Her research interests are multi-attribute evaluation processes and diagnostic decision making. [*Pieter Baan Centre, Forensic Psychiatric Observation Clinic, Gansstraat 170, 3582 EP Utrecht, The Netherlands.*]

Teci Hill is a Ph.D. student at the Department of Psychology at Stockholm University, Sweden. Her current research concerns status-quo decisions. [*Department of Psychology, University of Stockholm, S-106 91 Stockholm, Sweden.*]

Oswald Huber is Professor of Psychology in the University of Fribourg, Switzerland. His research interests include process tracing studies in multi-attribute and risky decision making, and multi-stage decisions. [*Department of Psychology, University of Fribourg, rue de Faucigny 2, CH-1701 Fribourg, Switzerland.*]

Niklas Karlsson is a graduate student in Psychology at Göteborg University, Sweden, working on a thesis in behavioural decision making. He is interested in the time parameters of decisions, in particular how decisions change with prior experience. [*Department of Psychology, Göteborg University, Haraldsgatan 1, S-413 14 Göteborg, Sweden.*]

Anna Blom Kemdal is a doctoral student of Psychology at Stockholm University, Sweden. Her research deals with decision making in naturalistic contexts and with the role of perspectives in attitude formation. [*Department of Psychology, University of Stockholm, S-106 91 Stockholm, Sweden.*]

José Kerstholt works as a research scientist at the Department of Information Processing of TNO Human Factors Research Institute, Soesterberg, The Netherlands. She received her Ph.D. in Psychology from the University of Amsterdam in 1996. Her research interests include basic and applied research on dynamic decision processes, time pressure effects, fatigue and supervisory control. [*Department of Information Processing, TNO Human Factors Research Institute, Kampweg 5, PO Box 23, 3769 ZG Soesterberg, The Netherlands.*]

Pieter Koele is Senior Lecturer in Judgement and Decision Making in the Faculty of Psychology at the University of Amsterdam, The Netherlands. He is Judgement and Decision Making Editor of *Acta Psychologica*, and has written journal articles and book chapters on statistics, psychometrics, subjective probability and decision making. [*Faculty of Psychology, University of Amsterdam, Roetersstraat 15, 1018 WB Amsterdam, The Netherlands.*]

Anton Kühberger received his Ph.D. from the University of Salzburg, Austria, and is currently Assistant Professor of Psychology at the University of Salzburg. His areas of interest are judgement and decision making. [*Institute of Psychology, University of Salzburg, Hellbrunnerstr. 34 A-5020 Salzburg, Austria.*]

Maria Lewicka is an Associate Professor at the Faculty of Psychology, University of Warsaw, Poland. Her research and theoretical interests include processes of evaluation, the interrelationship between affect and cognition, human rationality and cognitive biases, and affective disorders (depression). [*Faculty of Psychology, University of Warsaw, Stawki 5/7, PL00–183 Warsaw, Poland.*]

John Maule is Senior Lecturer in Management Decision Making at Leeds University Business School. His research interests are in the effects of mood, emotion and time pressure on decision making and informed decision making in patients. [*Leeds University Business School, University of Leeds, 11 Blenheim Terrace, Leeds LS2 9JT, UK.*]

Henry Montgomery is Professor of Cognitive Psychology at Stockholm University, Sweden. His present research concerns the role of perspectives and perspective shifts in decision making and attitude formation. [*Department of Psychology, University of Stockholm, S-106 91 Stockholm, Sweden.*]

Jeroen Raaijmakers is Professor of Psychology at the University of Amsterdam, The Netherlands, and Director of the Graduate Research Institute for Experimental Psychology (EPOS). He received his Ph.D. in Psychology from the University of Nijmegen in 1979. [*Faculty of Psychology, University of Amsterdam, Roeterstraat 15, 1018 WB Amsterdam, The Netherlands.*]

Rob Ranyard is Reader in Psychology at Bolton Institute of Higher Education, UK. His research interests includes process tracing studies of decisions under risk, qualitative studies of financial decision making and analyses of how important decisions are communicated. [*Psychology Subject Group, Bolton Institute of Higher Education, Deane Road, Bolton BL3 5AB, UK.*]

Joakim Romanus is a graduate student in Psychology working on a thesis in behavioural decision making at the University of Göteborg, Sweden. He is interested in the time parameters of decisions, in particular how decisions change with prior experience. [*Department of Psychology, Göteborg University, Haraldsgatan 1, S-413 14 Göteborg, Sweden.*]

Marcus Selart is Lecturer in Psychology at Göteborg University, Sweden. His research centres on the psychology of thinking and reasoning and, in particular, issues related to process tracing methods. [*Department of Psychology, Göteborg University, Haraldsgatan 1, S-413 14 Göteborg, Sweden.*]

Ola Svenson has been Professor of Psychology at Stockholm University, Sweden, since 1993. Before that he was Professor of Psychology at Lund University. His research interests include cognitive psychology, decision processes, human factors and risk analysis. [*Department of Psychology, University of Stockholm, S-106 91 Stockholm, Sweden.*]

Karl Halvor Teigen is Professor of Cognitive Psychology at the University of Tromsø, Norway. He was educated at the University of Oslo and for several years held various academic positions at the University of Bergen. His main publications are on subjective probability judgements, but he has also carried out studies on social cognition, cognitive motivation, and the history of psychology. [*Department of Psychology, University of Tromsø, N-9037 Tromsø, Norway.*]

Bas Verplanken is an Associate Professor in Social Psychology at the University of Nijmegen, The Netherlands. His current research interests are in the areas of attitude theory, social cognition and decision making. [*Department of Psychology, University of Nijmegen, PO Box 9104, 6500 HE Nijmegen, The Netherlands.*]

Dan Zakay received his Ph.D. in Cognitive Psychology from the Department of Psychology at Tel-Aviv University, Israel. He currently holds the title of Associate Professor at Tel-Aviv University. His research interests are in decision making, judgement and subjective time. [*Department of Psychology, the University of Tel-Aviv, Ramat-Aviv, Israel.*]

Acknowledgements

The editors are very grateful to Sheila Buckthorpe of Bolton Institute for her patience and skill in the preparation of the final typescript. We also thank the following for their constructive and critical reviews of draft chapters: Tommy Gärling, Oswald Huber, Pieter Koele, Maria Lewicka, Henry Montgomery, Bas Verplanken and Dan Zakay.

The following have been reprinted by courtesy of their copyright holders:

Figure 1.1, page 7, © 1979 The Econometric Society.
Figure 4.2, page 64, © 1997 Academic Press.
Figure 4.2, page 63, © 1997 Academic Press.
Extract from *The House at Pooh Corner* by A.A. Milne, page 112, published by Methuen Childrens Books 1974, © 1974 Reed Consumer Books Ltd.

Part I

Fundamentals

Introduction to Part I

This book comprises a set of chapters which have been especially written for this volume and which offer a description and a critical evaluation of important research on the psychology of decision making. The chapters examine the nature of the psychological processes underlying decision making and the problems that people face in their everyday decisions. The authors' approach is concerned with explaining how decisions are made in terms of motives, cognitive processes and mental representations. They draw on the insights of cognitive psychology to analyse the decision into more elementary processes. As such, this is a descriptive approach that can be contrasted with the normative and mathematical theories that have dominated much psychological and economic thinking in the study of decision making. The emphasis is on the analysis of what individuals actually do rather than on comparisons with idealised optimal or rational decision makers. The decision process is considered to be one that is extended in time: it involves a series of information search, judgement and evaluation processes which are followed by further post-decision processes that serve to help people to adjust to the implications of their decisions and to understand their own goals and values. It is recognised that decisions are made within a social context and need to be justified to oneself and to others. In a similar vein the question of helping people to improve their decisions is approached from considerations of how they actually make them, rather than from a narrow focus on discrepancies between actual and idealised decisions.

The chapters cover and summarise important decision research up to 1996. The intention is that the volume should serve as a source book for those who want to update their knowledge about research within the descriptive decision making approach. In addition, the book presents some of the most recent results of the authors' own decision making research.

Part I consists of two chapters. The first, by Crozier and Ranyard, provides an introduction to the volume by identifying the themes and issues which characterise contemporary research on decision making from a cognitive perspective. It traces the origins and development of this approach since the 1950s, and introduces some of the key theoretical and empirical issues facing it.

Many everyday decisions fall into the category of multiattribute choice problems in which conflicts across a set of attributes can be identified. For example, consumer purchases usually involve a conflict between price and quality. In Chapter 2, Harte and Koele discuss process tracing research into multiattribute decision making and raise important methodological and psychometric issues. First they give an overview of the main research paradigms in this area based on the analysis of information search patterns and verbal protocols. The authors draw a distinction between research intended to describe individual decision processes, and research aimed at testing hypotheses about factors influencing them. They go on to make valuable recommendations of research designs which will yield more reliable descriptions of individual decision processes and more powerful tests of factors influencing these processes. Process tracing techniques are illustrated and discussed in several subsequent chapters. Selart, and Kemdal and Montgomery (Chapters 4 and 5) analyse verbal data while Lewicka and Huber (Chapters 6 and 9) summarise studies which monitor information search. Taken together, then, Chapters 1 and 2 provide the background for the chapters which follow and set them in a broader context.

Chapter 1

Cognitive process models and explanations of decision making

Ray Crozier and Rob Ranyard

Decision making is fundamental to modern life in its individual, collective and corporate aspects. Individuals in the developed world are faced with personal decisions to an extent that previous generations would have found difficult to imagine. A combination of economic, social and technological developments has produced a situation where people have to make important decisions about their relationships and family life, their health, and their education and careers. They are involved in the management of their personal finances as home owners and consumers. Decisions are also fundamental at a societal level. The ballot box is central to democratic political systems as is the jury to the legal system. Business and financial institutions are faced daily with decisions about investment, research and development, and deployment of resources in a complex and uncertain environment.

It is perhaps the social and economic significance of decisions that has resulted in the considerable influence upon psychological approaches to the study of decision making of concepts from other disciplines, in particular, economics. The concepts of utility and subjective probability and theories that account for their integration have shaped psychological enquiry and influenced its research paradigms.

Subjectively expected utility (SEU) theory is a model of rational behaviour, originating in economics and mathematics. This assumes that decisions should be reached by summing over the set of alternatives the utility of each alternative weighted by the subjective probability of its occurrence. Its elegance and authoritative status provide an incentive for decision makers to apply it to their own situation. Nevertheless, the value of utility maximisation as a normative choice principle was criticised, for example, by Simon (1957), who argued that people can successfully adapt to their environment by identifying actions that are merely satisfactory for their goals. He proposed the alternative normative principle of satisficing: take the first course of action that is satisfactory on all important aspects. He argued that this principle could be applied without sophisticated powers of discrimination and evaluation, powers that humans do not possess. He thus developed the concept of bounded rationality, which incorporates the basic assumption that rationality is relative to the information processing capacities of the decision maker. We return to this point below.

Moreover, the status of SEU as a model that describes how people actually make decisions did not receive unequivocal support from empirical studies. Edwards and Tversky (1967: 123) summarised the early research as follows:

> These studies . . . generally show consistent, orderly, rational performance. The SEU model is clearly wrong in detail; certain invariances, that should exist if it were right, do not exist. But the sizes of the discrepancies indicate that no one is likely to lose his shirt by making bets that grossly deviate from rationality – whether rationality is defined as maximization of SEU or even as maximization of expected value.

Much of this initial phase of psychological research was concerned with issues of measuring utility and subjective probability. Later research explored empirical findings that one and the same decision problem could produce different decisions either because of variation in the ways in which it was presented or because different response measures were used, even though these were supposed to be equivalent indices of preferences (see Selart, Chapter 4). These findings were difficult to explain in terms of a behavioural model of rational behaviour.

One approach to reducing these discrepancies between behaviour and the SEU theory has been to develop fresh theories that provide a better account of some of these findings. Such theories can be described as 'structural', in that they relate decisions to structural characteristics of the decision problem. One of the most influential of these has been prospect theory proposed by Kahneman and Tversky (1979). This theory assumed that, in well-defined risk problems, stated probabilities are translated into subjective weights according to the function shown in Figure 1.1 (Kahneman and Tversky, 1979: 283). If the weighting function followed the diagonal line shown on the graph, then decision weights would correspond exactly to stated outcome probabilities. Prospect theory proposes, however, that for very low probabilities weights are higher, but otherwise they are lower than stated probabilities. Kahneman and Tversky note that the function does *not* represent subjective estimates of probability; rather, it reflects the weight given to well-defined risky prospects in preferential choice situations. The overweighing of very low probabilities predicts some aspects of gambling and insurance behaviour, and the general slope of the function reflects the sensitivity of preference to changes in outcome probability. This treatment of well-defined probabilities is one reason why prospect theory represents a significant advance over SEU theory as a

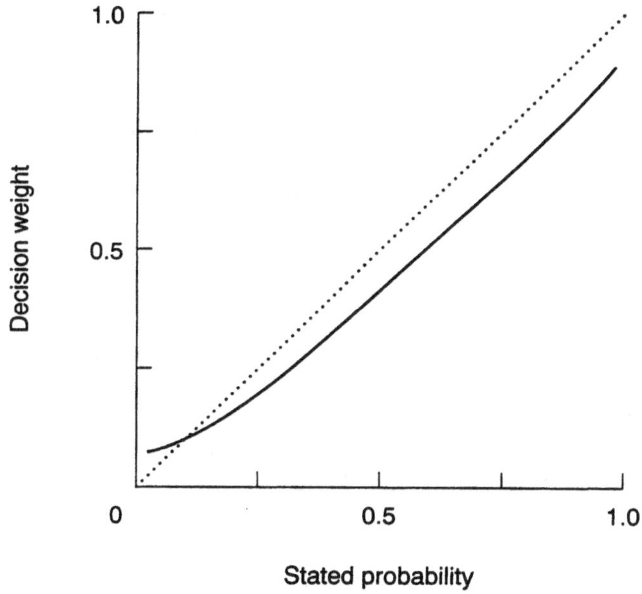

Figure 1.1 Prospect theory's probability weighting function

descriptive model of risky decision making. The concept of the decision weight is more coherent than the notion implicit in SEU theory that people distort stated probabilities when they have no good reason to do so. Prospect theory also included a major advance in the way evaluations of outcomes were conceptualised and, in general, it provided a parsimonious account of subjects' behaviour on several experimental tasks that was difficult to explain in terms of the SEU theory.

The erosion of the dominant role played by SEU theory in decision research coincided with changes in psychology more generally. In particular, behaviourist approaches, with their emphasis on the discovery of functional relationships between task variables and behavioural outcomes, were displaced by cognitive psychology. One form of explanation that has been influential in cognitive psychology is the 'information processing' model that sets out a sequence of mental operations that takes place between the presentation of a stimulus and the execution of a response. This trend in psychology also had an impact upon research into decision making, particularly in the development of the 'process' approach. This is characterised by Svenson (1996: 252) as follows:

> In process approaches the researcher follows and draws conclusions about the psychological process from problem presentation to decision through collecting process tracing measures, such as information search

and think aloud protocols. Hypotheses and theories based on process approach data can later be tested in new process or structural approaches.

The remainder of this chapter examines implications of the process approach for the study of decision making and briefly considers issues that have arisen in research that has been influenced by this approach.

PROCESS STUDIES OF DECISION MAKING

First, we consider the implications of this approach for the methods used to study decision making. It is noteworthy that Svenson's characterisation assigns a central place to process tracing methods. Second, we identify some significant features of process explanations of decision making. We suggest that these features include: (a) an emphasis upon the temporal dimension of decision making, that is, the decision process is regarded as extended in time; (b) a revitalisation of, and a fresh role for, the concept of decision rule that is associated with the picture of an adaptive decision maker, drawing upon a range of possible strategies in order to reach a decision; (c) the notion that decision makers change their representation of the problem in order to reach a decision. Finally, we consider some trends that can be identified in cognitive psychology that are also evident in decision research. The first of these is a concern with the ecological validity of laboratory methods and the extent to which findings from experimental methods can be generalised to the 'real world'. The second trend involves the forging of closer links between cognitive and social psychology. The third is an awareness of the important role of affect in cognitive processes.

Process tracing methods

Although some research has used the recording of eye movements in an attempt to capture the information that is sought by decision makers (e.g., Russo and Rosen, 1975), the most frequently used methods have been the information board technique and think aloud protocols. The information board displays information that is relevant to a decision on a number of cards that are arranged on a display that takes the form of an alternatives × attributes matrix (such matrices can also be displayed on a computer, with the participant selecting information by moving and clicking the mouse). For example, the rows of the matrix can refer to a set of alternative apartments and the columns to attributes, such as cost of rent, distance from workplace, size of rooms, and so on. The participant in the study requests information by asking for the information on cards to be made visible, and the sequence of cards requested can be recorded. Attempts can be made to identify the decision strategies adopted by the participants and to test hypotheses about information search on the basis of these sequences (see, for example, Payne, 1976; Koele and Westenberg, 1995). The influence of task variables upon information search can be investigated. For example, Lewicka (Chapter 6) reports evidence that decisions where the goal is to accept one alternative from a set (e.g., to appoint a candidate for a post or to select an article for publication) tend to produce more inspection of the attributes of particular alternatives whereas decisions to reject an alternative produce more inspection of different alternatives on one attribute. In a further example, Maule and Edland (Chapter 11) report that increasing time pressure upon decisions results in more attention being paid to important attribute information about each alternative and, more generally, produces increased use of attribute-based processing relative to alternative-based processing.

The collection of verbal protocols by asking participants to 'think aloud' while making a decision has been controversial, since it can be interpreted as representing a return to previously discredited methods of introspection. Hence, it can elicit criticism on the grounds of 'reactivity', where the instruction to verbalise changes the process that is the subject of investigation. However, seminal reports by Ericsson and Simon (1980, 1993) set out conditions under which the collection of concurrent verbal protocols could avoid such problems, and a considerable body of research has now used this approach to study decision processes (Ford *et al.*, 1989; Montgomery and Svenson, 1989; Westenberg and Koele, 1994; Payne, 1994).

It is essential to distinguish process tracing via verbal protocols from qualitative approaches or methods of content analysis that have attracted considerable interest among psychologists in recent years. The verbal protocols are treated as *data*, that is, specific predictions are made about their contents on the basis of process theories. For example, a hypothesis can be tested about the frequency of references to the alternative that is eventually chosen at different points in the decision process. As is the case with information board methods, attempts are made to infer decision strategies from the protocols and to study the influence of task variables. The process approach raises many methodological issues, but we do not pursue these here, as they are examined in depth in the following chapter by Harte and Koele. Finally, it will be evident from the empirical studies reported throughout this volume that the cognitive approach is not restricted to these process tracing methods; a range of experimental methods are used to test hypotheses and to explore decision phenomena.

The temporal dimension

The decision process is regarded as extended in time. One way to construe this is to consider that the process can be divided into a number of phases or stages. These phases can be generated by task analysis. For example, decisions require information so it is only a small step to propose an information acquisition phase. Alternatively, the phases can be generated by theory. Prospect theory assumed that a problem formulation stage involving framing and editing processes precedes an evaluation stage. Montgomery's (1983) dominance structuring theory proposed that decision making is a search for a dominance structure, an attempt to find a representation of the decision problem such that one alternative is 'dominant', i.e., it is superior to all others on at least one attribute and is not inferior to any alternative on any of the other attributes. Search for dominance was hypothesised to go through four phases (Montgomery, 1989: 24–5): pre-editing – establishing relevant decision alternatives and attributes; finding a promising alternative; testing whether this promising alternative dominates the other alternatives; dominance-structuring, or transforming the psychological representation of alternatives so that dominance can be achieved. Svenson (1992, 1996; see Chapters 3 and 13, this volume) has developed differentiation and consolidation theory, which also proposes four stages in the decision process: detection of the decision problem; processes of differentiation of an initially chosen alternative from the other alternatives; the decision stage; the post-decision consolidation stage, to support the implementation of the decision and to protect the decision maker from regret at having made the wrong decision.

Svenson's theory assigns considerable weight to post-decision processes; not only are they viewed as important in their own right, for providing a complete picture of how decisions are reached, but they also influence the pre-decision differentiation phase. In order to protect against potential regret, differentiation processes have to be sufficiently rigorous to distinguish one alternative clearly from the others or, in the contemporary political cliché, to 'keep clear blue water' between them. The study of consolidation processes extends the time frame of decisions. It also recognises that decisions are often meaningful events in the course of someone's life, not isolated 'problems' that can be resolved once and for all.

Theories that emphasise post-decision processes also draw attention to the importance of justification processes in decision making. A justification may be defined as an argument constructed to support the position that one's decision is or was the correct one. The concept of justification has played a part in several approaches to decision making (Crozier, 1989); for example, Slovic (1975) has proposed that the ease with which a rule may be justified may be an important factor in determining its selection, and Montgomery (1983) has characterised decision making as 'a search for good arguments'. Montgomery (1983) identified a good argument with the dominance principle: if a decision could be structured in such a way that one alternative could be said to dominate another, then this would be particularly easy to argue for. In more recent theorising, as we have seen above, post-decision justification influences the pre-decision phase in that the decision maker evaluates any promising decision alternatives, at least in part, by imagining how justifiable they will be in the future.

Time affects decisions in many ways. Once the study of decision making is re-inserted into a temporal dimension, a number of issues are raised. One concerns the interdependence of decisions taken at different times. The outcomes of past actions can influence future actions. The degree of confidence in a past decision can influence one's approach to future decisions, an issue explored by Zakay (Chapter 14). One 'decision' may in fact be a sequence of decisions, each influencing the next. Alternatively, decisions may be 'dynamic' in that the situation in which the decision is to be made is not static but is always changing, and the *timing* of a decision can become an important factor (Kerstholt and Raaijmakers, Chapter 12). Their chapter studies the control of complex systems, but the issue of timing is a general one, involved in many situations from dating to the purchase and selling of shares. Presumably all decisions are dynamic in the sense that their context must inevitably be changing and 'static' decisions are simply ones where their dynamic nature is less salient. Finally, time limitations place constraints upon many decisions and influence the selection of strategies. One benefit of adopting an information processing approach is that it enables the researcher to frame questions about which phases in the decision process are affected by moderating factors such as time pressure. Issues related to the temporal dimension are investigated in several chapters in this volume, particularly in Part IV.

Decision rules

Models like SEU and prospect theory assume that decision making is a mechanical procedure. In particular, they assume that the rules for combining probabilities and outcome values are invariant across contexts. Cognitive researchers have adopted an alternative approach, whereby decision makers are conceived as having a number of strategies for making decisions available in their repertoire (Beach and Mitchell, 1978; Huber, 1989; Payne *et al.*, 1993; Svenson, 1979). The choice of a particular strategy or decision rule will be influenced by task considerations and/or by individual habits or preferences. Rather than simply following procedures, the decision maker is flexible in approach and will vary his or her behaviour, perhaps balancing the effort that needs to be expended on the problem with the requirements for accurate decisions (Payne *et al.*, 1993).

Svenson (1979) provided an influential taxonomy of decision rules. He took rules of several kinds and classified them in terms of the demands that they make upon the cognitive system. Such rules vary in the cognitive demands that they make, for example, in whether or not compensatory judgements have to be made across attributes. Thus, the dominance principle can be construed as a non-compensatory rule requiring that, for each attribute independently, the attractiveness of a decision aspect is measured only on an ordinal scale. The SEU model and prospect theory can be construed as complex, cognitively demanding rules involving compensation between attributes and across alternatives. The key point is that subjects are not bound by rules but use them in an adaptive fashion. Payne *et al.* (1993) reviewed a wide selection of evidence of context-dependent changes in decision behaviour and showed that much of it could be explained by decision rule selections. However, there has always been a strand of cognitive theory which has argued that the notion of decision rule selection is insufficient in itself.

The representation of decision information

As we have seen, decision making is represented as a process extended over time which can be divided into a number of stages or phases, one of which might be an evaluation phase involving decision rule selection. Many models and theories propose that presented information is restructured prior to the evaluation stage. For example, prospect theory assumes a problem formulation stage involving framing and editing processes. Huber (1986, 1989) assumed that people actively restructure decision problems via complex sequences of elementary information operations known as structuring plans. Other models have assumed that people change from one decision rule to another during the pre-decision phase (e.g., Payne, 1980; Beach, 1990).

At least three types of restructuring information have been identified and are considered to be important in decisions involving well-defined risks: first, the framing or coding of outcomes as gains or losses relative to some reference level, as proposed by prospect theory. It is usually assumed that the gains or losses displayed in a gamble in laboratory studies are evaluated relative to the status quo. Second is the grouping by similarity of elements of the choice problem. For example, Ranyard (1987) observed that people sometimes made choices among several gambles in two stages: at the first stage they put similar alternatives into groups and chose the best from each group; at the second stage, they chose from those alternatives selected at the first stage. The third type of restructuring operation is the *editing* operation that has been identified for gambles (e.g., Huber, 1989; Payne *et al.*, 1984; Ranyard and Crozier, 1984). For example, segregation, cancellation and combination heuristics are important elements of prospect theory (Kahneman and Tversky, 1979).

Ranyard (1995) investigated a reversal of preference between compou-nd gambles and their equivalent standard forms and found evidence that people applied generalisations of two of prospect theory's editing heuristics. The first is the cancellation-by-similarity heuristic. The analysis of verbal reports showed that people often cancel shared gamble components in a wider range of circumstances than is permitted by traditional utility theory. With standard gambles, they sometimes cancelled outcomes which were similar in value and probability, as well as ones that were identical. Furthermore, as Tversky and Kahneman (1981, 1987) have observed, people sometimes cancel common elements of compound gambles rather than conjoining them with the other elements. Neither of these uses of cancellation is strictly allowed by normative utility theory. However, Birnbaum and McIntosh (1996) failed to find evidence of cancellation of common components in gambles. The pattern of preferences shown by their subjects was incompatible with both SEU and cumulative prospect theory (see Kühberger, Chapter 8, for a description of this theory).

The second editing operation investigated by Ranyard (1995) was the amalgamation heuristic, an extension of prospect theory's combination operation to the combination of similar outcomes. In this heuristic, which is applicable to standard gambles with at least three outcomes, outcomes are grouped by similarity and their probabilities are combined. Ranyard concluded that the observed reversal of preference between compound and simple gambles occurred because subjects simplified the information presented using these heuristics. Compound gambles were routinely simplified using the cancellation heuristic whereas their equivalent standard forms were routinely simplified by the amalgamation heuristic, and sometimes by the cancellation-by-similarity heuristic. These operations produce quite different mental representations of the two gamble isomorphs, which explains the reversal of preference.

These restructuring heuristics can be understood in terms of the decision maker's need to simplify a cognitively demanding task. The notion that decision makers select a strategy on the basis of a *cost–benefit analysis*, at least in part, is a common one (e.g., Beach and Mitchell, 1978). The restructuring of information plays a more fundamental role in both Montgomery's and Svenson's theories. According to Montgomery (1983), where no alternative achieves dominance over the others, decision makers must impose a dominance structure on the decision problem. In Svenson's theory, a decision can only be reached if differentiation processes ensure that one alternative is perceived as sufficiently more attractive than the others. The theories differ in that Svenson proposes that several different decision rules can be involved in the differentiation process, depending on characteristics of the task and the decision maker (Svenson, 1996: 254), whereas Montgomery's theory emphasised the dominance rule.

Representation processes are involved in the evaluation phase of the decision process in many ways, as exemplified in several chapters of this volume, particularly in Part II. The same information can appear different to the decision maker depending on the perspective that he or she takes (Kemdal and Montgomery, Chapter 5) or the degree or kind of involvement that he or she has in a particular decision (Verplanken and Svenson, Chapter 3).

One of the more subtle forms of representation is the mental account, introduced to explain a number of anomalies in financial decision making. Tversky and Kahneman (1981: 457) illustrate such an anomaly in the 'jacket and calculator' problem:

> Imagine that you are about to purchase a jacket for $125 and a calculator for $15. The calculator salesman informs you that the calculator you want to buy is on sale for $10 at the other branch of the store, located 20 minutes' drive away. Would you make a trip to the other store?

Only 29 per cent of subjects responded that they would make the trip, but when the problem was rephrased so that the prices of jacket and calculator were reversed, with the calculator being $125 in one store and $120 in the other, 68 per cent were prepared to make the trip. Although the change in price of calculator ($5) is the same in both forms of the problem, respondents tended to represent it differently. This has been interpreted as being due to the mental account for the transaction that is primed by the problem. Kahneman and Tversky proposed three different types of accounts (see Gärling *et al.*, Chapter 10), and Ranyard and Abdel-Nabi (1993) were able to draw upon choice data and verbal protocols to distinguish explanations of the jacket and calculator problem in terms of these three types. Thaler (1985, 1993; Shefrin and Thaler, 1988) has used the term 'mental account' somewhat differently, to describe the implicit, on-going accounting systems that people develop to manage their financial transactions. He hypothesised that people have multiple accounts and are guided by the budgetary restrictions of the account(s) that they have identified as relevant. One function of mental accounts in Thaler's sense is to simplify sequences of income and expenditure changes over time. Successive gains or losses may be integrated into the same mental account or segregated into separate ones, depending on the situation (these operations of integration and segregation are examples of editing processes discussed earlier). Gärling *et al.* (Chapter 10) review the extensive research that has been carried out on segregation and integration and discuss alternative cognitive and motivational factors influencing such mental accounting processes. Studies inspired by the notion of accounts provide further evidence for the role of cognitive representations in the evaluation of decision alternatives and they illustrate the limitations of models that suggest that a single scale of utility can summarise people's preferences.

SOME TRENDS IN COGNITIVE DECISION RESEARCH

We now consider briefly some trends in cognitive psychology that have also had some impact upon decision research. The first of these is a concern with the ecological validity of laboratory methods and the extent to which findings from experimental methods can be generalised to decision making in natural settings. The legacy of SEU is evident in the reliance of much research upon the 'gamble' as a task for studying decision making. Here, the experimental subject makes a choice between gambles involving explicit amounts of money to be won or lost with probabilities that are expressed in terms of odds or depicted as the ratio of winning to losing segments on a roulette wheel. In many respects, this has been the prototypical task in psychological studies of decision making. Yet the gambles are typically stripped of many of the features of 'real-life' gambling and it is arguable whether the conditions of presentation serve to exclude many of the psychological responses that characterise risk taking. Ethical concerns about the possibility of subjects losing their money as well as practical considerations – researchers can rarely afford to act as a banker to cover their own potential losses – mean that the wins and losses involved tend to be either hypothetical or else merely token amounts of money. Tests of models often require that the subject 'plays' a large number of gambles one after the other, and it can be argued that this repetition of the task, typically without any feedback as to the outcomes of the gambles, further reduces the ecological validity of the task. Indeed, decision researchers are rarely interested in gambling behaviour in its own right and have seldom investigated how it is carried out in natural settings; rather, this activity tends to be studied by researchers adopting different theoretical perspectives.

Of course, gambles can 'stand for' or be metaphors for a range of types of decisions. Preferences for one outcome rather than another, notions of gains and losses, and uncertainty about whether one event or another will occur characterise many, perhaps all, real-life decisions. After all, even a mundane decision that seems to require only a straightforward expression of individual preference, for example, whether you should purchase a black jacket or a blue jacket, often calls into question your preferences or reveals uncertainties about the future – 'Will I like it when I get it home?'; 'Will the colour match my trousers?'; 'How durable is it going to be?' Casting a decision like this into the terminology of SEU theory is possible, but much recent research has queried whether this offers the best approach to describing and explaining how decisions are made outside the laboratory. Rather than a research strategy that assimilates preferences and uncertainties to a paradigm of rational behaviour, it might be more fruitful to describe them as they function in real-life decisions.

Fischhoff (1996) asked subjects for recollections of decisions that had been important to them. The majority of these decisions involved focus on a single option, e.g., whether to give up smoking, and there was little explicit comparison of different options. This contrasts with the tasks typically set in the laboratory, where subjects are asked to choose among options. There was little mention of uncertainties, again an issue that has been a focus of decision research. Huber (Chapter 9) brings out explicitly many of the differences between laboratory gambles and decision problems in natural settings. In the gamble, the investigator provides a problem structure for the subject whereas, in natural decisions, the structure may have to be found; the gamble makes no demands upon the subject's knowledge about factors involved in the decision; the outcomes of the gamble are deliberately arranged to be beyond the subject's control, whereas in 'real life' the decision maker has some measure of real or imagined control or, at any rate, seeks for it. Research into problem solving has shown that perceived control over outcomes is an important determinant of whether a problem solver persists at a difficult task and it predicts success at such tasks (Bandura, 1990). The question of controllability is also an important factor in counterfactual thinking (Mandel and Lehman, 1996) and hence might be related to post-decision regret. Huber summarises the differences between these two kinds of situation: 'Naturalistic decisions are ill-structured problems in knowledge-rich domains, where causal relations and attributions and the decision maker's control beliefs are present.'

There is now evidence of a growing interest in decisions in more natural settings (e.g., Klein *et al.*, 1993) and this is represented in several chapters in this volume. For example, Kemdal and Montgomery (Chapter 5) interviewed participants about important personal decisions that they had made; the decisions nominated by participants concerned their careers, important financial commitments, and social relationships. Svenson and Hill (Chapter 13) investigate students' choices of academic programmes, choices that can have far-reaching implications for their careers. Other chapters examine psychological constructs that are relevant to the 'reality' of decisions. Verplanken and Svenson (Chapter 3) look at the influence of different kinds of involvement upon decision processes. Teigen and Brun (Chapter 7) argue that judgements of risk are influenced by 'whatever makes the event appear life-like, substantial, or psychologically real'.

A second trend that has had some impact on decision research involves the forging of closer links between cognitive and social psychology. Post-decision processes provide a good example here. One of the seminal theories of social psychology has been Festinger's (1957) theory of cognitive dissonance. After a decision has been made, any attractive attributes of the rejected alternatives (or negative aspects of the chosen alternative) remain a potential source of psychological tension since they are discrepant with the recognition that a particular alternative has been chosen. According to Festinger, psychological 'work' is required to reduce this tension, and this has been investigated within several experimental paradigms. More recent psychological research in this tradition has explored 'counterfactual' thinking (Miller *et al.*, 1991) and associated emotions of regret and self-reproach. Larrick (1993) has related post-decision regret to self-presentation processes and the protection of self-esteem. Verplanken and Svenson (Chapter 3) discuss the potential influence of impression-relevant involvement on decision making. Post-decision dissonance was neglected for many years, but the process approach to decision making has revived interest in this topic. Additionally, it has made fresh contributions. For example, Svenson's differentiation and consolidation theory has provided a more detailed analysis of attractiveness restructuring than is found in dissonance theory.

A third trend is driven by recognition that cognitive research has paid insufficient attention to *affect*. Mood and emotion have been shown to influence a range of cognitive processes (Blaney, 1986; Hamilton *et al.*, 1993; Schwarz *et al.*, 1991). Abelson (1963) distinguished between 'hot' and 'cold' cognition in order to contrast motivated errors (like the attractiveness restructuring proposed by dissonance theory) with those that are due to information overload or cognitive biases. Decision research has tended to emphasise 'cold' cognition, comparing behaviour with the prescriptions of models of rationality. Discrepancies are interpreted in terms of limitations on the capacity of the cognitive system to cope with information. Particular decisions may be consequences of adopting specific frames (as in the Asian disease problem – see Kühberger, Chapter 8), or of systematic bias, for example errors in probabilistic thinking, as in the neglect of base rate information in reaching conclusions in the light of evidence (Nisbett and Ross, 1980). Lewicka (Chapter 6) provides a review of evidence for two kinds of utilities – cognitive and emotional – where evaluations are either 'rooted in descriptions of evaluated objects or ... mere expressions of emotional attitudes'. Her review covers research in topics like impression formation and the mere exposure effect that have been the focus of social psychological enquiries as well as research in decision making. She concludes that both types of utilities have their place in decision making but that evidence suggests that positive utilities have a more emotional character whereas negative utilities are 'colder'.

CONCLUDING REMARKS

In this chapter we have attempted to identify important themes and issues in the cognitive process approach to decision making. We have touched upon many questions that are examined in greater depth in the different chapters of this volume. The success of any approach is evident from the insights it offers into the complexity of human decision making. It should suggest fresh answers to established problems in the field and it should pose new questions. We believe that the cognitive process approach has much to offer with respect to these criteria, and this is amply demonstrated in the following chapters. Several of them review important recent decision research and therefore serve as a source book for those who want to update their knowledge. Other authors have focused on presenting the most recent results of their own process research. In both cases, the chapters afford the reader an opportunity to explore significant developments in this exciting period in decision research.

ACKNOWLEDGEMENT

We are grateful to Ola Svenson for his comments on an earlier draft.

REFERENCES

Abelson, R.P. (1963) 'Computer simulation of "hot" cognition', in S.S. Tomkins and S. Messick (eds) *Computer Simulation of Personality*, New York: Wiley.

Bandura, A. (1990) 'Conclusion: reflections on nonability determinants of competence', in R.J. Sternberg and J. Kolligian, Jr (eds) *Competence Considered*, New Haven: Yale University Press.

Beach, L. (1990) *Image Theory: Decision Making in Personal and Organizational Contexts*, Chichester: Wiley.

Beach, L.R. and Mitchell, T.R. (1978) 'A contingency model for the selection of decision strategies', *Academy of Management Review*, 3: 439–49.

Birnbaum, M.H. and McIntosh, W.R. (1996) 'Violations of branch independence in choices between gambles', *Organizational Behavior and Human Decision Processes*, 67: 91–110.

Blaney, P.H. (1986) 'Affect and memory: a review', *Psychological Bulletin*, 99: 229–46.

Crozier, W.R. (1989) 'Postdecisional justification: the case of De Lorean', in H. Montgomery and O. Svenson (eds) *Process and Structure in Human Decision Making*, Chichester: Wiley.

Edwards, W. and Tversky, A. (1967) *Decision Making*, Harmondsworth: Penguin.

Ericsson, K.A. and Simon, H.A. (1980) 'Verbal reports as data', *Psychological Review*, 87: 215–51.

Ericsson, K.A. and Simon, H.A. (1993) *Protocol Analysis: Verbal Reports as Data* (2nd edn), Cambridge, MA: MIT Press.

Festinger, L. (1957) *A Theory of Cognitive Dissonance*, Evanston, IL: Row Peterson.

Fischhoff, B. (1996) 'The real world: what good is it?', *Organizational Behavior and Human Decision Processes* 65: 232–48.

Ford, J.K., Schmitt, N., Schechtman, S.L., Hults, B.M. and Doherty, M.L. (1989) 'Process tracing methods: contributions, problems and neglected research questions', *Organizational Behavior and Human Decision Processes* 43: 75–117.

Hamilton, D.L., Stroessner, S.J. and Mackie, D.M. (1993) 'The influence of affect on stereotyping: the case of illusory correlations', in D.M. Mackie and D.L. Hamilton (eds) *Affect, Cognition, and Stereotyping: Interactive Processes in Group Perception*, New York: Academic Press.

Huber, O. (1986) 'Decision making as a problem solving process', in B. Brehmer, H. Jungermann, P. Lourens and G. Sevon (eds) *New Directions in Research on Decision Making*, Amsterdam: North–Holland.

Huber, O. (1989) 'Information-processing operators in decision making', in H. Montgomery and O. Svenson (eds) *Process and Structure in Human Decision Making*, Chichester, Sussex: Wiley.

Kahneman, D. and Tversky, A. (1979) 'Prospect theory: an analysis of decision under risk', *Econometrica*, 47: 263–91.

Klein, G.A., Orasuna, J., Calderwood, R. and Zsambok, C.E. (eds) (1993) *Decision Making in Action: Models and Methods*, Norwood, NJ: Ablex.

Koele, P. and Westenberg, M.R.M. (1995) 'A compensation index for multiattribute decision strategies', *Psychonomic Bulletin and Review*, 2: 398–402.

Larrick, R.P. (1993) 'Motivational factors in decision theories: the role of self-protection', *Psychological Bulletin*, 113: 440–50.

Mandel, D.R. and Lehman, D.R. (1996) 'Counterfactual thinking and ascriptions of cause and preventability', *Journal of Personality and Social Psychology*, 71: 450–63.

Miller, D.T., Turnbull, W. and McFarland, C. (1991) 'Counterfactual thinking and social perception: thinking about what might have been', in M. Zanna (ed.) *Advances in Experimental Social Psychology*, 23: 305–31, San Diego, CA: Academic Press.

Montgomery, H. (1983) 'Decision rules and the search for a dominance structure: towards a process model of decision making', in P.C. Humphreys, O. Svenson and A. Vari (eds) *Analyzing and Aiding Decision Processes*, Amsterdam: North-Holland.

Montgomery, H. (1989) 'From cognition to action: the search for dominance in decision making', in H. Montgomery and O. Svenson (eds) *Process and Structure in Human Decision Making*, Chichester: Wiley.

Montgomery, H. and Svenson, O. (eds) (1989) *Process and Structure in Human Decision Making*, Chichester: Wiley.

Nisbett, R.E. and Ross, L. (1980) *Human Inference: Strategies and Shortcomings of Social Judgment*, Engelwood Cliffs, NJ: Prentice-Hall.

Payne, J.W. (1976) 'Task complexity and contingent processing in decision making: an information search and protocol analysis', *Organizational Behavior and Human Performance*, 16: 366–87.

Payne, J.W. (1980) 'Information processing theory: some concepts and methods applied to decision research', in T.S. Wallsten (ed.) *Cognitive Processes in Choice and Decision Behavior*, Hillsdale, NJ: LEA.

Payne, J.W. (1994) 'Thinking aloud: insights into information processing', *Psychological Science*, 5: 241–52.

Payne, J.W., Bettman, J.R. and Johnson, E.J. (1993) *The Adaptive Decision Maker*, New York: Cambridge University Press.

Payne, J.W., Laughhunn, D.J. and Crum, R. (1984) 'Multiattribute risky choice behavior: the editing of complex prospects', *Management Science*, 11: 1350–61.

Ranyard, R. (1987) 'Cognitive processes underlying similarity effects in risky choice', *Acta Psychologica*, 64: 25–38.

Ranyard, R. (1995) 'Reversals of preference between simple and compound risks: the role of editing heuristics', *Journal of Risk and Uncertainty*, 11:159–75.

Ranyard, R. and Abdel-Nabi, D. (1993) 'Mental accounting and the process of multiattribute choice', *Acta Psychologica*, 84: 161–77.

Ranyard, R. and Crozier, W.R. (1984) 'Reasons given for risky judgement and choice: a comparison of three tasks', in P.D. Humphries, O. Svenson and A.

Vari (eds) *Analyzing and Aiding Decision Processes*, Amsterdam: North-Holland.

Russo, J.E. and Rosen, L.D. (1975) 'An eye fixation analysis of multiattribute choice', *Memory and Cognition*, 3: 267–76.

Schwarz, N., Bless, H. and Bohner, G. (1991) 'Mood and persuasion: affective states influence the processing of persuasive communications', *Advances in Experimental Social Psychology*, 24: 161–99.

Shefrin, H. and Thaler, R.H. (1988) 'The behavioral life-cycle hypothesis', *Economic Inquiry*, 26: 609–43.

Simon, H.A. (1957) *Models of Man*, New York: John Wiley.

Slovic, P. (1975) 'Choice between equally valued alternatives', *Journal of Experimental Psychology: Human Perception and Performance*, 1: 280–7.

Svenson, O. (1979) 'Process descriptions of decision making', *Organizational Behavior and Human Performance*, 23: 86–112.

Svenson, O. (1992) 'Differentiation and Consolidation Theory of human decision making: a frame of reference for the study of pre- and post-decision processes', *Acta Psychologica*, 80: 143–68.

Svenson, O. (1996) 'Decision making and the search for fundamental psychological regularities: what can be learned from a process perspective?', *Organizational Behavior and Human Decision Processes*, 65: 252–67.

Thaler, R.H. (1985) 'Mental accounting and consumer choice', *Marketing Science*, 4: 1199–214.

Thaler, R.H. (1993) 'Mental accounting matters', paper presented at the 14th Research Conference on Subjective Probability, Utility and Decision Making, Aix-en-Provence, August 1993.

Tversky, A. and Kahneman, D. (1981) 'The framing of decisions and the psychology of choice', *Science*, 211: 453–8.

Tversky, A. and Kahneman D. (1987) 'Rational choice and the framing of decisions', in R. Hogarth and M. Reder (eds) *Rational Choice: The Contrast Between Economics and Psychology*, Chicago: University of Chicago Press.

Westenberg, M.R.M. and Koele, P. (1994) 'Multi-attribute evaluation processes: methodological and conceptual issues', *Acta Psychologica*, 87: 65–84.

Chapter 2

Psychometric and methodological aspects of process tracing research

Johanna M. Harte and Pieter Koele

Judgement and decision making behaviour can be studied from various perspectives. The most common distinction is between the normative and the descriptive approach. In the normative approach the decision problem is well defined and there exist axiomatic theories that prescribe which decision a rational person should take in order to maximise some goal. The descriptive approach, on the other hand, is not so much interested in what rational subjects should do, but what 'real' subjects actually do. Its primary aim is to understand and to explain how individuals process available information in order to arrive at a judgement or a choice. Descriptive decision science does not consider individual differences in decision making as deviations from optimal behaviour, but it views them as conceptually relevant differences that should be explained by, among others, motivational and cognitive factors.

Process tracing research is one of the ways in which descriptive decision science is trying to monitor the cognitive process that leads from information input to judgement or decision outcome. In this chapter we intend to focus on process tracing research dealing with multiattribute evaluation problems, a topic that has received considerable attention over the last decades (Westenberg and Koele, 1994).

Multiattribute evaluation situations are defined by the following components. There is a *judge*, and there is a set of *alternatives* (objects or actions) about which information is available on a number of *attributes* (relevant characteristics of the alternatives; they are also called *dimensions* or *criteria*). The information about an alternative on an attribute is called an *attribute value*, or *aspect*. The judge has to consider the information in order to reach some conclusion about the alternatives, in terms of their overall (subjective) value, attractiveness, or suitability.

The way in which the judge has to express his or her opinion about the attractiveness of the alternatives depends on the nature of the task. In some tasks the 'best' alternative has to be chosen, whereas in other tasks alternatives have to be categorised or judged. Several studies (e.g., Billings and Scherer, 1988; Westenberg and Koele, 1990, 1992; Montgomery *et al.*,

1994) have shown that it is important to distinguish between these different types of response mode. Because this distinction is not essential for the issues to be discussed in this chapter, we will not go into a further consideration of it and use the terms 'decision', 'judgement' and 'evaluation' interchangeably.

Many real-life situations can be modelled as a multiattribute evaluation problem, for instance the selection of job applicants or the choice of the most suitable treatment for a patient. The major research question in multiattribute decision studies is how judges handle the available attribute information in order to arrive at a decision. It must be understood that there is no normative 'correct' way to do this, nor an alternative that is absolutely the 'best' one. The question is not whether a judge is right in some way, but how the judge, as an individual, deals with the problem. Decision research distinguishes itself in this sense from problem solving research, in which subjects are presented with problems that mostly have one logically correct solution. Both areas have a common interest, the cognitive information processing strategy leading to a response (either a decision or a solution), and, as will be discussed later on in this chapter, share some important research techniques.

RESEARCH TECHNIQUES

The two major approaches in studying multiattribute decision processes are the structural modelling approach and the process tracing approach. In structural modelling studies the subject is requested to give an evaluation of each alternative, based on all available attribute information. This attribute information (the aspects of each alternative) is seen as the input of the evaluation process, and the evaluations as the output. When an algebraic model is fitted on these input–output data, a formal description of the evaluation process is obtained. In many of these studies subjects are asked to give a numerical evaluation of each alternative, and a model is fitted by means of multiple regression analysis.

Structural modelling studies have been performed to study the process of evaluating job applicants (Einhorn, 1971), jobs (Reilly and Doherty, 1989), consumer products (Einhorn *et al.*, 1979), houses (Onken *et al.*, 1985; Lindberg *et al.*, 1989), performance (Brannick and Brannick, 1989) and companies (Slovic *et al.*, 1990).

New developments shifted towards a more cognitive-oriented point of view, process tracing. The initiators (e.g., Payne, 1976; Svenson, 1979) felt a growing dissatisfaction with the use of algebraic models as the representation of a cognitive process. Payne (1976) advocated the study of information search and acquisition in order to obtain insight into the cognitive evaluation process, and he introduced process tracing techniques, based on the techniques used in human problem solving research

(Newell and Simon, 1972). The emphasis in the process tracing approach is on information search and combination during the decision process, rather than on the input and output variables that precede and follow the process. Therefore, data are collected during the decision process (Svenson, 1979), and particular attention is paid to which information is searched, in which order it is searched, and how the searched information is combined in order to reach a decision.

The process tracing approach has been applied to various decision problems, including decisions about houses (Billings and Marcus, 1983; Kerstholt, 1992), job applicants (Billings and Scherer, 1988), consumer products (Olshavsky, 1979; Verplanken and Weenig, 1993), performance (Williams *et al.*, 1985) and travel mode choice (Aarts *et al.*, 1997).

There are two major process tracing techniques, *verbal protocols* and *information boards*. The verbal protocol technique requires the subjects to 'think aloud' as they work on the decision problem. The tape-recorded data are transcribed into separate statements and the researcher codes the verbal statements using a coding scheme. Subsequently, the coded statements are used to test hypotheses about the decision process, or to generate such hypotheses in an exploratory way when they are not available beforehand.

Much discussion has been devoted to the validity of think aloud protocols. Russo *et al.* (1989) distinguish two forms of invalidity: reactivity and non-veridicality. A protocol is reactive if the verbalisation influences the way in which the main task is performed, and it is non-veridical if it does not accurately reflect the process under study. Ericsson and Simon (1980, 1993) conclude that reactivity does not have a substantial impact on the validity of think aloud data: thinking aloud tends to slow down the process, but it does not change the sequence of thoughts during the process. Non-veridicality of the protocols depends, according to Ericsson and Simon, on the decision task the subjects have to perform while thinking aloud. To ensure confidence in the veridicality it should be investigated experimentally. This is quite complicated because one needs knowledge about the actual process in order to establish the degree of non-veridicality of the protocols. One way to overcome this problem is to compare the results of the analyses of verbal protocols with the results of other techniques that try to capture the same aspects of the cognitive process. Biggs *et al.* (1993) and Harte and Koele (1995) demonstrated that with the decision tasks they used verbal protocols appear to have a satisfactory degree of correspondence with other data describing the decision process.

Verbal protocols can also be obtained retrospectively, by requesting subjects to tell the researcher afterwards what they thought during the decision process. In this way any effect of reactivity is circumvented. However, as there is room for interpretation and forgetting between the actual process and the verbalisation of the process, retrospective protocols quite often appear to be incomplete (Fidler, 1983; Svenson, 1989).

The information board technique, which is often used to study tasks in which the most attractive alternative has to be selected from a set of alternatives, requires the subject to ask or search for information explicitly. The information board displays the information that is relevant to the decision situation on a number of cards, which are arranged in an alternative × attribute matrix. Initially, the information is not visible. The subject has to seek the information by turning around cards or opening envelopes that contain cards (Payne, 1976). Information boards can also be computerised, by letting subjects open the information cells they want to explore by moving the cursor on the screen and 'clicking the mouse'. In such a computerised information board task, search pattern data can be stored on file immediately. A few studies identify search patterns by recording the subjects' eye movements when they are presented with a board on which all information is visible. Eye movements provide data on the specific information the subject is looking for, and also on the sequence in which it is searched (e.g., Russo and Rosen, 1975). However, this technique is only accurate when the number of attributes and alternatives is very small (see Svenson, 1979).

Information boards allow the subject's information search pattern to be traced easily. On the basis of this pattern several variables can be derived which give insight into the decision making process, for instance whether the information has been searched mainly by alternative or by attribute. These variables have also been used as indications of particular decision strategies, like the elimination by aspects strategy or the additive difference strategy (Tversky, 1969, 1972). It must be kept in mind that this is a form of inductive reasoning with doubtful validity: different strategies may lead to the same search pattern, so one cannot link a specific search pattern to a single decision strategy.

It is not surprising that the two approaches, structural modelling and process tracing, that study the decision process from different points of view, have their own specific (dis)advantages and provide a different kind of information about the process. Structural modelling has been criticised for the fact that it does not give a realistic presentation of the process (Payne *et al.*, 1978; Svenson, 1979; Ford *et al.*, 1989; Maule and Svenson, 1993). The reason for this is that the focus of the structural modelling techniques is on the input and the output of the process and not on the process itself. Moreover, the simple algebraic models used in multiple regression analysis are very robust and ignore non-linear aspects of the process. Nevertheless, structural modelling techniques can provide important information about the process by fitting mathematical models, which can show how important the attrib-utes have been during the decision process and how information from different attributes is combined into an overall judgement (Brehmer, 1994).

Process tracing techniques, on the other hand, focus on the process itself and not on the relation between the attribute values and the final evaluations. From data gathered during the process, which pieces of information have been used and how they have been used can be traced. To obtain a realistic, detailed and complete representation of the actual evaluation process, process tracing seems to be more suitable than structural modelling (see Svenson, 1996). A main problem with process tracing is that conclusions are usually based on only one observation; data are derived from the evaluation of only one decision problem and the impact of measurement error is disregarded. As Einhorn *et al.* (1979) state, process tracing techniques allow for the possibility that irrelevant details or inconsistencies in the process are taken for systematic rules and heuristics. It is this feature of the process tracing paradigm that will be discussed in the remainder of this chapter.

DESCRIBING DECISION PROCESSES

In studies in which process tracing techniques are used to examine the decision making process, a subject usually receives only one decision problem. During the decision making one observes by means of the process tracing technique what information is used and in what order, obtaining in this way some kind of description of the process. However, the fact that conclusions about decision processes are drawn on the basis of only one decision problem per subject leads to a problem, even in cases in which the researcher is only interested in the way a particular decision problem is handled. Providing one problem to a subject, and thus studying one process per subject, means that only one observation per subject is obtained. As a consequence, it is not possible to separate measurement error from the 'true' decision process.

The idea of a true decision process originates from Classical Test Theory. This theory, which provides a framework for the construction and analysis of psychological tests, states that a subject's score on a test is the sum of the subject's true score and an error component (Crocker and Algina, 1986). The true score is the degree to which the subject possesses the characteristic which the test intends to measure. Measurement of this characteristic can, however, never provide an exact representation of the true score as every type of measurement is affected by error. Two types of error can be distinguished: systematic error and random error. Systematic error is the result of some particular characteristic of the test (e.g., item bias) or the subject (e.g., visual impairment), and therefore results in systematic deviations of a subject's test score from his or her true score. Random error affects a subject's score because of chance happenings (e.g., computer failures, a subject's physical and mental fitness) unrelated to the construct being measured. It may affect the subject's test score in either a positive or a negative direction; it is uncorrelated with the true score and its mean is zero.

These concepts from Classical Test Theory not only hold for measurement by means of psychological tests but for any kind of measurement, including measurement of multiattribute decision processes. The true decision process is the way the subject actually processes information and arrives at a decision. The pattern in which information is gathered, which is in fact an observation or measurement of the decision process, will never be an exact copy of the true process because there will always be some impact of error. Systematic error may be caused by characteristics of the decision task (e.g., information presentation mode), of the subject (e.g., cognitive ability), and of the context in which the decision is made (e.g., time pressure). Within the area of multiattribute decision making much research has been devoted to these types of effects. Overviews of these studies are provided by Payne (1982), Ford *et al.* (1989), Payne *et al.* (1993) and Harte (1995).

Apart from systematic error there will also be random error having an effect on the registration of the decision process. The aim of multiattribute decision research is to reveal the true information processing strategy a subject intends to apply. It can be assumed this true information processing strategy is influenced by random fluctuations, such as the inspection of an unintended cell of an information board by the accidental clicking of the mouse, or the occurrence of factors outside the experimenter's control that momentarily disturb the subject's concentration.

The existence of this error component seems to be ignored within the process tracing paradigm. This is in contrast with the structural modelling paradigm. If, for example, an algebraic model is fitted on the decision making process, the subject has been requested to evaluate a large number of alternatives. Subsequently, the parameters of the model are determined in such a way that the model shows the best fit on the input (the attribute values) and the output (the evaluations) of the process. Deviations of the actual evaluations from the model predictions are regarded as random error. As a result an indication of the impact of random error is provided by the goodness of fit of the model on the data. In process tracing research, where only one decision problem per subject is studied, the impact of the random error component is unknown. For the analysis of verbal protocols as well as the information display board technique this leads to problems with the interpretation of the results.

If verbal protocols are gathered, the most precise description of an individual's decision process can be obtained by constructing a process model. Process models, which have frequently been used in research on problem solving (see Newell and Simon, 1972; VanLehn, 1989; Anderson, 1989), describe how the process proceeds from an initial state of knowledge through a sequence of states of knowledge to a particular goal state. When it is given data as input, such a model should be able to produce output in the way the process under study is supposed to do. Harte *et al.* (1994) distinguish seven different steps in the construction of a process model. In the first and second step a model is formulated on the basis of available knowledge and theories about decision strategies, as well as cognitive constraints of the human mind. Decision strategies, like, for example, the linear strategy, the conjunctive strategy, the elimination by aspects strategy, and the additive difference strategy can be used as a basis for the models. In the third step a link between this model and the text of the think-aloud protocol is made by means of a coding scheme. In steps four and five the protocols are collected, transcribed and segmented into statements, which are subsequently coded according to the coding scheme in the sixth step. The seventh and last step, comparing the coded protocol with predictions from the psychological model, is by far the most complicated step. If the coded statements of the protocols are in perfect accordance with the model and thus also appear in the same sequence, it can be concluded that the model is a good representation of the process. In practice such a result will seldom be found. The experimenter will always be confronted with several differences between the coded protocol and the model, and for every difference he or she has to decide whether or not the model has to be adjusted. A difference with the model can also be caused by characteristics of the particular decision problem; the subject can deviate from his or her true strategy on the basis of some remarkable, unexpected attribute values, that occurred only by chance. Since the impact of such random variations is not known, decisions to adjust the model are often made intuitively. Determining the fit of a model is therefore a very difficult job.

The absence of an error theory also complicates the interpretation of the results obtained with the information board. With this technique the information in the cells that are opened by the subject is considered to be the information used during the process, and the order of opening is seen as the order of processing this information. On the basis of this pattern of gathering information, several variables are derived that describe certain characteristics of the decision process. Variability of search and the compensation index (Koele and Westenberg, 1995) give an indication of the degree of compensation between attribute values within alternatives. Depth of search describes the percentage of information used, and pattern of search (Payne, 1976) shows whether information is processed per alternative or per attribute. The pattern in which cells are opened will, however, depend not only on the strategy the subject applies. A subject might, for example, have the intention to open first all cells for the attribute regarded as the most important one. For the alternatives with high scores on this attribute he or she subsequently opens the remaining cells to check the other attribute values. The alternative with the highest overall attribute values is selected. When the attribute values have been randomly selected by the experimenter, as is usually the case, it might happen that all alternatives have very low values on the one attribute the subject intended to use to screen the alternatives. In that case the subject has to use information on other, less important attributes in order to screen the alternatives, and the experimenter consequently does not obtain a description of the 'true' decision process of this subject. Since the subject usually receives only one decision problem, the values of the information board variables are based on only one observation of the decision process. The impact of chance on these variables is unknown.

HYPOTHESIS TESTING

Despite the problems described in the previous section, process tracing techniques have successfully been applied to discovering more about decision processes. In many studies verbal protocols or the information display board have been used to test hypotheses about the way subjects process information (see Ford *et al.*, 1989).

An example of a study in which think-aloud protocols were used to investigate decision processes is described in Svenson (1989). In this study two types of statements, absolute evaluations and comparative evaluations, were counted in different parts of the process. It appeared that according to the results of the total group of subjects, comparative statements increased towards the very end of the process. Also by counting several types of statements in different parts of the process, the study of Bettman and Park (1980) showed that in the early phases there is more processing per attribute while later phases are dominated by processing per alternative. Effects on the process caused by the context in which the decision is made have been investigated by comparing frequencies of certain statements in think-aloud protocols that were obtained in different conditions. Svenson and Karlsson (1986) examined whether an attribute was mentioned more often by subjects who participated in a condition in which an attribute was presented numerically than by those who made their decision in a condition in which it was presented verbally. Isen and Means (1983) wanted to know whether a positive feeling state affects the decision process. They found that the protocols of subjects whose state was manipulated in a positive way (by being complimented on their performance on a foregoing task), contained fewer references to attributes than the protocols of subjects in the control condition.

The information display board has frequently been used to test hypotheses about decision processes. One of the main topics in experimental studies using the information display board is whether the process is compensatory, for example whether during the process high values on some attributes can compensate for low values on other attributes. Many of these studies aimed to investigate the effect of characteristics of the task on the degree of compensation within the process. An example of such a characteristic is the complexity of the task, which is defined by the number of alternatives and attributes. Several studies have shown by means of the information display board that decision processes of subjects in conditions with larger information display boards are less compensatory (see, e.g., Biggs *et al.*, 1985; Klayman, 1985; Nichols-Hoppe and Beach, 1990; Westenberg and Koele, 1990, 1992; Kerstholt, 1992). Another characteristic of the decision task is the way in which information about the alternatives are presented. In the studies of Bettman and Kakkar (1977), Herstein (1981) and Sundström (1987) it was shown that, in the condition in which the organisation of the information display board was alternative-salient, subjects process information differently from those in the condition in which it was presented attribute-salient.

Testing differences between conditions or between parts of the decision process, as in the studies described above, allows important information about decision processes to be obtained. Such studies give insight into the effects of characteristics of the task on the process, the effects caused by the context in which a decision is made, and more, generally, how decision processes develop. In all studies, however, the results have been aggregated over subjects as if subjects are replicates of each other. This circumvents the problem of measurement error because it may be assumed that over groups of subjects its mean is zero. Nevertheless, the statistical techniques (t-tests, analyses of variance) used to test hypotheses about systematic effects of experimental manipulations compare the variance of the means of the experimental conditions (between-groups variance) to the pooled variance within conditions (within-groups variance). Only when the between-groups variance is sufficiently larger than the within-groups variance the null hypothesis of no effect is rejected (see Winer *et al.*, 1991). In order to have a test with a high power (the probability of correctly rejecting the null hypothesis; see Koele, 1982), it is important to have a within-groups variance that is as small as possible.

Within-groups variance consists of two components: individual differences and measurement error. Of course, individual differences cannot be reduced; they exist, and as such are worth investigating in their own right. In the next section it will be shown how the other component of within-group variance, measurement error, can be reduced, and how this results in more powerful tests.

CONCLUDING REMARKS

The main purpose of descriptive decision making research is to describe the true decision process of an individual as accurately as possible. According to Classical Test Theory, a subject's true score is interpreted as the mean of a large number of observed scores of that subject in repeated testing on the same test or on strictly parallel forms of the test (Crocker and Algina, 1986). A subject's true decision process can, by analogy with Classical Test Theory, be approximated by means of repeated measurements. For that reason, it is necessary to present the subject with a series of decision problems that can be regarded as parallel forms.

For the interpretation of verbal protocols such a series of decision problems can be very useful. The experimenter who is confronted with a discrepancy between the model and the protocol has the opportunity to examine other protocols from the same subject in which similar decisions were made. This will reveal whether the discrepancy is just a coincidence, or a fundamental and consistent part of the subject's way of processing information. An experimenter might, for example, hypothesise that a subject making a choice between alternatives first uses the most important attribute to simplify the problem by rejecting alternatives that do not meet a minimum threshold on this attribute. In the think-aloud protocol it might appear that the subject indeed simplifies the problem in this way but on the basis of the values on an attribute other than the one the experimenter expected. Consequently, the experimenter might adjust the decision model. If, however, more protocols are gathered, it might appear that using this other attribute was exceptional behaviour caused by the fact that all alternatives in the choice set were almost equally attractive according to the most important attribute. Although the decision whether or not to adjust the model will always be a difficult one, much more information on which to base this decision is available when more protocols of the same subject on similar problems are available.

In a study by Harte *et al.* (1996) a series of information display boards was used. This series was presented on a computer screen; after the subject had made a choice on an information board, a new board appeared on the screen. The information boards differed only according to the attribute values. The series of similar problems was used to obtain estimates of subjects' attribute weights, but such a series of boards can of course also be used to calculate the mean values of other information board measures like variability and pattern of search. In this way one obtains estimates of the true scores on these measures that contain considerably less error than the estimate based on just one observation, because the efficiency of a point estimator increases as a linear function of the number of observations on which it is based; or in other words, when the number of observations increases with a factor k, the variance of the estimator decreases with a factor k.

A series of decision problems should not be too long. One of the conditions for obtaining a valid think-aloud protocol is that task performance is not automatic (Ericsson and Simon, 1993). If the subject has to solve many similar problems, he or she gets too familiar with the task and task performance will become an automatic process. When performing a task automatically, the subject is not completely aware of what he or she is actually doing. As a consequence, a verbal report of what is going on in the mind will not contain a complete view of how the decision is made. Moreover, regardless of the technique used, it is important that the subject remains motivated till the end of the series. This leads to a problem, because on the one hand the experimenter aims to gather as much information as possible, while on the other hand the subject has to stay motivated. Harte *et al.* (1996) carried out a pilot study before their main experiment, in order to find out the number of information boards a subject can handle before getting demotivated or irritated; for this particular task it proved to be ten information boards. In other experimental situations the number of repeated measurements might have to remain smaller, but even in these cases it is useful to take repeated measurements, because, as mentioned before, obtaining for instance four observations instead of one already decreases the variance of the estimator by a factor of four.

Apart from this psychometric approach to reducing error reduction there are also methodological ways of reducing error variance, for instance by using within-subjects designs: testing the same subject on all treatment levels of the experimental manipulation. In this way it is possible to separate the individual differences from the within-groups variance. Such designs also have the advantage that they allow the experimenter to study the effect of manipulations within the same subject, by relating changes in decision process measures to other subject characteristics. This method combines the experimental investigation into the effect of manipulations on groups of subjects with a more correlational approach to explain individual differences in decision processes.

The use of within-subjects designs is not without problems, because a subject's behaviour may be influenced by various aspects of the experimental design and procedure, such as the order in which the manipulations are administered, the probably lengthy and tiresome experimental session, and the desire to please (or tease) the experimenter by responding in a manner that confirms (or disconfirms) the apparent experimental hypothesis. These threats to the internal validity of the experiment (see Campbell and Stanley, 1966) should be considered seriously when the experiment is being designed.

We have argued in this chapter that by using repeated measurements on the same subject the experimenter has the opportunity to obtain a more stable, reliable description of an individual's decision process, because a substantial part of measurement error can be removed from the measures describing this process. This error reduction has also advantages when experimental designs are being used to study the influence of certain factors like information presentation and task complexity on the decision process, because it increases the power of the statistical tests executed to test hypotheses about this influence. By using repeated measurements on the same subjects one has the possibility of obtaining reliable descriptions of individual decision processes and powerful tests of contextual and other influences on the decision process.

REFERENCES

Aarts, H., Verplanken, B. and van Knippenberg, A. (1997) 'Habit and information use in travel mode choices', *Acta Psychologica,* 96: 1–14.

Anderson, J.R. (1989) 'A theory of the origins of human knowledge', *Artificial Science*, 40: 313–51.

Bettman, J.R. and Kakkar, P. (1977) 'Effects of information presentation format on consumer information acquisition strategies', *Journal of Consumer Research*, 3: 233–40.

Bettman, J.R. and Park, C.W. (1980) 'Effects of prior knowledge and experience and phase of the choice process on consumer decision processes: a protocol analysis', *Journal of Consumer Research*, 7: 234–48.

Biggs, S.F., Bedard, J.C., Gaber, B.G. and Linsmeier, T.J. (1985) 'The effects of task size and similarity on the decision behavior of bank loan officers', *Management Science*, 31: 970–87.

Biggs, S.F., Rosman, A.J. and Sergenian, G.K. (1993) 'Methodological issues in judgment and decision-making research: concurrent verbal protocol validity and simultaneous traces of process', *Journal of Behavioral Decision Making*, 6: 187–206.

Billings, R.S. and Marcus, S.A. (1983) 'Measures of compensatory and noncompensatory models of decision behavior: process tracing versus policy capturing', *Organizational Behavior and Human Performance*, 31: 331–52.

Billings, R.S. and Scherer, L.L. (1988) 'The effects of response mode and importance on decision-making strategies: judgement versus choice', *Organizational Behavior and Human Decision Processes*, 41: 1–19.

Brannick, M.T. and Brannick, J.P. (1989) 'Nonlinear and noncompensatory processes in performance evaluation', *Organizational Behavior and Human Decision Processes*, 44: 97–122.

Brehmer, B. (1994) 'The psychology of linear judgment models', *Acta Psychologica*, 87: 137–54.

Campbell, D.T. and Stanley, J.C. (1966) *Experimental and Quasi-Experimental Designs for Research*, Chicago: Rand McNally & Company.

Crocker, L. and Algina, J. (1986) *Introduction to Classical and Modern Test Theory*, New York: Holt, Rinehart & Winston.

Einhorn, H.J. (1971) 'Use of nonlinear, noncompensatory models as a function of task and amount of information', *Organizational Behavior and Human Performance*, 6: 1–27.

Einhorn, H.J., Kleinmuntz, D.N. and Kleinmuntz, B. (1979) 'Linear regression and process-tracing models of judgement', *Psychological Review*, 86: 465–85.

Ericsson, K.A. and Simon, H.A. (1980) 'Verbal reports as data', *Psychological Review*, 87: 215–51.

Ericsson, K.A. and Simon, H.A. (1993) *Protocol Analysis: Verbal Reports as Data* (rev. edn), Cambridge, MA: MIT Press.

Fidler, E.J. (1983) 'The reliability and validity of concurrent, retrospective, and interpretative verbal reports: an experimental study', in P. Humphreys, O. Svenson and A. Vari (eds) *Analyzing and Aiding Decision Processes*, Amsterdam: North-Holland.

Ford, J.K., Schmitt, N., Schechtman, S.L., Hults, B.M. and Doherty, M.L. (1989) 'Process tracing methods: contributions, problems and neglected research questions', *Organizational Behavior and Human Decision Processes*, 43: 75–117.

Harte, J.M. (1995) *Multiattribute Evaluation Processes: Evaluation Types and Research Techniques*, Amsterdam: Faculty of Psychology Dissertation Series.

Harte, J.M. and Koele, P. (1995) 'A comparison of different methods for the elicitation of attribute weights: structural modeling, process tracing, and self-reports', *Organizational Behavior and Human Decision Processes*, 64: 49–64.

Harte, J.M., Koele, P. and van Engelenburg, G. (1996) 'The estimation of attribute weights in a multiattribute choice situation', *Acta Psychologica*, 93: 37–55.

Harte, J.M., Westenberg, M.R.M. and van Someren, M.W. (1994) 'Process models of decision making', *Acta Psychologica*, 87: 95–120.

Herstein, J.A. (1981) 'Keeping the voter's limits in mind: a cognitive process analysis of decision making in voting', *Journal of Personality and Social Psychology*, 40: 843–61.

Isen, A.M. and Means, B. (1983) 'The influence of positive affect on decision-making strategy', *Social Cognition*, 2: 18–31.

Kerstholt, J.H. (1992) 'Information search and choice accuracy as a function of task complexity and task structure', *Acta Psychologica*, 80: 185–97.

Klayman, J. (1985) 'Children's decision strategies and their adaptation to task characteristics', *Organizational Behavior and Human Decision Processes*, 35: 179–201.

Koele, P. (1982) 'Calculating power in analysis of variance', *Psychological Bulletin*, 92: 513–16.

Koele, P. and Westenberg, M.R.M. (1995) 'A compensation index for multi-attribute decision strategies', *Psychonomic Bulletin and Review*, 2: 398–402.

Lindberg, E., Gärling, T. and Montgomery, H. (1989) 'Differential predictability of preferences and choices', *Journal of Behavioral Decision Making*, 2: 205–19.

Maule, A.J. and Svenson, O. (1993) 'Theoretical and empirical approaches to behavioral decision making and their relation to time constraint', in O. Svenson and A.J. Maule (eds) *Time Pressure and Stress in Human Judgment and Decision Making*, New York: Plenum Press.

Montgomery, H., Selart, M., Gärling, T. and Lindberg, E. (1994) 'The judgment-choice discrepancy: noncompatibility or restructuring?', *Journal of Behavioral Decision Making*, 7: 145–55.

Newell, A. and Simon, H.A. (1972) *Human Problem Solving*, Englewood Cliffs, NJ: Prentice-Hall.

Nichols-Hoppe, K.T. and Beach, L.R. (1990) 'The effects of test anxiety and task variables on predecisional information search', *Journal of Research in Personality*, 24: 163–72.

Olshavsky, R.W. (1979) 'Task complexity and contingent processing in decision making: a replication and extension', *Organizational Behavior and Human Performance*, 24: 300–16.

Onken, J., Hastie, R. and Revelle, W. (1985) 'Individual differences in the use of simplification strategies in a complex decision-making task', *Journal of Experimental Psychology: Human Perception and Performance*, 11: 14–27.

Payne, J.W. (1976) 'Task complexity and contingent processing in decision making: an information search and protocol analysis', *Organizational Behavior and Human Performance*, 16: 366–87.

Payne, J.W. (1982) 'Contingent decision behavior', *Psychological Bulletin*, 92: 382–402.

Payne, J.W., Bettman, J.R. and Johnson, E.J. (1993) *The Adaptive Decision Maker*, Cambridge: Cambridge University Press.

Payne, J.W., Braunstein, L. and Carroll, J.S. (1978) 'Exploring predecisional behavior: an alternative approach to decision research', *Organizational Behavior and Human Performance*, 22: 17–44.

Reilly, B.A. and Doherty, M.E. (1989) 'A note on the assessment of self-insight in judgment research', *Organizational Behavior and Human Decision Processes*, 44: 123–31.

Russo, J.E., Johnson, E.J. and Stephens, M.L. (1989) 'The validity of verbal protocols', *Memory and Cognition*, 17: 759–69.

Russo, J.E. and Rosen, L.D. (1975) 'An eye fixation analysis of multialternative choice', *Memory and Cognition*, 3: 267–76.

Slovic, P., Griffin, D. and Tversky, A. (1990) 'Compatibility effects in judgment and choice' in R.M. Hogarth (ed.) *Insights in Decision Making: A Tribute to Hillel J. Einhorn*, Chicago: University of Chicago Press.

Sundström, G.A. (1987) 'Information search and decision making: the effects of information displays', *Acta Psychologica*, 65: 165–79.

Svenson, O. (1979) 'Process descriptions of decision making', *Organizational Behavior and Human Performance*, 23: 86–112.

Svenson, O. (1989) 'Eliciting and analysing verbal protocols in process studies of judgement and decision making', in H. Montgomery and O. Svenson (eds) *Process and Structure in Human Decision Making*, Chichester: Wiley.

Svenson, O. (1996) 'Decision making and the search for fundamental psychological regularities: what can be learned from a process perspective?', *Organizational Behavior and Human Decision Processes*, 65: 252–67.

Svenson, O. and Karlsson, G. (1986) 'Attractiveness of decision alternatives characterized by numerical and non-numerical information', *Scandinavian Journal of Psychology*, 27: 74–84.

Tversky, A. (1969) 'Intransitivity of preferences', *Psychological Review*, 76: 31–48.

Tversky, A. (1972) 'Elimination by aspects: a theory of choice', *Psychological Review*, 79: 281-99.

VanLehn, K. (1989) 'Problem solving and cognitive skill acquisition', in M.I. Posner (ed.) *Foundations of Cognitive Science*, Cambridge, MA: MIT Press.

Verplanken, B. and Weenig, M.W.H. (1993) 'Graphical energy labels and consumers' decisions about home appliances: a process tracing approach', *Journal of Economic Psychology*, 14: 739–52.

Westenberg, M.R.M. and Koele, P. (1990) 'Response modes and decision strategies', in K. Borcherding, O.I. Larichev and D.M. Messick (eds) *Contemporary Issues in Decision Making*, Amsterdam: North-Holland.

Westenberg, M.R.M. and Koele, P. (1992) 'Response modes, decision processes and decision outcomes', *Acta Psychologica*, 80: 169–84.

Westenberg, M.R.M. and Koele, P. (1994) 'Multi-attribute evaluation processes: methodological and conceptual issues', *Acta Psychologica*, 87: 65–84.

Williams, K.J., DeNisi, A.S., Blencoe, A.G. and Cafferty, T.P. (1985) 'The role of appraisal purpose: effects of purpose on information acquisition and utilization', *Organizational Behavior and Human Decision Processes*, 35: 314–39.

Winer, B.J., Brown, D.R. and Michels, K.M. (1991) *Statistical Principles in Experimental Design*, (3rd edn), New York: McGraw-Hill, Inc.

Part II

Values and involvement

Introduction to Part II

The chapters in Part II are concerned with understanding how people evaluate decision alternatives. In traditional decision research it was assumed that values could be described by a single value or utility function. Recent approaches consider this to be a much too simple approach. Instead of one commensurate scale of utility, more scales have to be considered that are used in different ways by decision makers. How people assign values is a question that is not restricted to decision research but has also been important in social psychology, for example in research into attitude formation and change, and into psychological aesthetics. Forging links between cognitive and social psychological perspectives is a common theme in these chapters. Another theme is the rejection of the decision maker as a passive and dispassionate processor of information, like the stereotyped accountant whose book contains columns detailing profits and losses. Rather, the decision maker is actively searching for meaning, is seeking for, and testing hypotheses about what would produce an outcome that 'feels right' and that can be justified. Information is not simply analysed, it is restructured and viewed from shifting perspectives.

Making the right decision is the principal concern of decision makers for there is often much at stake. A decision may be irreversible, its consequences can be serious and far-reaching, and it is often made in the public eye where one's actions are open to scrutiny. Decisions vary in their seriousness and in the extent to which they are involving. One can envisage a continuum from crucial, literally life or death decisions, to mundane choices, for example, which video to rent. It seems plausible that decision processes are affected by the degree of involvement in a decision. This may lead, for example, to varying amounts of effort being expended upon assessing alternatives. Verplanken and Svenson (Chapter 3) explore the influence of involvement, drawing upon classifications of different types of involvement made by social psychologists and Svenson's Differentiation and Consolidation theory of decision making. Their chapter explores the effects of three different kinds of involvement at different stages in the decision process. More specifically, it examines effects upon identification of the decision problem and processes of differentiation and consolidation. Differentiation processes function to separate the alternatives until one alternative is sufficiently more attractive to enable a decision to be made. Differentiation continues after the decision (consolidation processes) in order to support the chosen alternative and to protect the decision maker from dissonance and regret. The authors argue that the three kinds of involvement have different motivational bases and hence affect decision processes in different ways.

The complexity of the issues involved in measuring 'values' is evident in Chapter 4, where Selart examines content and task effects upon different assessments of the attractiveness of decision alternatives. Research has shown that theoretically similar response measures may not provide equivalent indices of people's preferences and utility functions. For example, a subject might be asked to respond to a pair of gambles, each comprising a payoff (an amount of money to win) with a specific probability, either by making a choice of one gamble over the other or by nominating a price that he or she would accept for buying or selling each gamble. However, subjects often exhibit a pattern of behaviour where they choose one gamble but demand a higher selling price for the other. This 'preference reversal' is influenced by the response mode, in that subjects seem to attach more weight to the payoff when they nominate a price than when they make a choice. One plausible explanation for this is that it reflects the compatibility between payoff and response – both are expressed in monetary terms.

Selart examines alternative versions of the compatibility hypothesis. He argues that compatibility effects are related to how information is structured and organised at both stimulus input and output stages in the decision process. His chapter reports suggestive evidence from verbal protocol analysis that different decision strategies are 'primed' by the range of values and by response modes. This research demonstrates the effectiveness for exploring decision phenomena of a combination of approaches involving both traditional measures of preference and process tracing methods.

Kemdal and Montgomery (Chapter 5) propose that evaluation processes are based on the adoption of particular perspectives with regard to decision alternatives. Specific attributes of alternatives can appear either as 'figure' or 'ground' depending on the evaluative perspective that is adopted. The particular perspective taken is related to the target of a person's identification, the congruence between identification and the attributes of an alternative, and the extent to which the person is committed to any one alternative. In an empirical study, subjects' retrospective accounts of significant personal decisions were coded for the frequencies of references to circumstances, actions, beliefs, preferences and emotions. Subjects attached great weight to the circumstances in which the decision was taken and the actions undertaken, and they did not focus solely on beliefs and preferences. Subjects who expressed satisfaction with their decisions reported more emotions in total concerning the situation prior to the decision whereas those who regretted the decision referred to more emotions (particularly negative emotions of guilt and regret) after the decision had been made. These differences in the verbal protocols of subjects who were satisfied or regretted their decision are interpreted in terms of Montgomery's Perspective theory.

Lewicka (Chapter 6) considers evidence for two types of utilities. Her contrast between emotional and cognitive types recalls Zajonc's seminal distinction between preferences and inferences. She associates these with two types of evaluation, 'diagnostic', that arrive at evaluative judgements on the basis of assessment of specific attributes of alternatives, and 'prospective', that are based upon more global, undifferentiated attitudes towards alternatives. For example, one might reach a decision by writing down the advantages and disadvantages of each course of action and choosing the one with the most favourable profile. Alternatively one might have a kind of 'gut feeling' about an alternative, a feeling that is difficult to analyse or to explain to others, but which influences how one assesses specific attributes of that alternative. Indeed, listing the attributes can simply lead to inaction rather than a decision; as Lewicka argues, prospective evaluations may be 'preconditions for commitment'. They are also useful in the post-decision phase, to support what Svenson describes as consolidation processes. Lewicka relates her analysis of these types of evaluations to empirical findings of differences in information acquisition strategies between decisions where the goal is to accept an alternative (e.g., choose the best candidate for a job) and those where the goal is to reject an alternative (e.g., screen out unsatisfactory candidates).

Fundamental goals of the cognitive perspective are to identify ways in which decision processes are adaptive and to emphasise that strategies are not only selected in response to task and environmental demands but are also influenced by personal characteristics of decision makers such as their involvement in the decision, their commitments to particular courses of action and their need to justify their actions to themselves and to others. The chapters in this section illustrate diverse and significant approaches to realising these goals.

Chapter 3

Personal involvement in human decision making

Conceptualisations and effects on decision processes

Bas Verplanken and Ola Svenson

Decisions vary widely in importance for the decision maker. Many decisions are unimportant, such as everyday purchases. Such choices are routine actions, which need little thought. Other decisions are more important, and evoke active reasoning aimed at acquiring a satisfactory representation of attractiveness of options. Decisions may be important for many reasons. For instance, decisions are important when high costs are involved (e.g., buying a house), or when an outcome has far-reaching consequences (e.g., the choice of a career). A decision may also be important when it relates to a significant opinion or emotional value (e.g., voting for a political party). Motivation has received little attention in process approaches to decision making research (Larrick, 1993), and so has the role of involvement (e.g., Ford *et al.*, 1989). In this chapter we discuss effects that various types of involvement may have in individual decision making processes.

In a general sense, involvement in an issue, product, or decision is often considered as a motivational factor that affects the cognitive effort that individuals expend on a problem, and on strategies that are used to form a judgement or make a decision. However, such a general characterisation of the construct is incomplete at best, and does not take into account the multifaceted nature of involvement. Indeed, a number of frameworks have been developed, in particular in the domain of consumer behaviour, that differentiate between a variety of types of involvement (e.g., Bloch and Richins, 1983; Greenwald and Leavitt, 1984; Houston and Rothschild, 1978; Mittal and Lee, 1989; Zaichkowsky, 1985). In social psychology there is a long tradition of research on attitudes and persuasion, in which involvement has an important role. Johnson and Eagly (1989) presented a meta-analysis on effects of involvement on attitude change. They distinguished between three types of involvement, i.e., *value-relevant involvement*, *outcome-relevant involvement*, and *impression-relevant involvement* and found evidence to suggest that each type relates differently to persuasion and attitude change.

In this chapter we attempt to extrapolate Johnson and Eagly's (1989) findings to a decision making context, in particular to decision processes as these are described in Svenson's (1992) Differentiation and Consolidation Theory of decision making. Although Johnson and Eagly's (1989) analysis is confined to persuasion and attitude change, their analysis is a useful framework for elaborating on the role of involvement in decision making processes for a number of reasons. First, the distinction between the three types of involvement is relevant in many decision making contexts. Second, Johnson and Eagly's (1989) meta-analysis suggests that the three types of involvement result in different types of information processing, and, as we will argue, may have corresponding effects on decision making processes. Third, the meta-analysis is based on a substantial amount of empirical evidence stemming from different research traditions in social psychology. These reasons make this perspective more attractive for the present purpose compared to, for instance, the consumer behaviour-oriented perspectives that were cited above. In the following, the different types of involvement are discussed, followed by an outline of the theory of Differentiation and Consolidation. Then the two perspectives are integrated.

THREE TYPES OF INVOLVEMENT

Johnson and Eagly (1989) discuss involvement in terms of self-relevance, and define the construct as 'the motivational state induced by an association between an activated attitude and some aspect of the self-concept' (Johnson and Eagly, 1989: 293). Their meta-analysis is based on research in three traditions in social psychology, i.e., social judgement theory (e.g., Sherif and Cantril, 1947; Sherif and Hovland, 1961), dissonance theory (Zimbardo, 1960) and the dual-process persuasion research tradition (Chaiken, 1987; Petty and Cacioppo, 1986). In each tradition involvement was operationalised differently, and in fact referred to different aspects of the self-concept, and thus to different motivational states.

In the social judgement perspective, the self or 'ego' consists of a set of enduring attitudes that define a person, for instance in terms of biological drives, personal and social values, or status within groups or institutions. When any stimulus or situation is related to this frame of reference, an accompanying attitude is said to be characterised by a high level of 'ego involvement' (Sherif and Cantril, 1947). Accordingly, *value-relevant involvement* refers to the psychological state that is created by the activation of attitudes that are linked to important values. In the social judgement perspective the structure of an attitude is described by three ranges or 'latitudes': positions that one finds acceptable, positions that one rejects and positions towards which one is indifferent (i.e., latitudes of acceptance, rejectance and non-commitment, respectively).

The theory suggests that ego involvement enhances latitudes of rejectance. Consequently, high ego involvement attitudes are supposed to be less easily influenced, because message positions are more likely to fall into latitudes of rejectance compared to low ego involvement attitudes. Johnson and Eagly's (1989) meta-analysis confirms that value-relevant involvement inhibits persuasion.

The second type of involvement, *impression-relevant involvement*, was introduced as 'response involvement' by Zimbardo (1960). It refers to self-presentation motives in contexts where someone expresses an attitude. Impression-relevant involvement increases to the extent that someone expects that expressing an attitude has consequences for impressions that other people have of her/him. Impression-relevant involvement can be regarded as a concern with holding a position that is defensible in front of potential evaluators (Leippe and Elkin, 1987). Although Johnson and Eagly's (1989) meta-analysis contained a limited number of studies that manipulated impression-relevant involvement, they found that this involvement type tends to reduce persuasion.

The third type of involvement, *outcome-relevant involvement*, is rooted in the current cognitive-oriented research on persuasion (Chaiken, 1987; Petty and Cacioppo, 1986). It refers to the degree that situations or issues pertain to attaining desirable outcomes. Johnson and Eagly (1989) restrict this involvement type to issues that are unfamiliar and which are unlikely to be linked to important values or to a context of social evaluation, so as to distinguish them from value-relevant and impression-relevant involvement issues. Outcome-relevant involvement is supposed to lead to message-relevant thinking, for instance thorough scrutiny of the merits of presented arguments in a persuasive message. In line with this assumption, the meta-analysis provides strong evidence to suggest that the quality of presented arguments moderates the relationship between outcome-relevant involvement and attitude change. Given that a highly outcome-involved person expends much effort in attending to the content of a presented message, he or she will be persuaded by strong, but not by weak, arguments, whereas argument strength is less likely to influence low involvement persons' attitudes.

Johnson and Eagly (1989) speculate about *processes* that underlie the involvement-attitude patterns. For instance, following the social judgement approach, the perception of a communicator's attitude position is supposed to be contrasted (i.e., it is seen as a position that is more discrepant from one's own) when it falls in the latitude of rejection, which is more likely at high levels of ego involvement. Generally, at high levels of value-relevant involvement, information processing is likely to be biased conforming to one's own attitude position and values. Thus, one may attend less to information that is inconsistent with activated values, or perceive discrepant positions as ones that are less objective.

Persuasion processes related to outcome-relevant involvement have been particularly documented in the research tradition of current persuasion models (Chaiken, 1987; Petty and Cacioppo, 1986), which are rooted in the cognitive response approach (Greenwald, 1968). High outcome-relevant involvement is related to relatively objective scrutiny of information. This analytical processing mode, which is relatively effortful, is aimed at revealing the strengths and weaknesses of presented information so as to be able to respond appropriately in obtaining the best outcome.[1]

In contrast to the former types of involvement there is little empirical work that revealed attitude change processes related to impression-relevant involvement. Leippe and Elkin (1987) found that, like outcome-relevant involvement, impression-relevant involvement instigates high levels of attention. However, unlike outcome-relevant involvement, high impression-relevant involved participants did not show evidence of systematic processing. Impression-involved persons' processing goal is often to gain information about possible positions, rather than an evaluation of arguments. In anticipating an unknown public, for instance, one may look for a moderate, defensible and flexible position. Or, in case a future interaction with known positions is expected, one may look for arguments that are helpful in creating an appropriate image. This may lead to biased processing of available information (Chen *et al.*, 1996).

DIFFERENTIATION AND CONSOLIDATION THEORY OF DECISION MAKING

In order to theorise about effects of the three types of involvement on decision making, we use Svenson's (1992, 1996) Differentiation and Consolidation Theory of decision making (Diff Con Theory) as a framework. In this theory the decision making process is modelled as one in which a choice option is gradually differentiated from other alternatives, until it is judged sufficiently superior in attractiveness to be chosen. The theory not only focuses on this pre-choice differentiation path, but also considers post-decision consolidation processes. A basic assumption is that the decision maker's goal is not only to choose the best option, but to choose the option that will remain the best option in the post-decision future. An option that is not well enough differentiated from its competitors may result in, for instance, a reversal of preference, or negative feelings such as uncertainty, regret, or envy. Table 3.1 presents an overview of the theory.

According to Diff Con Theory, a decision process starts with identifying decision alternatives, attributes and goals. Once the decision problem is defined, various types of differentiation processes may take place.

Table 3.1 Phases in Differentiation and Consolidation Theory

Phase	*Stage*	*Process*
Recognition of decision problem	Identification of alternatives	Perceptual and cognitive identification
	Goal elicitation	Involvement elicitation
Differentiation	Screening	Goal adaptation
	Editing	Holistic differentiation
	Selection of reference and/or preliminary alternative	
	Differentiation	Process and structural differentiation
		Problem restructuring
Decision		
Consolidation	Post-decision consolidation	Process and structural differentiation
	Implementation of decision	Problem restructuring
	Post-implementation consolidation	
	Outcome	
	Post-outcome consolidation	

Decision makers start with screening the available options, and attempt to eliminate options that do not qualify for further consideration. A quick holistic process may select a preliminary choice candidate. *Holistic differentiation* thus comprises a quick classification, which occurs automatically, intuitively, and thus beyond the decision maker's awareness (Beach, 1990). Differentiation criteria may stem from, for instance, experience with similar decisions, intuitive use of schemas, comparison with an exemplar or prototype, or explicit demands or restrictions in the decision context. Holistic differentiation may thus be sufficient for making a decision, lead to a set of alternatives that deserve further consideration, provide a preliminary choice that is further tested or an alternative that serves as a reference in the process that follows.

The second type of differentiation is *process differentiation.* Given that a decision maker has a set of alternatives, further differentiation may be accomplished by processing information about the options. Such information may be retrieved from memory, or acquired externally. In this phase one alternative is gradually differentiated so as to become the chosen one. Various processing strategies may be used, which is referred to as *decision rule differentiation*. Application of decision rules creates information about the degree of superiority of one alternative over another. A large variety of decision rules have been described in the decision making literature (see, e.g., Abelson and Levi, 1985; Bettman *et al.*, 1991; Payne, 1976; Svenson, 1979). Some rules result in elimination of alternatives early in the selection process. For instance, according to the conjunctive rule, all alternatives that do not meet a given criterion level on an attribute are eliminated from the choice set. Other rules comprise a relatively effortful evaluation of all alternatives. For instance, following the weighted additive rule, pros and cons of alternatives are weighted by the importance of the attributes, and the option is chosen that has the most favourable weighted score. In general, rules that allow decision makers to make trade-offs between attribute values (compensatory strategies) are cognitively more effortful than rules that do not allow compensation, such as the conjunctive rule. Decision strategies typically comprise combinations of rules, which are often utilised in a bottom-up, constructive and adaptive fashion (cf. Payne *et al.*, 1992).

Some rules need criteria to be set by the decision makers, for example criteria of rejection in the conjunctive rule, or criteria of acceptance in the disjunctive rule. In the disjunctive rule an alternative is chosen that exceeds a certain criterion level of attractiveness on an attribute. Such criteria may be varied during the process of applying a rule, and may thus be used as a tool in accomplishing sufficient differentiation, which is known as *criterion differentiation.*

In contrast to most decision-theoretic approaches, the interpretation of decision rules in Diff Con Theory not only acknowledges the rules' power to select one alternative as superior, it views decision rules as tools to establish the degree of superiority of one alternative over others. For instance, the conjunctive rule provides information about how far from the pass–fail criterion alternatives are. Decision rules and criterion differentiation are processes that ultimately differentiate one option sufficiently from its competitors.

In conjunction with the application of decision rules, changes in the representation of the decision problem also take place, called *structural differentiation.* Structural differentiation refers to changes in one's representation of the choice problem. Structural differentiations are of four types, i.e., restructuring of (1) attractiveness, (2) attribute importance, (3) the interpretations of facts and (4) the decision problem.

Attractiveness restructuring comprises revision of attractiveness of attribute values of options. Also, a decision maker may ascribe different degrees of importance to attributes so as to support a preliminary choice. This is denoted as *importance restructuring*. Facts may be differently interpreted, reinterpreted, or misinterpreted during the decision process, i.e., *facts restructuring*. This may especially occur to the extent that facts are uncertain, or information is ambiguous. Finally, the decision problem as such may be changed into *problem restructuring*. For instance, in unstructured decision contexts one may look for new alternatives in addition to evaluating present options. Structural differentiation mechanisms, and in particular attractiveness and attribute importance restructuring, are related to decision rule and criterion differentiation. Like the latter processes, the goal of structural differentiation is to achieve sufficient differentiation such that one alternative can be chosen.

Once a decision is made, Diff Con Theory postulates that differentiation mechanisms continue to operate, which is referred to as *consolidation* of the decision. After a choice is made, differentiation of the chosen option and its competitors is further increased, so as to minimise the occurrence of regret (Loomes and Sugden, 1982) or cognitive dissonance (Festinger, 1957). Consolidation comprises many of the differentiation principles that were described for the pre-decision phase. Thus, once a decision has been made, the decision maker may also engage in holistic, process and structural differentiation processes. For instance, attractiveness restructuring may take place by increasing the attractiveness difference between the chosen and non-chosen alternative on one or more attributes (Svenson and Benthorn, 1992).

ON EFFECTS OF INVOLVEMENT ON DECISION MAKING PROCESSES

We now consider how each involvement type may relate to decision making processes. Specifically, we discuss how value-relevant, outcome-relevant and impression-relevant involvement may affect identification of the decision problem, and holistic, process and structural differentiation and consolidation.

Identifying the decision problem

Involvement is important in the very first stage of the decision process, when the decision maker identifies the problem, and searches for choice alternatives and relevant attributes in relation to the decision goals. Each involvement type is related to a particular decision goal. In high value-relevant involvement contexts, decision makers are motivated to make decisions that are in accordance with activated values, or at least not to violate them. These values are also likely to guide the identification of alternatives and relevant attributes. For instance, Christian parents who select a pre-school for their child may consider certain alternatives (Catholic, Protestant, or state schools), but may not even be aware of the existence of Muslim schools. On the other hand, high outcome-relevant and high impression-relevant involvement decision makers, although they have different motives, are likely to search for all relevant alternatives and attributes, so as to be sure to include all relevant options.

Holistic differentiation

At low levels of any type of involvement, decision makers may tend to engage in holistic differentiation, which provides a differentiated representation of the decision problem at relatively low cognitive costs. Low involvement information processing typically comprises the use of readily available category-based judgements (Fiske and Neuberg, 1990), simple heuristics (Chaiken *et al.*, 1989; Petty and Cacioppo, 1986), or habit-based responses (Verplanken *et al.*, in press). Such processing results in quick categorisations of choice options, or leads to an immediate choice.

It can be argued that holistic differentiation is not confined to low involvement contexts. In high value-relevant involvement decisions, holistic differentiation is also conceivable. Activated values may provide cues that allow for quick categorisation processes, which characterise holistic differentiation, by evoking schemas. A schema can be defined as 'a cognitive structure that represents knowledge about a concept or type of stimulus, including its attributes and the relations among these attributes' (Fiske and Taylor, 1991: 98). Schemas may provide readily available value-related labels, which make quick categorisations easy. For instance, health-related schemas may provide a consumer who has strong health values with food categories ('junk food', 'sweets', 'low fat products') in the supermarket. Schemas also trigger readily available attractiveness judgements, which may thus lead to an immediate differentiated representation (Sujan, 1985). Schemas also tend to minimise perceived differences among category members, and to maximise differences between members and non-members, and thus help categorisation. In sum, under conditions of high value-relevant involvement value-related schemas may guide differentiation and (preliminary) choices.

The occurrence of holistic differentiation under conditions of high impression-relevant involvement depends on the type of evaluation context that is expected. When the decision maker expects to face an audience with unknown standpoints, taking a moderate, defensible decision is the optimal strategy. In that case holistic differentiation is less likely. On the other hand, when the decision maker knows *how* he or she will be evaluated, this criterion can be used in a holistic differentiation process, leading to categorisation of alternatives, and a (preliminary) choice. For instance, a politician who plans to address an audience that has a certain interest easily determines which topics are suitable to discuss and which are not.

Holistic differentiation is least likely to occur in high outcome-relevant involvement contexts. The analytic processing mode that this involvement type elicits is not compatible with quick categorisation processes of holistic differentiation. Moreover, the typical highly outcome-involved decision maker will not want to drop alternatives too early in the process.

Process differentiation

Decision rules represent powerful differentiation processes. By applying one or more rules, the decision maker reaches a judgement about the decision problem that allows for making a sustainable choice. It is conceivable that the three types of involvement strongly affect the use of decision rules, attributes and selection criteria.

Generally, when involvement in a decision is low, simple decision rules are likely (e.g., the satisficing or the lexicographic rule). These rules are non-compensatory, requiring little mental effort, and may yet result in a satisfactory decision, given that accuracy motives are not strongly present (Payne *et al.*, 1988).

In high value-relevant involvement decisions, effort is expended on mapping the decision maker's values and goals on the problem. As long as this mapping is not clear, acceptance criteria (e.g., in a conjunctive rule) may be relaxed, in order not to drop potentially valuable alternatives. As soon as a satisfactory mapping is accomplished, values may determine the strictness of the cut-off criteria, which are used to maintain or reject alternatives (cf. the notion of latitudes of rejection in social judgement theory). In the example of religious parents looking for an appropriate school, they may use the number of hours per week of religious teaching as a selection criterion. When value-relevant involvement is high, the screening phase is likely to result in a small set of strictly selected options, which are in accordance with the activated values. If these options are equally attractive according to the values that are at stake, a compensatory strategy (e.g., the weighted additive rule) may be used to select the best option. Strict screening may also lead to keeping one alternative, which is thus chosen.

In high outcome-relevant involvement decisions, it can be expected that if a conjunctive strategy is used to screen alternatives, criteria will be lenient so as not to drop alternatives too early. When buying a house, for example, one may wish to consider all available houses that fall within the financial limits. The resulting set will be larger than in high value-relevant involvement situations, and an early preliminary choice less likely. Given the general finding that outcome-relevant involvement leads to systematic information processing, the use of compensatory rules is likely under those conditions. Such rules ensure high accuracy, albeit at the expense of cognitive effort.

Involvement in how a decision will be seen by significant others necessitates a dual evaluation of a decision problem (i.e., from one's own as well as from the other's perspective). Therefore, in a high impression-relevant involvement decision context the decision maker will keep a large set of options open for consideration, when the need for a moderate or compromise decision is expected. The criterion in a conjunctive type of elimination process may then be less strict. Having to consider impression-relevant information may induce the consideration of two perspectives (one's own and the other's), thereby using up resources for complex compensatory rule applications. When the real or imagined audience's position is well known in advance, rules that comprise selective search (e.g., the lexicographic rule, or elimination-by-aspects rule) will result in a satisfactory differentiation and choice.

There are other aspects of process differentiation that might be influenced by involvement. Process differentiation comprises consideration of information about choice options. This information may be available in memory, or may have to be acquired. In either case, value-relevant involvement in particular may affect the search for information. A value structure provides a framework that guides, or perhaps biases, the search for information. For instance, the health-involved consumer may be alert to product information about chemical additives, while other, possibly important, information is neglected. Values may also affect the interpretation and evaluation of information, for instance by determining which evaluative labels one uses to judge 'facts'. For instance, the health-involved consumer may judge information about the percentage of fat in cheese on a scale ranging from unhealthy (high percentages) to healthy (low percentages), whereas others may interpret the same percentages as creamy versus tasteless. Such effects are less likely in high outcome-relevant and impression-relevant involvement decisions.

An important element in process differentiation is that at some point in the process a preliminary choice is tested against alternatives, and gradually differentiated so as to become the chosen alternative. Involvement may be related to the readiness to give up a preliminary choice, and to select another candidate. It can be expected that, compared to high outcome-relevant and impression-relevant involvement contexts, in high value-relevant involvement conditions commitment to a preliminary choice is stronger, as it is made early in the process and backed up by activated values.

On the other hand, in high outcome-relevant decisions, dropping a preliminary choice depends on a less committed, more objective, evaluation of its merits compared to what is known about alternative options. In a high impression-relevant decision process, commitment to a preliminary choice is likely to be low, because decision makers should be able to switch easily to options that better fit the goal of a favourable impression on other people.

Finally, in so far as involvement is related to decision rule choice, it can be expected that at high involvement levels, in particular value-relevant and outcome-relevant involvement, decision makers will adapt differently from less involved persons to cognitive demands that are related to task and decision context, for example task complexity or time pressure. Involvement may overrule people's natural tendency to adapt to decision problem complexities. Verplanken (1993), for instance, found that participants who had a relatively strong chronic motivation to expend cognitive effort on a task (i.e., who were high in 'need for cognition') were less adaptive to time pressure than participants with less such motivation.

Structural differentiation

Structural differentiation refers to changes in representations of decision problems, which may concern attractiveness of aspects, attribute importance, facts, or the problem as such. Because the representations of decision alternatives are contingent on the decision maker's goals, representations are likely to be modelled according to goals that are elicited by the three involvement types.

Involvement type will be related to aspect attractiveness restructuring. The involvement type-related goals (adhering to a value, accuracy, and eliciting an appropriate impression, respectively) provide the frame of reference for attractiveness judgements, and thus for attractiveness restructuring. The same holds for attribute importance restructuring. The involvement-related goal structures may determine which attributes are used in a process of restructuring, for instance in changing relative importance of an attribute that makes a preliminary chosen alternative more attractive.

Facts restructuring is likely at very high levels of involvement, in particular in high value-relevant involvement decisions. Strong value-driven motives to support an alternative may be backed up by a biased interpretation of reality. For instance, the religious parents who select a school for their child may think that lessons on religion in state schools are used for atheistic indoctrination. This type of restructuring typically obstructs discussions on value-laden decisions. Both high outcome- and high impression-involvement are less likely to lead to attractiveness and facts restructuring, the former because of the evoked accuracy motive, the latter because of the expected confrontation with others.

Some decision problems bring about problem restructuring resulting in alternative ways of representing the decision problem, for instance by finding new attributes, creating new alternatives, or modifying old ones. This kind of fundamental restructuring may bolster a preliminary choice, which is likely in high value-relevant involvement decisions. It may also lead to a completely new representation, one that produces a new choice candidate. This situation may be expected at very high levels of outcome-relevant involvement decisions, when the decision maker is unable to solve the problem satisfactorily according to the course of action followed so far. In that case a relatively objective and creative fresh look at the problem is needed.

Consolidation

Diff Con Theory states that differentiation processes continue to operate after the decision is made. It can be expected that the extent to which such consolidation is needed is related to the level of involvement and the outcome (Benthorn, 1994; Cooper and Fazio, 1984; Svenson and Malmsten, in press). Unimportant decisions, such as routine choices, do not need consolidation, whereas this is more likely for important decisions.

When impression-relevant situations are temporary, there will be little post-choice consolidation. When impression-management concerns are long-lasting (e.g., a person who buys a pretentious car in order to show off), consolidation can be expected. At high value-relevant and outcome-relevant involvement levels the need for consolidation will be relatively strong. The impact of value-relevant and outcome-relevant involvement on post-decision consolidation processes will largely parallel the principles for pre-decision differentiation processes.

EMPIRICAL EVIDENCE

The ideas outlined so far concerning possible effects of value-, impression- and outcome-relevant involvement on decision making processes are tentative, and need to be empirically tested. However, existing studies that investigated effects of these or related motivations in judgement and decision making tasks may provide circumstantial evidence for some of our arguments. In the following, such evidence is discussed for each of the involvement types.

Effects of value-relevant involvement

There is a substantial literature in the domain of game theory, which describes how people behave in situations like the Prisoner's Dilemma (e.g., Dawes, 1980). One finding is that individual differences in value orientations are related to behaviour in such games. More specifically, and important for the present discussion, individuals' value orientation determines how a particular choice situation is defined, for instance in terms of personal profits (as an 'individualist' would do) or collective interests (as a co-operatively oriented individual would do). Van Vugt *et al.* (1995), for instance, found that participants' pre-measured social value orientation determined the way they defined travel mode choice problems as either environmental problems (other-oriented participants), or as accessibility problems (self-oriented participants).

Values also directly affect the decision makers' attributes weights. For instance, Hughes *et al.* (1976) showed that value orientations were related to attribute weights in decisions concerning the building of a nuclear power plant. Judge and Bretz (1992) found that, in a job selection study, participants were more likely to choose jobs that called for values that matched their own. Apparently, values provided a functional framework that guided participants' decisions. This was also demonstrated by Feather (1995), who found that values were related to the attractiveness of choice alternatives that matched those values, and thus to choices. Verplanken *et al.* (1997) demonstrated how primed values may affect attribute weights and choices.

Values are also involved in post-decision consolidation processes. In particular, one may assume that when important values are involved, decisions may affect one's self-image. Protection of self-image has been found to be a powerful post-decisional motive. For instance, Steele (1988) arranged for some participants to be protected from feeling post-decisional regret by reminding them about something good about themselves, and found that they rationalised less after a decision than participants who were not protected. Evidence of effects of personal involvement on post-decisional restructuring can also be found in research into cognitive dissonance. If a decision has aversive consequences for the decision maker, for instance missing an attractive option, this may induce cognitive dissonance. Dissonance is only induced when the individual is personally responsible for her/his behaviour, and when the person is sufficiently involved, for instance when important values are threatened. Cognitive restructuring may follow in such a way that the state of discomfort is relieved (e.g., Cooper and Fazio, 1984; Festinger, 1957).

In sum, there are several lines of research that illustrate the way values can affect various elements of the decision process in ways that we have suggested. The studies above suggest that value-relevant involvement plays an important role in defining the problem, the selection and implementation of decision strategies, and in post-decision consolidation.

Effects of impression-relevant involvement

Effects of an expected audience have been widely studied in a variety of contexts. Most manipulations of this kind are denoted as accountability demands. Although their research was not aimed at comparing different motivational states, Tetlock and colleagues have shown that accountability demands have profound effects on how people process information and respond (e.g., Tetlock, 1983). Generally, if individuals know which responses will be favourably evaluated, they shift their views toward those responses. If such responses are not known, they tend to engage in multidimensional and relatively complex information processing, so as to prepare for flexible response capability.

Accountability may thus lead to the use of more analytical judgement and decision modes, as has been found in a number of studies (e.g.,

Hagafors and Brehmer, 1983; McAllister *et al.*, 1979). However, in line with our thoughts concerning effects of impression-relevant involvement, it seems that the accountable individual's responses, and thus the way information is processed, depend on the justification criteria to which he or she anticipates being subjected. In other words, information processing is not more complex *per se* under conditions of accountability, but is functional in meeting the expected justification. Simonson and Nye (1992), for instance, demonstrated that participants under accountability conditions exhibit normatively correct, as opposed to biased, responses in decision tasks, when they expect these responses to be positively evaluated by the researchers, and when the normatively correct response was seen as easier to justify. When the correct responses were not known, accountability did not reduce the occurrence of biased responses.

Some studies provide evidence to suggest that accountability demands may lead to more information search, but not necessarily to more complex choice rules (Nichols-Hoppe and Beach, 1990; Verplanken *et al.*, in press). These results may also be interpreted as indications of strategic preparations for the justification phase, and not necessarily of more complex decision making.

Effects of outcome-relevant involvement

As has been repeatedly demonstrated in persuasion research, some studies on decision making provide evidence to suggest that when decisions have personal consequences, decision makers tend to engage in relatively complex and analytical processing. Billings and Scherer (1988), for instance, found that outcome-involved decision makers searched more information, whereas low involvement participants employed more intradimensional and variable search patterns, suggesting the use of non-compensatory strategies. Klayman (1985) also found that, given sufficient memory capacity and a complex choice problem, children used more complex choice strategies when the topic was perceived as important. Christensen-Szalanski (1978) found that participants who were paid more exhibited more complex problem solving strategies. Finally, in a field study among farmers, Gensch and Javalgi (1987) found respondents' use of compensatory or non-compensatory choice rules a function of measured personal relevance of the decision topic.

CONCLUDING REMARKS

Whereas common sense may tell us that personal involvement affects decision processes, the message of the present chapter is that such a statement is too simple, and requires more careful consideration. The basis of our argument is that personal involvement may refer to different constructs. Each involvement type has a different motivational basis, and thus elicits different processing goals. Drawing upon Johnson and Eagly's (1989) meta-analysis in the area of persuasion and attitude change, we distinguished motivations that are related to adhering to enduring values, attaining desirable outcomes, and presenting oneself in a socially desirable way. We argued that decision processes should also be influenced by these different motives. Processes related to value-relevant involvement can be expected to be selective and biased. High outcome-relevant involvement decisions will trigger accuracy-driven processes that are relatively objective, but cognitively demanding. Impression-relevant involvement processes are aimed at keeping the decision maker informed about useful positions, so as to be flexible in the expected social interaction.

We have presented some empirical support for our arguments. However, it is clear from a review of the existing literature that motivational factors have received little attention in research on decision making processes (Ford *et al.*, 1989; Larrick, 1993). We therefore need empirical research that explicitly addresses the phenomena that we discussed. This may become a promising line of research, which may lead to a deeper understanding of human decision making.

NOTE

1 The claim that value-relevant and outcome-relevant involvement are conceptually distinct constructs, and lead to different processes, was challenged by Petty and Cacioppo (1990), and was further commented on by Johnson and Eagly (1990). However, although this is an important discussion, for the present purposes we do not elaborate on it, and draw on Johnson and Eagly's (1989) original conclusions.

ACKNOWLEDGEMENTS

The authors thank Anders Johansson for his contribution in retrieving relevant literature, and Ray Crozier, Johanna Harte, Rob Ranyard and two reviewers for their helpful comments on earlier drafts of this chapter.

REFERENCES

Abelson, R.P. and Levi, A. (1985) 'Decision making and decision theory', in G. Lindzey and E. Aronson (eds) *Handbook of Social Psychology,* (3rd. edn), vol. 1, New York: Random House.

Beach, L.R. (1990) *Image Theory: Decision Making in Personal and Organizational Contexts*, New York: Wiley.

Benthorn, L.J. (1994) 'On post-decision processes', Unpublished doctoral dissertation, University of Lund, Sweden.

Bettman, J.R., Johnson, E.J. and Payne, J.W. (1991) 'Consumer decision making', in T.S. Robertson and H.H. Kassarjian (eds) *Handbook of Consumer Behavior*, Englewood Cliffs, NJ: Prentice-Hall.

Billings, R.S. and Scherer, L.L. (1988). 'The effects of response mode and importance on decision-making strategies', *Organizational Behavior and Human Decision Processes*, 41: 1–19.

Bloch, P.H. and Richins, M.L. (1983) 'A theoretical model for the study of product importance perceptions', *Journal of Marketing*, 47: 69–81.

Chaiken, S. (1987) 'The heuristic model of persuasion', in M.P. Zanna, J.M. Olson and C.P. Herman (eds) *Social Influence: The Ontario Symposium*, vol. 5, Hillsdale, NJ: Erlbaum.

Chaiken, S., Liberman, A. and Eagly, A.H. (1989) 'Heuristic and systematic information processing within and beyond the persuasion context', in J.S. Uleman and J.A. Bargh (eds) *Unintended Thought*, New York: Guilford Press.

Chen, S., Shechter, D. and Chaiken, S. (1996), 'Getting at the truth or getting along: accuracy- versus impression-motivated heuristic and systematic processing', *Journal of Personality and Social Psychology*, 71: 262–75.

Christensen-Szalanski, J.J.J. (1978) 'Problem solving strategies: a selection mechanism, some implications and some data', *Organizational Behavior and Human Performance*, 22: 307–23.

Cooper, J. and Fazio, R.H. (1984) 'A new look at dissonance theory', *Advances in Experimental Social Psychology*, 17: 229–66.

Dawes, R.M. (1980) 'Social dilemmas', *Annual Review of Psychology*, 31: 169–93.

Feather, N.T. (1995) 'Values, valences and choice: the influence of values on the perceived attractiveness and choice of alternatives', *Journal of Personality and Social Psychology*, 68: 1135–51.

Festinger, L. (1957) *A Theory of Cognitive Dissonance*, Stanford, CA: Stanford University Press.

Fiske, S.T. and Neuberg, S.L. (1990) 'A continuum of impression formation, from category-based to individuating processes: influences of information and motivation on attention and interpretation', *Advances in Experimental Social Psychology*, 23: 1–74.

Fiske, S.T. and Taylor, S.E. (1991) *Social Cognition*, (2nd edn), New York: McGraw-Hill.

Ford, J.K., Schmitt, N., Schechtman, S.L., Hults, B.M. and Doherty, M.L. (1989) 'Process tracing methods: contributions, problems, and neglected research questions', *Organizational Behavior and Human Decision Processes*, 43: 75–117.

Gensch, D.H. and Javalgi, R.G. (1987) 'The influence of involvement on disaggregate attribute choice models', *Journal of Consumer Research*, 14: 71–82.

Greenwald, A.G. (1968) 'Cognitive learning, cognitive response to persuasion, and attitude change', in A.G. Greenwald, T.C. Brock and T.M. Ostrom (eds) *Psychological Foundations of Attitudes*, New York: Academic Press.

Greenwald, A.G. and Leavitt, C. (1984) 'Audience involvement in advertising: four levels', *Journal of Consumer Research*, 11: 581–92.

Hagafors, R. and Brehmer, B. (1983) 'Does having to justify one's judgments change the nature of the judgment process?', *Organizational Behavior and Human Performance*, 31: 223–32.

Houston, M.J. and Rothschild, M.L. (1978) 'Conceptual and methodological perspectives on involvement', in S. Jain (ed.) *Research Frontiers in Marketing: Dialogues and Directions*, Chicago: American Marketing Association.

Hughes, G.D., Rao, V.R. and Alker, H.A. (1976) 'The influence of values, information, and decision orders on a public policy decision', *Journal of Applied Social Psychology*, 6: 145–58.

Johnson, B.T. and Eagly, A.H. (1989) 'Effects of involvement on persuasion: a meta-analysis', *Psychological Bulletin*, 106: 290–314.

Johnson, B.T. and Eagly, A.H. (1990) 'Involvement and persuasion: types, traditions, and the evidence', *Psychological Bulletin*, 107: 375–84.

Judge, T.A. and Bretz, R.D., Jr (1992) 'Effects of work values on job choice decisions', *Journal of Applied Psychology*, 77: 261–71.

Klayman, J. (1985) 'Children's decision strategies and their adaptation to task characteristics', *Organizational Behavior and Human Decision Processes*, 35: 179–201.

Larrick, R.P. (1993) 'Motivational factors in decision theories: the role of self-protection', *Psychological Bulletin*, 113: 440–50.

Leippe, M.R. and Elkin, R.A. (1987) 'When motives clash: issue involvement and response involvement as determinants of persuasion', *Journal of Personality and Social Psychology*, 52: 269–78.

Loomes, G. and Sugden, R. (1982) 'Regret theory: an alternative theory of rational choice under uncertainty', *Economic Journal*, 42: 805–24.

McAllister, D.W., Mitchell, T.R. and Beach, L.R. (1979) 'The contingency model for the selection of decision strategies: an empirical test of the effects of significance, accountability, and reversibility', *Organizational Behavior and Human Performance*, 24: 228–44.

Mittal, B. and Lee, M.-S. (1989) 'A causal model of consumer involvement', *Journal of Economic Psychology*, 10: 363–89.

Nichols-Hoppe, K.T. and Beach, L.R. (1990) 'The effects of test anxiety and task variables on predecisional information search', *Journal of Research in Personality*, 24: 163–72.

Payne, J.W. (1976) 'Task complexity and contingent processing in decision making: an information search and protocol analysis', *Organizational Behavior and Human Performance*, 16: 366–87.

Payne, J.W., Bettman, J.R. and Johnson, E.J. (1988) 'Adaptive strategy selection in decision making', *Journal of Experimental Psychology: Learning, Memory, and Cognition*, 14: 534–52.

Payne, J.W., Bettman, J.R. and Johnson, E.J. (1992) 'Behavioral decision research: a constructive processing perspective', *Annual Review of Psychology*, 43: 87–131.

Petty, R.E. and Cacioppo, J.T. (1986) *Communication and Persuasion: Central and Peripheral Routes to Attitude Change*, New York: Springer-Verlag.

Petty, R.E. and Cacioppo, J.T. (1990) 'Involvement and persuasion: tradition versus integration', *Psychological Bulletin*, 107: 367–74.

Sherif, M. and Cantril, H. (1947) *The Psychology of Ego Involvements: Social Attitudes and Identifications*, New York: Wiley.

Sherif, M. and Hovland, C.I. (1961) *Social Judgment: Assimilation and Contrast Effects in Communication and Attitude Change*, New Haven, CT: Yale University Press.

Simonson, I. and Nye, P. (1992) 'The effect of accountability on susceptibility to decision errors', *Organizational Behavior and Human Decision Processes*, 51: 416–46.

Steele, C.M. (1988) 'The psychology of self-affirmation: sustaining the integrity of the self', *Advances in Experimental Social Psychology*, 21: 261–302.

Sujan, M. (1985) 'Consumer knowledge: effects on evaluation strategies mediating consumer judgments', *Journal of Consumer Research*, 12: 31–46.

Svenson, O. (1979) 'Process descriptions of decision making', *Organizational Behavior and Human Performance*, 23: 86–112.

Svenson, O. (1992) 'Differentiation and Consolidation Theory of human decision making: a frame of reference for the study of pre- and post-decision processes', *Acta Psychologica*, 80: 143–68.

Svenson, O. (1996) 'Decision making and the search for fundamental psychological regularities: what can be learned from a process perspective?', *Organizational Behavior and Human Decision Processes*, 65: 252–67.

Svenson, O. and Benthorn, L.J. (1992) 'Consolidation processes in decision making: post-decision changes in attractiveness of alternatives', *Journal of Economic Psychology*, 13: 315–27.

Svenson, O. and Malmsten, N. (in press) 'Post-decision consolidation over time as a function of gain or loss of an alternative', *Scandinavian Journal of Psychology*.

Tetlock, P.E. (1983) 'Accountability and the complexity of thought', *Journal of Personality and Social Psychology*, 45: 74–83.

van Vugt, M., Meertens, R. and van Lange, P. (1995) 'Car versus public transportation? The role of social value orientations in a real-life social dilemma', *Journal of Applied Social Psychology*, 25: 258–78.

Verplanken, B. (1993) 'Need for cognition and external information search: responses to time pressure during decision making', *Journal of Research in Personality*, 27: 238–52.

Verplanken, B., Aarts, H. and van Knippenberg, A. (in press) 'Habit, information acquisition, and the process of making travel mode choices', *European Journal of Social Psychology*.

Verplanken, B., Sas, I., Harte, J.M. and Svenson, O. (1997) 'Motivated decision making: effects of primed values on multiattributive choice processes', Unpublished manuscript.

Zaichkowsky, J.L. (1985) 'Measuring the involvement construct', *Journal of Consumer Research*, 12: 341–52.

Zimbardo, P.G. (1960) 'Involvement and communication discrepancy as determinants of opinion conformity', *Journal of Abnormal and Social Psychology*, 60: 86–94.

Chapter 4

Aspects of compatibility and the construction of preference

Marcus Selart

One of the most powerful concepts for understanding and aiding judgements and decisions is compatibility. There are several reasons for this. To begin with, compatibility has an impact on many types of perceptual and motor performances. This is because the difficulty of a specific task depends on the particular sets of stimuli and responses that are used in it. Of special importance is how the stimuli and responses are paired with each other. For instance, many studies in cognitive psychology have revealed that subjects' responses are faster and more accurate if they are compatible with the stimuli. Consequently, as has been pointed out by Shafir (1995), subjects' responses to a pair of lights assigned to a pair of keys are faster and more accurate if the left light is assigned to the left key and the right light to the right key (Fitts and Seeger, 1953; Wickens, 1984). Furthermore, a pointing response is faster than a vocal response when a visual stimulus is presented, whereas the reverse holds true when the stimulus consists of an auditory message (Brainard *et al.*, 1962). Compatibility between stimulus and responses has also been shown to be salient for a broad range of other perceptual and motor performance tasks (see, e.g., Kornblum *et al.*, 1990 and Proctor and Reeve, 1990, for reviews).

It has recently been shown that the compatibility between input and output is also a factor in how people construct their preferences in reasoning and decision making. Shafir (1995) has argued that compatibility may contribute to a broad range of biases, including confirmatory biases (Barsalou, 1992), congruence biases (Baron, 1994), verification biases (Johnson-Laird and Wason, 1970) and matching biases (Evans, 1984, 1989). It is argued that violations of the normative principles underlying these forms of biases are due to people's tendency to focus on those instances that are more compatible with the instructions or with the tested hypotheses. An implication of these assumptions is that compatibility between the way in which decision alternatives are described and the way responses are expressed has an impact on how preferences are finally constructed (see, e.g., Slovic, 1995, for a review).

The preference reversal phenomenon has to a large extent contributed to the understanding of the role of compatibility in cognition and decision (Slovic and Lichtenstein, 1983). A preference reversal is said to occur when an individual prefers one alternative in one procedure, but reveals a different preference order in another procedure. For instance, it has been shown that subjects who are presented with two normatively equivalent gambles with the same expected value often make a choice of the gamble with the higher probability. At the same time they indicate a higher selling price for the one with the higher pay-off. Consequently, making a choice between two gambles seems to involve other psychological processes than when the alternatives are being priced separately. The idea of compatibility was introduced as a possible explanation of the preference reversal phenomenon. Compatibility seemed to be able to explain why naming a prize for the gambles was dependent on the pay-off information to such a large extent. Lichtenstein and Slovic (1973) suggested that the compatibility between an attribute and the actual response has an impact on that attribute's influence when the response is made. This reasoning eventually resulted in the *scale compatibility hypothesis*, which states that the weight of a stimulus attribute in a decision or a judgement is increased by its compatibility with the response mode (see, e.g., Slovic *et al.*, 1990; Tversky, 1977; Tversky *et al.*, 1988). The hypothesis finds support in process tracing studies that have shown that response scales may prime the attention to the compatible attribute: pricing judgements prime attention to the amount to be won just as rating scales prime the attention to probabilities (Schkade and Johnson, 1989). In line with this, Chapman and Johnson (1994) reported that scale compatibility occurs if an anchor and a preference judgement are expressed on the same scale. It was also shown by Chapman and Johnson (1995) that semantic categorisation is an important feature of scale compatibility. In life expectancy evaluations, health items were preferred to commodities, whereas in monetary evaluations commodities were preferred to health items.

A parallel line of reasoning emanates from the results of Slovic (1975). In this study, subjects were instructed to make a choice between two equally attractive alternatives. The participants first matched different pairs of alternatives, in that they equated the values of the alternatives of each pair (see below for details of this procedure). Later on, they were instructed to make a choice between the matched alternatives. Slovic found that subjects did not make their choices at random, but instead tended to choose the alternative that dominated on the most important attribute. This reasoning led to the introduction of the *prominence hypothesis* (Tversky *et al.*, 1988), which implies that the most important or prominent attribute looms larger in choice than in matching. The hypothesis thereby asserts that people tend to make choices according to the most important dimension, but they match options by comparing trade-offs along dimensions. For instance, Tversky *et al.* (1988) demonstrated that the majority of their subjects chose the alternative that dominated on the prominent attribute, even though subjects in a parallel matching task favoured the other alternative.

Tversky *et al.* (1988) suggested that different heuristics or computational schemes may have been triggered in the two types of task. The qualitative nature of choice was seen as more likely than the quantitative nature of matching to lead to a preference for the alternative that dominated on the prominent attribute. This idea was elaborated by Fischer and Hawkins (1993), who suggested that the prominence effect was not restricted to choice and matching, but could be generalised to any comparison between qualitative and quantitative preference tasks. They termed their notion the *strategy compatibility hypothesis.*

TOWARDS A STRUCTURE COMPATIBILITY MODEL

This chapter aims to present a new cognitive model of compatibility which has been briefly introduced elsewhere (Selart, 1996; Selart *et al.*, 1997). It argues that significant compatibility effects can be attributed to how the information is structured and organised in input and output.

As may be seen in Figure 4.1, the model assumes that a compatibility test between the output and the input initially takes place (1). Here, whether the information structure in input is compatible with the information structure of the response mode in output is tested. This test has implications for the selection of decision strategy (2). A lack of compatibility will result in the use of a non-compensatory strategy, whereas compatibility between input and output will lead to the use of a compensatory strategy. The use of decision strategy will in turn affect both the evaluation of the decision outcomes (3) and the implementation of the judgement or decision (4).

Building on the results of Payne (1982) and Hawkins (1994), it is suggested that two general classes of variables play a major part in how subjects construct their preferences. These are task and context effects. Task effects can be related to manipulations of the general structure of the decision, including response mode, number of options or attributes, time pressure and presentation constraints (Bettman, 1982; Klayman, 1985; Russo and Dosher, 1983). Context effects, on the other hand, are connected to manipulations of the content of the decision problem, involving attribute values, similarity of alternatives, attribute covariation, and overall attractiveness of alternatives (Casey, 1991; Johnson *et al.*, 1988; Stone and Schkade, 1991).

Among the task variables, response mode has perhaps been most investigated. As was shown above, earlier models of compatibility emphasised the idea that response mode may either enhance the weight of the

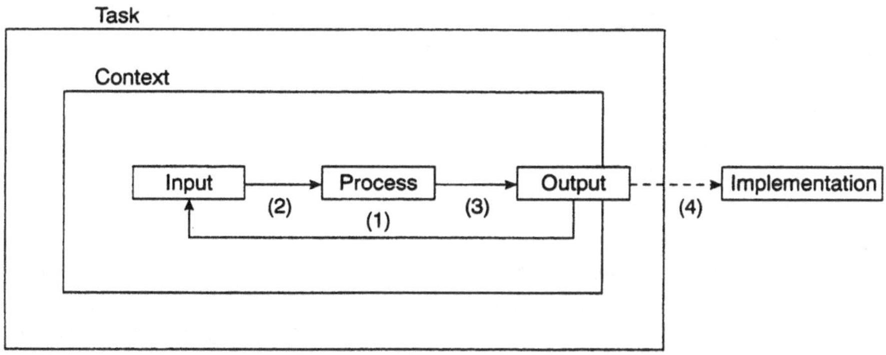

Figure 4.1 A conceptual model of structure compatibility

compatible value attribute (scale compatibility) or prime a particular decision strategy (strategy compatibility). These are alternative explanations of how the response mode in output affects the input (1). The structure compatibility model takes as its point of departure that there are decisions and judgements that prime the same decision strategy because of the compatibility between input and output. An important implication of this is that prominence effects may also occur in judgements. Empirical findings reveal that prominence effects are not restricted to choices. It has been amply shown that the prominent attribute looms larger also in preference ratings (Fischer and Hawkins, 1993; Montgomery *et al.*, 1994; Selart, 1996; Selart *et al.*, 1997; Selart *et al.*, 1994). That is, subjects rate the alternative that dominates on the prominent attribute as more attractive despite the fact that both alternatives have previously been judged as equally attractive in a matching procedure. Hence, it is assumed that the prominence effect cannot be explained in terms of different strategies evoked by judgements and decisions in a general sense. Instead, it is proposed that the prominence effect is due to differences in compatibility between the required output and the structure of input information.

Similar ideas, emphasising the role of structure compatibility, have been put forward by Schkade and Kleinmuntz (1994), who suggest that organisation of elements strongly influences information acquisition strategies. Creyer and Johar (1995) have also noted that task characteristics such as the number of attributes used to describe alternatives influence the prominence effect. We think that similar task demands in choices and preference ratings display a common organisational principle that is different from the one used in matching. There is also research indicating that compatibility effects may be produced by manipulation of the context. For instance, Parducci (1968, 1974) has shown that different scale continua may influence how a given stimulus is being weighted and judged. One of the findings in his studies was that subjects judged a particular pay-off as satisfying in one such scale continuum but unsatisfying in another. Mellers and Cooke (1994) reported that attribute range influenced the perception of attribute values. It was shown that the effects of a given attribute were greater when presented within a narrow range than within a wide range. This held true for both single-attribute and multiattribute judgements. For example, a monthly rent of $400 seemed worse in a narrow rent range than in a wide rent range.

In this chapter it is assumed that the range of values in the attribute levels of a decision task influences the prominence effect: wide ranges are assumed to increase the effect whereas narrow ranges are thought to decrease it. The rationale behind this notion is that wide ranges stimulate the use of a lexicographic decision strategy, whereas narrow ranges facilitate the use of an additive strategy. Moreover, it must be pointed out that neither the scale compatibility hypothesis nor the strategy compatibility hypothesis predicts any effects of value ranges.

In the following sections of the chapter, structure compatibility is demonstrated in two empirical studies of preferences. A description of the cognitive processes involved is also given in one of the studies where a verbal protocol analysis is performed.

STUDY 1: MATCHING, PREFERENCE AND VALUE RANGE

In many studies a paradigm has been used in which subjects' response outcomes in a matching task are directly compared with their preference statements in choice (e.g., Tversky *et al.* 1988). Building on the model used by Slovic (1975) we, however, let subjects first perform a matching task, in which they were instructed to make pairs of alternatives equally attractive (Selart, 1996). We then let subjects state their preferences for the alternatives to see whether, for instance, they were choosing at random or whether a bias in terms of a prominence effect could be detected.

A new feature of this study was that the value ranges between the attribute levels were manipulated both in the matching task and in the preference task. Thus, in the matching task values on both attributes were expressed on a scale ranging from 0 to 100. The alternatives were constructed by systematically varying the range between the highest and the lowest value on each attribute in steps of 5, 10, 15, 20 or 25 (see Table 4.1). The subjects were undergraduate students at Göteborg University. They were asked to imagine that they were suffering from a disease, and in each problem a pair of treatments were shown. Their task was to provide a missing value so that the options were experienced as equally attractive. The order in which the missing attribute levels were presented was counterbalanced. In the analysis of the matching task we calculated the mean weight ratios between the dimensions in which the mean differences between each attribute were divided.[1] These results revealed that the attribute which we had hypothesised to be experienced as the more important one in fact also turned out to be the prominent one. However, an analysis of variance yielded no reliable effects of value range.

In a subsequent experiment, the mean weight ratios obtained in the matching task were used to construct new sets of stimulus alternatives. In this experiment, subjects' preferences were elicited in terms of choices and preference ratings. Also in these tasks the value ranges between the attribute levels were subject to manipulation, as can be seen in Table 4.2.

The instructions were the same as in the matching task, except that subjects were asked to choose between or to rate the options. Choices and preference ratings were scored equivalently, by means of a recoding

Table 4.1 Examples of stimuli used in the matching task (Study 1)

	Value ranges				
Pair	*05*	*10*	*15*	*20*	*25*
1	X_1 30 30 35	X_1 30 30 40	X_1 30 30 45	X_1 30 30 50	X_1 30 30 55
2	35 X_2 30 35	40 X_2 30 40	45 X_2 30 45	50 X_2 30 50	55 X_2 30 55
3	35 30 X_3 35	40 30 X_3 40	45 30 X_3 45	50 30 X_3 50	55 30 X_3 55
4	35 30 30 X_4	40 30 30 X_4	45 30 30 X_4	50 30 30 X_4	55 30 30 X_4

Notes:
1 X_1 Highest value on the prominent attribute missing
2 X_2 Lowest value on the prominent attribute missing
3 X_3 Lowest value on the non-prominent attribute missing
4 X_4 Highest value on the non-prominent attribute missing

Table 4.2 Examples of stimuli used in the preference task (Study 1)

Value ranges	*Options*	*Prominent attribute*	*Non-prominent attribute*
Narrow	Treatment A	41[1]	36
	Treatment B	36	46
Narrow	Treatment A	42	37
	Treatment B	37	47
Wide	Treatment A	41	1
	Treatment B	1	78
Wide	Treatment A	42	2
	Treatment B	2	79

Note: 1 The values of the prominent and the non-prominent attributes are expressed on a scale ranging from 0 (very low) to 100 (very high)

procedure. In this procedure, preferences for the alternative which dominated on the prominent attribute and preferences for the alternative which was dominated on the same attribute received identical scores in both procedures.

Prominence effects were found in all conditions, that is, both for choices and ratings (see Figure 4.2). The results also revealed that the prominence effect was reliably weaker when the value range was narrow than when it was wide.

One may ask why the manipulation of the value ranges had an impact on the prominence effect in these preference tasks, while it did not affect the mean weight ratios in the matching task. A possible explanation might be that if the range of values is wide between the attribute levels in, for instance, the choice task, then subjects to a greater extent really must 'make a choice between the dimensions', and then the prominent attribute becomes more salient. If, on the other hand, the ranges are narrow in the choice task, then a trade-off between the dimensions will be facilitated, leading to the use of a compensatory decision strategy. The same reasoning applies to preference ratings in which the structure of the task is similar to the one in choice. However, in the matching task this 'either/or' conflict is not to the same extent increased by the wide value ranges.

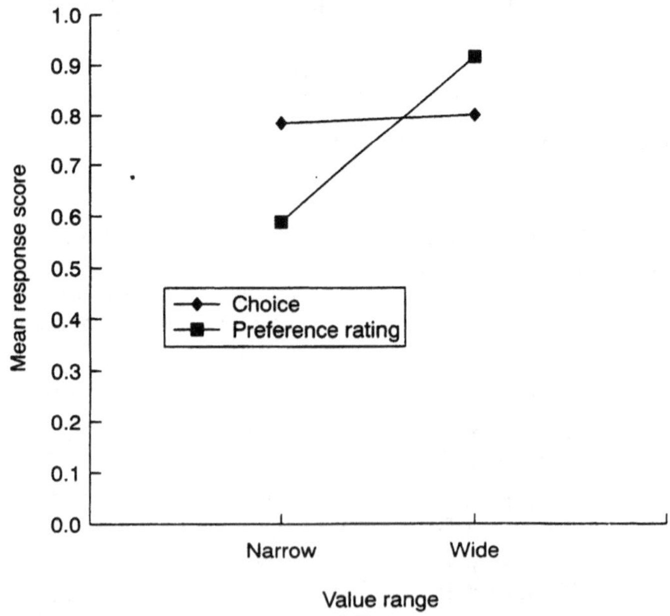

Figure 4.2 Mean response scores for different value ranges in Study 1

STUDY 2: A VERBAL PROTOCOL ANALYSIS

Another issue which must be discussed is how this suggested notion of structure compatibility can be measured. Generally, it may be argued that the ratio between the attention given to the input and the output of a task may provide such a measure. But when considering the matching task/preference task anomaly, perhaps subjects also pay more attention overall to the attribute levels in the matching task than they do in a preference task. If so, then this lower degree of attention could explain the presence of the prominence effect. It may also be plausible to assume that subjects give a more balanced amount of attention to both attributes in the matching task, and that in this task they also compare the attribute levels more often than they do in a preference task.

In order to test these ideas, we designed another study in which the use of verbal protocols was introduced (Selart *et al.*, 1997). Silent control conditions were also conducted (see Russo *et al.*, 1989, for a discussion). The matching task and the preference tasks were constructed and analysed in much the same way as in the first study. An extension was that in the present study we also used acceptance decisions as a complement to choices and preference ratings. Undergraduate students at Göteborg

Table 4.3 Attribute levels of choice problems (medical treatments) presented to subjects (Study 2).

	Attribute	*Option 1*	*Option 2*
1	*Medical care* (1–100)	65	54
	Freedom from disturbance (1–100)	47	62
2	*Health improvement* (1–100)	61	52
	Comfort (1–100)	48	64
3	*Efficiency* (1–100)	56	47
	Pain relief (1–100)	46	58
4	*Medical skill* (1–100)	59	42
	Freedom from fees (1–100)	35	55
5	*Food value* (1–100)	66	51
	Size of food portions (1–100)	49	63
6	*Protection against relapse* (1–100)	55	40
	Program shortage (1–100)	35	52
7	*Medical follow-up* (1–100)	56	43
	Freedom from encroachment (1–100)	28	59
8	*Communication with staff* (1–100)	66	51
	Leisure (1–100)	46	63

Note: Prominent attribute in italics

University once again served as subjects. The problems which were used are shown in Table 4.3. For each problem, we predicted that one attribute would be prominent and the other one non-prominent.

Our predictions about the salience of these attributes were confirmed, technically, since the mean weight ratios of the matching task were higher than 1.0 for every condition, with some variation (see Table 4.4).

Prominence effects were revealed in all preference tasks, that is, all levels reliably differed from the chance level of 0.50 (Table 4.5).

The processing of the verbal protocols followed a procedure which has been developed in previous research (e.g., Harte *et al.*, 1994; Svenson, 1989; see also Chapter 2). Each statement was coded with respect to (a) which of the alternatives, if any, it referred to; (b) which of the attributes, if any, it referred to; and (c) whether subjects compared two attribute levels or attended to a single attribute level. The results are displayed in Table 4.6.

The analysis of the verbal protocols revealed that the prominence effects obtained in the preference tasks were accompanied by a lower degree of attention to the attribute levels. Subjects also compared attribute levels less frequently in the preference tasks than in the matching task. However, the enhanced attention to the prominent attribute that should have been found in the preference tasks was not as clear-cut.

Still, both the generality of the prominence effect in the preference tasks and the obtained process differences between the matching task and the preference tasks reveal that different kinds of decision strategies seem to be involved in the two kinds of tasks, leading to prominence effects in the preference tasks.

Table 4.4 Mean ratios of weights for prominent and non-prominent attributes in the matching task by preference task (Study 2)

	Choice	*Acceptance decision*	*Preference rating*
Think-aloud condition	1.05	1.24	1.11
Silent condition	1.28	1.32	1.36

Table 4.5 Mean response scores for choice, acceptance decision and preference rating (Study 2)

	Response mode		
	Choice	*Acceptance decision*	*Preference rating*
Think-aloud condition	0.86	0.72	0.70
Silent condition	0.83	0.76	0.68

Table 4.6 Means of attention to attribute levels in the think-aloud condition (Study 2)

	Prominent option		*Non-prominent option*	
	Prominent attribute	*Non-prominent attribute*	*Prominent attribute*	*Non-prominent attribute*
Choice condition				
Matching task				
Attribute levels compared	3.75	3.67	3.58	3.83
Attribute levels attended singly	0.25	0.50	0.47	0.58
Preference task				
Attribute levels compared	1.00	0.58	0.50	0.08
Attribute levels attended singly	0.67	0.75	0.17	0.42
Acceptance decision condition				
Matching task				
Attribute levels compared	2.83	2.67	2.75	2.92
Attribute levels attended singly	2.50	1.08	1.17	2.33
Preference task				
Attribute levels compared	1.17	1.00	1.08	0.92
Attribute levels attended singly	0.58	0.17	0.75	0.67
Preference rating condition				
Matching task				
Attribute levels compared	4.83	3.33	4.17	2.83
Attribute levels attended singly	3.00	2.50	1.58	3.75
Preference task				
Attribute levels compared	1.00	0.75	1.67	1.42
Attribute levels attended singly	1.58	0.83	1.17	1.00

The observed process differences also provide an example of how the issue of compatibility can be studied with cognitive data. These data suggest that a low degree of attention to the attribute levels, especially in terms of performed comparisons, seems to be crucial for the prominence effect.

DISCUSSION

In this chapter, it has been shown that structure compatibility effects can be attributed to manipulations both of the task and the context. In two studies, manipulations of the task showed that prominence effects may occur in both choices and preference ratings. This finding was in line with the model which states that choices and preferences involve the same processing mechanism, which is different from the one used in the matching task. Neither the scale compatibility nor the strategy compatibility hypotheses can explain this finding. The scale compatibility hypothesis (Tversky *et al.*, 1988) prescribes the absence of a prominence effect in the rating condition during the described circumstances. This is because the attribute levels used in the present studies ranged from 1 to 100 for both the prominent and the non-prominent attributes, as did the response scales for preference ratings. This should have resulted in a more equal weighting of the attributes in preference ratings than in choices, according to the hypothesis. The failure of the hypothesis corroborates earlier findings that suggest that scale compatibility may operate more readily if prominence effects are absent. The strategy compatibility hypothesis (Fischer and Hawkins, 1993) also suggests a stronger prominence effect in choice, since different kinds of reasoning are assumed to be inherent in choices and judgements independently of the information structure: qualitative response modes are assumed to prime qualitative decision strategies, whereas quantitative response modes are assumed to prime quantitative decision strategies. These differences will in turn lead to differential weighting mechanisms in judgement and choice.

Context effects were investigated by the introduction of different value ranges in Study 1. It was found that, although different value ranges did not have an impact on the weights of the attributes in the matching task, they did affect the prominence effect in both choice and preference rating data. Neither the scale nor the strategy compatibility hypotheses make any context assumptions. However, recent models provided by Mellers and Cooke (1996) may suggest predictions which can be integrated into the model.

Furthermore, an analysis of verbal protocols in Study 2 revealed that subjects made more comparisons between the attribute levels in the matching task than they did in the preference tasks. This finding is in line with the predictions of the model, which assumes that the use of decision strategy should be influenced by the degree of structure compatibility. Similar results have been reported by Hawkins (1994). He tested a set of hypotheses of which a majority concerned processing differences (response time, fixation time) between choice and matching tasks. A computerised information board technique was used in the empirical investigation. First of all, the prominence effect was replicated. It was also found that the matching task in relation to choice had (i) longer total response times, (ii) acquisition of more information, and (iii) longer relative fixation times for the prominent attribute. Furthermore, it was found that a prominence effect between choice and matching could be attributed to relative attention paid to the prominent attribute in choice. These results show clear similarities with the ones obtained in our verbal protocol analysis in which matching and choice also were compared. However, our model also accounts for similar processing differences between matching and preference rating data.

Taken together, our results – and the empirical examples presented from other studies – indicate that it seems necessary to introduce a contingent weighting mechanism that assigns equal importance to input and output information. A structure compatibility model has therefore been proposed in which the importance of both task and context effects is emphasised. From a general point of view, it can be assumed that models of compatibility in judgement and decision must be complex in nature, allowing predictions based on the interaction of several factors. Task effects can be attributed to manipulations of the general structure of the decision, including response mode, number of options or attributes, time pressure and presentation constraints (Bettman, 1982; Klayman, 1985; Russo and Dosher, 1983). Context effects, on the other hand, can be connected to manipulations of the content of the decision problem, involving attribute values, similarity of alternatives, attribute covariation and overall attractiveness of alternatives (Casey, 1991; Johnson *et al.*, 1988, 1988; Stone and Schkade, 1991). It is suggested that the notion of structure compatibility will benefit from future research involving both these classes of variables.

NOTE

1 The analyses of the results rested on the assumption that

$$u_{P,p}+u_{P,np} = u_{NP,p}+u_{NP,np} \tag{1}$$

where $u_{P,p}$ and $u_{P,np}$ denote the attractiveness of the levels of the prominent and non-prominent attributes for the prominent option (with the highest value on the prominent attribute), and $u_{NP,p}$ and $u_{NP,np}$ the corresponding attractiveness of the levels of the prominent and non-prominent attributes for the non-prominent option. If the objective attribute levels are denoted x and it is assumed that $u_{i,j} = w_j x_{i,j}$ with w_j denoting the attribute weights, then by substitution in Equation 1:

$$w_p/w_{np} = (x_{NP,np} - x_{P,np})/(x_{P,p} - x_{NP,p}) \tag{2}$$

ACKNOWLEDGEMENTS

The preparation of this chapter was financially supported by grants to the author from the Swedish Council for Research in the Humanities and Social Sciences and from the Royal Swedish Academy of Sciences. I am grateful to the editors, to Tommy Gärling, to Kazuhisa Takemura and to an anonymous reviewer for useful comments.

REFERENCES

Baron, J. (1994) *Thinking and Deciding,* (2nd edn), New York: Cambridge University Press.

Barsalou, L.W. (1992) *Cognitive Psychology: An Overview for Cognitive Scientists,* Hillsdale, NJ: Erlbaum.

Bettman, J.R. (1982) 'A functional analysis of the role of overall evaluation of alternatives in choice processes', in A.A. Mitchell (ed.) *Advances in Consumer Research*, vol. 9, Ann Arbor, MI: Association for Consumer Research.

Brainard, R.W., Irby, T.S., Fitts, P.M. and Alluisi, E. (1962) 'Some variables influencing the rate of gain of information', *Journal of Experimental Psychology*, 63: 105–10.

Casey, J.T. (1991) 'Reversal of the preference reversal phenomenon', *Organizational Behavior and Human Decision Processes*, 48: 224–51.

Chapman, G.B. and Johnson, E.J. (1994) 'The limits of anchoring', *Journal of Behavioral Decision Making*, 7: 223–42.

Chapman, G.B. and Johnson, E.J. (1995) 'Preference reversals in monetary and life expectancy evaluations', *Organizational Behavior and Human Decision Processes*, 62: 300–17.

Creyer, E.H. and Johar, G.V. (1995) 'Response mode bias in the formation of preference: boundary conditions of the prominence effect', *Organizational Behavior and Human Decision Processes*, 62: 14–22.

Evans, J. St B.T. (1984) 'Heuristic and analytic processes in reasoning', *British Journal of Psychology*, 75: 451–68.

Evans, J. St B.T. (1989) *Bias in Human Reasoning: Causes and Consequences*, Hillsdale, NJ: Erlbaum.

Fischer, G.W. and Hawkins, S.A. (1993) 'Strategy compatibility, scale compatibility, and the prominence effect', *Journal of Experimental Psychology: Human Perception and Performance*, 19: 580–97.

Fitts, P.M. and Seeger, C.M. (1953) 'S–R compatibility: spatial characteristics of stimulus and response codes', *Journal of Experimental Psychology*, 46: 199–210.

Harte, J.M., Westenberg, M.R.M. and van Someren, M. (1994) 'Process models of decision making', *Acta Psychologica*, 87: 95–120.

Hawkins, S.A. (1994) 'Information processing strategies in riskless preference reversals: the prominence effect', *Organizational Behavior and Human Decision Processes*, 59: 1–26.

Johnson, E.J., Payne, J.W. and Bettman, J.R. (1988) 'Information displays and preference reversals', *Organizational Behavior and Human Decision Processes*, 42: 1–21.

Johnson-Laird, P.N. and Wason, P.C. (1970) 'A theoretical analysis of insight into a reasoning task', *Cognitive Psychology*, 1: 134–48.

Klayman, J. (1985) 'Children's decision strategies and their adaptation to task characteristics', *Organizational Behavior and Human Decision Processes*, 35: 179–201.

Kornblum, S., Hasbroucq, T. and Osman, A. (1990) 'Dimensional overlap: cognitive basis for stimulus–response compatibility – a model and taxonomy', *Psychological Review*, 97: 253–70.

Lichtenstein, S. and Slovic, P. (1973) 'Response-induced reversals of preference in gambling: an extended replication in Las Vegas', *Journal of Experimental Psychology*, 101: 16–20.

Mellers, B.A. and Cooke, A.D.J. (1994) 'Trade-offs depend on attribute range', *Journal of Experimental Psychology: Human Perception and Performance*, 20: 1055–67.

Mellers, B.A. and Cooke, A.D.J. (1996) 'The role of task and context in preference measurement', *Psychological Science*, 7: 76–82.

Montgomery, H., Selart, M., Gärling, T. and Lindberg, E. (1994) 'The judgment–choice discrepancy: noncompatibility or restructuring?', *Journal of Behavioral Decision Making*, 7: 145–55.

Parducci, A. (1968) 'The relativism of absolute judgment', *Scientific American*, 219: 84–90.

Parducci, A. (1974) 'Contextual effects: a range-frequency analysis', in E.C. Carterette and M.P. Friedman (eds) *Handbook of Perception*, vol. 2, New York: Academic Press.

Payne, J.W. (1982) 'Contingent decision behavior', *Psychological Bulletin*, 92: 382–402.

Proctor, R.W. and Reeve, T.G. (1990) *Stimulus–Response Compatibility: An Integrative Perspective*, Amsterdam: North-Holland.

Russo, J.E. and Dosher, B.A. (1983) 'Strategies for multiattribute binary choice', *Journal of Experimental Psychology: Learning, Memory, and Cognition*, 9: 676–96.

Russo, J.E., Johnson, E.J. and Stephens, D.L. (1989) 'The validity of verbal protocols', *Memory and Cognition*, 17: 759–69.

Schkade, D.A. and Johnson, E.J. (1989) 'Cognitive processes in preference reversals', *Organizational Behavior and Human Decision Processes*, 44: 203–31.

Schkade, D.A. and Kleinmuntz, D.N. (1994) 'Information displays and choice processes: differential effects of organization, form, and sequence', *Organizational Behavior and Human Decision Processes*, 57: 319–37.

Selart, M. (1996) 'Structure compatibility and restructuring in judgment and choice', *Organizational Behavior and Human Decision Processes*, 65: 106–16.

Selart, M., Gärling, T. and Montgomery, H. (1995) 'Compatibility and the use of information processing strategies', Manuscript.

Selart, M., Montgomery, H., Romanus, J. and Gärling, T. (1994) 'Violations of procedure invariance in preference measurement: cognitive explanations', *European Journal of Cognitive Psychology*, 6: 417–36.

Shafir, E. (1995) 'Compatibility in cognition and decision', in J. Busemeyer, R. Hastie and D.L. Medin (eds) *Decision Making from a Cognitive Perspective*, San Diego: Academic Press.

Slovic, P. (1975) 'Choice between equally valued alternatives', *Journal of Experimental Psychology: Human Perception and Performance*, 1: 280–7.

Slovic, P. and Lichtenstein, S. (1983) 'Preference reversals: a broader perspective', *American Economic Review*, 73: 596–605.

Slovic, P., Griffin, D. and Tversky, A. (1990) 'Compatibility effects in judgment and choice', in R.M. Hogarth (ed.) *Insights in Decision Making: A Tribute to Hillel J. Einhorn*, Chicago: University of Chicago Press.

Slovic, P. (1995) 'The construction of preference', *American Psychologist*, 50: 364–71.

Stone, D.N. and Schkade, D.A. (1991) 'Numeric and linguistic information representation in multiattribute choice', *Organizational Behavior and Human Decision Processes*, 49: 42–59.

Svenson, O. (1989) 'Eliciting and analysing verbal protocols in process studies of judgement and decision making', in H. Montgomery and O. Svenson (eds) *Process and Structure in Human Decision Making*, Chichester: Wiley.

Tversky, A. (1977) 'Features of similarity', *Psychological Review*, 84: 327–52.

Tversky, A., Sattath, S. and Slovic, P. (1988) 'Contingent weighting in judgment and choice', *Psychological Review*, 95: 371–84.

Wickens, C.D. (1984) *Engineering Psychology and Human Performance*, Columbus, OH: Merrill.

Chapter 5

Perspectives and emotions in personal decision making

Anna Blom Kemdal and Henry Montgomery

The growing interest in research on naturalistic decision making (Klein *et al.*, 1993) is presumably due to lack of correspondence between results from laboratory studies in decision making and the experience of making decisions. Decisions studied in laboratories often seem artificial and simple in comparison to the complexity of real-life decisions.

There is much research to be done before a coherent understanding is achieved of the interplay between factors involved in naturalistic decision making, particularly when it comes to personal decision making, i.e., relatively important decisions which people make in their private lives (Willén, 1994; Wolham, 1982). With a few exceptions, naturalistic studies have been limited to professional decision making (e.g., Klein *et al.*, 1993). The exceptional studies include research on adolescents' decision making (Fischhoff 1996), the decision to have a child (Willén, 1994), and different kinds of personal decisions (Karlsson, 1988).

Naturalistic studies of personal decisions are important for several reasons. Obviously, it is more interesting to people in general if the decisions studied are meaningful to them and if they can recognise themselves in the results of the research. Moreover, the results can contribute to decision theory by giving knowledge about other aspects of decision making than the frequently studied cognitive aspects, such as the importance of external circumstances, emotions and actions. Finally, it is possible to find out more about different types of decisions, e.g., personal vs. professional decisions or satisfying vs. regretted decisions.

In research in the area of personal decision making it is possible to draw on notions from descriptive decision theories. The present chapter draws on the notion that the relationship between a to-be-chosen alternative and the other available alternatives changes over time (Janis and Mann, 1977; Montgomery, 1983, 1994; Montgomery and Svenson, 1989; Svenson, 1992; Svenson and Hill, this volume). Below, we make a number of assumptions about personal decision making that are based on this notion.

1 Personal decision making involves attempts to structure and restructure available information in order to support the final choice.

Some scholars have claimed that the decision making process is not primarily focused on making the choice, but on finding arguments for defending a to-be-chosen alternative, to avoid the feeling of regret, and to be able to face others' critiques (e.g., Shepard, 1967; Slovic, 1975; Montgomery, 1983). In line with this claim, data show that the to-be-chosen alternative gradually is separated from other alternatives available (e.g., Montgomery and Svenson, 1989; Sedek *et al.*, 1993; Svenson and Hill, this volume). In Montgomery's (1983) Search for Dominance Structure (SDS) theory this process was called dominance structuring because it was assumed that the most common way to defend a decision is to find or create dominance, i.e., to find a representation in which the chosen alternative is better on at least one attribute and not worse on any attribute compared to the non-chosen alternative(s). In his Differentiation and Consolidation (Diff Con) theory, Svenson (1992; see also Svenson, 1996; Svenson and Hill, this volume) suggested that when a sufficiently high degree of differentiation between a to-be-chosen alternative and competitors is at hand, which does not necessarily coincide with dominance, then the decision maker is ready to make a choice. Differentiation is performed on the differentiation continuum, which is a hypothetical construct in the theory. There are different mediators of differentiation such as attractiveness differences and use of decision rules. Svenson further assumed that, after the decision has been made, post-decisional consolidation is performed in processes similar to those in pre-decisional differentiation. The data to be reported in the present chapter do not allow a comparison of the validity of SDS theory and Diff Con theory. However, the data may shed light on the general assumption in Diff Con theory as well as in SDS theory that decision makers attempt to separate clearly a preliminarily chosen alternative from its competitors. In the following, such attempts will be denoted as differentiation.

2 Personal decision making involves the adoption of perspectives which aid the decision maker to differentiate among the alternatives.

This assumption concerns the mechanism behind the structuring operations associated with differentiation among choice alternatives. Montgomery (1994) posited that the judgements made in a decision situation are constrained by the decision maker's (DM) evaluative perspective. The perspective is determined by (a) the DM's current subject identification (e.g., identification with ego-related interests, we-related interests, or other-related interests), (b) the congruence between features of a focused alternative and interests associated with the current subject identification, and (c) the DM's distance to (commitment to) an alternative.

The differentiation between choice alternatives is controlled by the conjunction of factors (a) and (b) and by factor (c). The first two factors determine the direction of the differentiation. Alternatives that are viewed as congruent with the current subject identification are assumed to be seen as controllable and trustworthy. The positive side of these alternatives is in the foreground. They are seen from an *inside perspective* in the sense that they are experienced as being located within the DM's action sphere. By contrast, incongruent alternatives are viewed as less controllable, less trustworthy, and, hence, they are viewed from their negative side. They are seen as independent of the DM and, in this sense, they are seen from an *outside perspective.* Factor (c), i.e., the DM's distance to different alternatives, is assumed to be negatively related to the size of the differentiation. That is, the greater the distance to the choice alternatives, the more balanced will the DM's view be of their good and bad sides.

3 Emotions are often important in personal decision making, before, during and after the decision.

Emotions may assist the DM to differentiate between choice alternatives in the following two ways. First, emotions may propel the DM to think and act in support of a to-be-chosen or already chosen alternative as well as in opposition to non-chosen alternatives (Bagozzi, 1992; Damasio, 1995; Frijda, 1986; Lewicka, 1990; Toda, 1980). For example, the emotion of anger may move the DM to choose destructive alternatives whereas the emotion of fear may induce the DM to avoid risky alternatives (Bagozzi, 1992). In this way, emotions may already be important at the start of the decision process in giving the process a certain direction. Sometimes this will happen in conflict with cognitively based preferences (Zajonc, 1980), but often DMs may succeed in adjusting their cognitions to be congruent with their emotions (Sjöberg, 1982). Second, emotions may give the DM positive or negative feedback about the current status of the differentiation process and in this way serve a monitoring function during the decision process as well as after the decision is made. During the decision process, the DM can feel good about the ongoing choice, implying that the decision process goes on smoothly, or the DM can feel anxiety or fear about what is going to happen, and maybe start feeling regret, or even going back to the start and making a new decision (Bagozzi, 1992). Emotional consequences after the decision are those that arise from making a 'good' or 'bad' decision: satisfaction, relief, regret, disappointment, and those that arise from publicly made decisions, e.g. pride or shame (Larrick, 1993; Gilovich and Husted Medvec, 1995).

Emotion appears to be a neglected issue in research on decision making in naturalistic contexts. For example, the term 'emotion' is missing in the subject index of the Klein *et al.*'s (1993) edited volume on naturalistic decision making. As indicated above, attempts have been made to examine the role of emotions in decision making (Bagozzi, 1992; Damasio, 1995; Janis and Mann, 1977; Toda, 1980; Zajonc, 1980), but we have not found any study systematically examining the role of specific emotions in personal decision making.

4 Personal decision making involves a dynamic interaction with the environment.

The decision process includes cycles of actions and reactions in relation to a changing environment (Brehmer, 1990; Klein, 1993; Orasanu and Connolly, 1993; Rasmussen, 1993). In order to deal with the decision problem and to find out more about the alternatives, the DM carries out strings of actions over time (Orasanu and Connoly, 1993). He/she also reacts to and copes with external events that occur during the decision process. Partly, cycles of actions and reactions have the character of action-feedback loops wherein the DM reacts to the consequences of actions that he/she has performed earlier in the decision process (Orasanu and Connoly, 1993).

Bringing the assumption that the DM attempts to separate clearly a preliminarily chosen alternative from its competitors into this picture of decision making suggests that the DM will carry out actions that aim at improving a promising alternative, but he/she may be less interested in doing so with other alternatives (Montgomery, 1993).

5 There are differences between satisfied and regretful DMs' pre- and post-decisional processes.

The four ideas concerning personal decision making mentioned above may have to be modified and specified when related to regretted decisions. It might be expected that regretful DMs, as compared to satisfied DMs: (a) in their pre-decisional processes are less active in their interaction with the environment (which may be related to regret because of the feeling that not everything was done to reach a good decision); (b) show less consolidation of their decision; and (c) have specific emotions other than regret (e.g., shame or guilt) after the decision has been made.

In the present study we collected retrospective reports of people's experience of important personal decisions. This method is rarely used in the field of decision making, perhaps because of the risk that subjects' memories of the decisions are not veridical (but see Lipshitz and Bar-Ilan, 1996). Research has shown that people reconstruct the past to make it more logical, sorting events in a causal chain, even if the events occurred rather randomly (Ross, 1989). On the other hand, in retrospect it may be easier to get the full picture of all the factors that have been of importance for the decisions. Moreover, concurrent reports may be biased inasmuch as people are unaware of factors that influence their actions (Nisbett and Wilson, 1977). Hence, ideally both retrospective and concurrent reports should be used to balance out biases associated with each method. In the present study, we took a first step to examine personal decisions by relying on retrospective reports.

METHOD

Subjects

Subjects were four men and seven women between 20 and 50 years of age. There were four museum employees, two students, one construction worker, one architect, one dance producer, one teacher and one archivist. They were all acquaintances of the interviewer, who was one of the authors. The advantage of this sampling was that the subjects felt comfortable talking to the interviewer and could be candid about how the decisions were made.

Procedure

The subjects described their decision(s) in two steps – first writing down the decision in their own words and a few days later in an interview. The reasons for this procedure were (a) to get a picture of the decisions before conducting the interview, as a help in planning the interview questions, and (b) to obtain a higher validity of the results by comparing two different kinds of data.

Written protocols

The subjects were requested to write about one or two important decisions that they were satisfied with or had regretted. Three subjects chose to describe two decisions and the others chose one decision. In the first six protocols, only one subject chose to describe a regretted decision. Therefore the remaining subjects were asked preferably to write about a regretted decision. After this change of the instruction, four of the remaining eight protocols described regretted decisions.

The subjects were instructed to describe the situation where the decision was made, including thoughts, feelings and actions before, during and after the decision. The protocols typically comprised 1,500 words.

Interviews

One of the authors (the one acquainted with the subjects) interviewed all the subjects. The interviews were semi-structured. The issues asked about were the same for all subjects, but the questions were open-ended, and there was an acceptance of expansions by both the interviewer and the interviewee.

The following issues were attended to in the interviews: the situation when the decision process started, available alternatives, advantages and disadvantages of the alternative(s), external events, influences from other people, responsibilities, personal abilities, moral values, preferences, emotions, intuitions, perspective(s) from which the alternative(s) was(were) seen, reasoning, beliefs, actions, and degree of satisfaction with the decision.

The interviews were tape-recorded and transcribed. The interviews lasted between 45 minutes and one and a half hours.

Coding the data

Three subjects described two decisions each; the remaining eight subjects described one decision. The decisions were divided into satisfying and regretted decisions. Two persons were satisfied with the consequences of their decisions, but regretted their way of making the decisions. Their decisions were included in the satisfied group.

The written protocols and interview protocols were divided into statements, each of which was judged as containing one idea (cf. Svenson, 1989). Each statement was coded in three respects, viz. with respect to (a) component of decision process, (b) phase of decision process, and (c) whether the statement was in favour or not of the chosen alternative.

Those categories that were used for coding decision components and also used in the data analysis are presented below. A few additional coding categories were used only in the codings but were omitted in the data analyses because they were applied in relatively few cases.

Circumstances

This category includes everything stable or out of the DM's control such as external events, environmental components, influences from other people, and stable qualities within the DM. Circumstances are relatively objective in the sense that people other than the DM may have access to the information referred to. Examples: 'There was an ad in the paper about a car for sale': 'My daughter thought it was a good idea'; 'I am a lazy person.'

Preferences

Preferences include what the DM wants and prefers, including wishes, dreams, hopes, goals and interests. They are goal-directed and concrete. Examples: 'I think freedom is more important than security'; 'I wanted to have my own car.'

Emotions

Emotions refer to moods and positive or negative reactions towards different situations, people and alternatives. Examples: 'It was a period of my life when I didn't feel very happy'; 'I liked her the moment I met her.'

The emotion statements were further coded into different types of positive and negative emotions. We could not find any classification of emotions which described all the different kinds of emotions we found in our decision protocols. The definitions below (which only include relatively frequent emotions that were used in the data analysis) are based on a combination of Ortony *et al.* (1988) and Rollenhagen's (1990) classifications of emotions, and our own modifications to make the definitions functional when coding emotion statements.

Positive emotions: Happiness (positive state of mind, e.g., satisfaction, pleasure, joy, comfort); Love/Liking (focus on positively valued object, e.g., appreciation, attraction, affection); Hope (focus on probable, but not certain, future positive situation, e.g., longing, optimism); Relief (focus on the absence of a negatively valued object).

Negative emotions: Unhappiness (negative state of mind, e.g., dissatisfaction, sadness, awkwardness, boredom); Hate/Dislike (focus on a negatively valued object, e.g., dislike, disgust); Fear (focus on a possible future negative situation with elements of uncertainty and lack of control, e.g., worry, anxiety, insecurity); Shame/Guilt, (own or others' negative evaluation of one's own person and/or actions); Regret (focus on the negative consequences of one's actions and the wish one had acted differently); and Ambivalence (difficulty of choosing between two or more possible future situations).

Actions

Actions correspond to the DM's active interaction with the environment and include local decisions, searching for information, talking to other people, making plans, and committing oneself. Examples: 'I promised to keep in touch'; 'I postponed visiting her'; 'I finally went to her place to see her.'

Beliefs

Beliefs refer to hypotheses and theories, e.g., about the consequences of the decision. Example: 'I thought I could resell the car for the same price I bought it.'

As mentioned above, each statement was also coded, if possible, with respect to different phases of the decision process: *before* the decision (initial situation), *during* the decision (i.e., the time period from the initial situation until the decision was made), and *after* the decision. Finally, each statement was coded as being in favour, not in favour, or neutral with regard to the chosen alternative. In the data analysis the two latter categories were collapsed into one category, denoted as not in favour of the decision since it was difficult to reach a satisfactory interjudge reliability with respect to the distinction between 'neutral' and 'not in favour'.

The codings were first carried out by two independent judges. Cases where the two judges disagreed on one or more categorisations (38 per cent of descriptive components, 40 per cent of time codings, 31 per cent of favourability codings) were coded by a third judge and those statements on which all three judges disagreed were coded by a fourth judge. Statements where all four judges disagreed on one or more categorisations (4 per cent of descriptive components, 2 per cent of time codings, 0 per cent of favourability codings) were not used in further data analyses. The same procedure was used for coding the specific emotions, but with three judges in total.

In addition to the relatively fine-grained codings described above, we made more global codings using entire decision making phases (i.e., before, during and after the decision) as coding units. These codings concerned the subject identification adopted by the DM in a given phase, i.e., ego, we, or other identification with respect to the chosen alternative or the non-chosen alternative(s). Results from this data analysis were previously presented in Montgomery (1994).

RESULTS

Decision problems

The decision problems selected by the subjects may be partitioned into the following groups, with regretted decisions marked by *: (1) moving decisions (moving to another town, moving to another town to be closer to work); (2) career decisions (starting university studies, quitting university studies, rejecting a job-offer, accepting a job-offer, starting a new career, trying a new job, producing an exhibition*); (3) economic decisions (buying a house, buying a car*, selling a piano*); and (4) decisions involving social relationships (getting a divorce, choosing not to contact a friend*, not helping a colleague with a job*).

Statistical data analysis

To get an overview of how the decision process developed across time for satisfied and regretful DMs, respectively, the following data analysis was carried out. For each decision protocol and each combination of time phase and favourability of decision, the proportion of statements referring to each descriptive component was computed by dividing the frequency of statements coded into a given category with the total number of statements in the entire protocol. These proportions were subjected to a 2 (group: satisfying vs. regretted decisions) × 3 (time: before, during and after) × 2 (favourability: favouring vs. non-favouring of the chosen alternative) analysis of variance (MANOVA) with repeated measures of the two latter factors. (Note, that this design is an approximation of the actual design, where the group factor was not consistently a between-subject factor inasmuch as this factor involved both between- and within-subject comparisons. This simplification of the actual design implied that significance tests involving the group factor are conservative, due to the fact that error variances for within-subjects factors are lower than for between-subjects factors.)

Overall frequencies of decision components

As can be seen in Table 5.1 (interview data) and in Table 5.2 (written protocols) the clearly most frequent decision component is Circumstances (34 per cent for satisfying, 32 per cent for regretted decision in interview protocols, 40 per cent vs. 44 per cent in written protocols). Preferences, Emotions, Actions and Beliefs occurred each in 5–17 per cent of the statements for satisfied and regretful DMs, respectively, in each of the two data sets. There does not seem to be any clear difference between the two data sets with respect to relative frequencies of different components. The greatest discrepancies were found for Preferences, which occurred more often in the interview data, and for Emotions, which were more often mentioned in the written protocols.

Preferences tended to be more common for satisfied than for regretful DMs although this tendency was significant only for interview data, $F(1,12) = 5.07, p < 0.05$ (written protocols). Emotions favouring the chosen alternative were also more common for satisfied DMs whereas there was an opposite tendency for regretful DMs. This pattern is substantiated by significant or marginally significant Group × Favourability interactions, $F(1,12) = 5.05$, $p < 0.05$ (interview data); $F(1,12) = 4.76$, $p = 0.05$ (written protocols). Circumstances are proportionately more common for regretful DMs (out of the coded statements) than was the case for satisfied DMs.

Differentiation

In both data sets, the proportions of statements favouring and not favouring the chosen alternative developed differently across time phases as shown by significant Time × Favourability interactions for total frequencies, $F(2,24) = 5.58$, $p = 0.01$ (written protocols) and $F(2,24) = 4{,}56$, $p < 0.05$ (interview data). For specific components, significant Time ×

Table 5.1 The five most frequent components (percentage of statements in the interviews)[1] of the decision process in favour (F) or not (~F) of the chosen alternative before, during and after the decision is made, for satisfied and regretful DMs

	Before		*During*		*After*		*Total*	
Components	*F*	*~F*	*F*	*~F*	*F*	*~F*	*F*	*~F*
Circumstances								
Satisfied	6	6	6	5	4	6	16	17
Regretful	5	4	8	4	4	7	17	15
Preferences								
Satisfied	4	2	3	1	3	1	10	4
Regretful	1	1	4	1	1	1	6	3
Emotions								
Satisfied	2	1	2	1	3	1	7	3
Regretful	0	1	2	1	1	3	3	5
Actions								
Satisfied	1	2	1	2	2	1	4	5
Regretful	0	2	4	1	1	2	5	5
Beliefs								
Satisfied	1	2	1	1	1	2	3	5
Regretful	2	0	2	1	1	3	5	4
Total								
Satisfied	14	13	13	10	13	11	40	34
Regretful	8	8	20	8	8	16	36	32
Grand total	22	21	33	18	21	27	76	66

Note: 1 There was a mean of 228 statements in the satisfied DMs' protocols and 179 in the regretful DMs' protocols

Favourability interactions were obtained for Circumstances (written protocols), $F(2,24) = 4.89$, $p < 0.05$ and actions (written protocols), $F(2,24) = 5.10$, $p < 0.05$.

To what extent do these time trends reflect differentiation and consolidation processes? The written protocols support the idea that there is an increasing differentiation between the alternatives in terms of the difference between proportion of statements favouring and not favouring the chosen alternative. Before the decision process started, components favouring and not favouring the decision were about equally common for both regretful and satisfied DMs, whereas in the written protocols the chosen alternative was clearly the favourite for satisfied DMs even before the decision started. During the decision process the chosen alternative was the favourite in both data sets and for both groups. After the decision the picture was less clear for both groups. They tended to mention more

Table 5.2 The five most frequent components (percentage of statements in the written protocols)[1] of the decision process in favour (F) or not (~F) of the chosen alternative before, during and after the decision is made, for satisfied and regretful DMs

	Before		*During*		*After*		*Total*	
Components	*F*	*~F*	*F*	*~F*	*F*	*~F*	*F*	*~F*
Circumstances								
Satisfied	16	7	4	4	5	4	25	15
Regretful	11	11	2	2	6	12	19	25
Preferences								
Satisfied	5	1	1	1	2	0	8	2
Regretful	1	2	1	0	0	2	2	4
Emotions								
Satisfied	5	1	2	2	5	2	12	5
Regretful	0	1	0	1	3	6	3	8
Actions								
Satisfied	4	1	1	1	0	1	5	3
Regretful	1	2	2	0	2	2	5	4
Beliefs								
Satisfied	3	1	1	0	0	0	4	1
Regretful	2	0	0	0	1	3	3	3
Total								
Satisfied	33	11	9	8	12	7	54	26
Regretful	15	16	5	3	12	25	32	44
Grand total	48	27	14	11	24	32	86	70

Note: 1 There was a mean of 177 statements in the satisfied DMs' protocols and 125 in the regretful DMs' protocols

circumstances and beliefs not in favour of the chosen alternatives, and the regretters mentioned more emotions not in favour. Thus, the difference in support of the chosen and non-chosen alternatives was decreasing for both groups after the decision was made, implying that the subjects did not show any consolidation (= no sign of increasing differentiation between chosen and non-chosen alternatives after the decision). Not surprisingly, the regretful DMs were particularly non-supportive of the chosen alternative after the decision, as substantiated by significant or marginally significant Group × Time × Favourability interactions for total frequencies, $F(2,24) = 5.79$, $p < 0.01$ (written protocols) and $F(2,24) = 3.22$, $p = 0.058$ as well as for Preferences (written protocols), $F(2,24) = 3.22$, $p = 0.058$, $F(2,24) = 2.95$, $p = 0.071$, Emotions (written protocols), $F(2,24) = 4.38$, $p < 0.05$, and Actions (written protocols), $F(2,24) = 5.62$, $p = 0.01$. However, it may be noted that the Group × Time

$\times$ Group interactions for Preferences and Emotions may also reflect the fact that these components tended to be more supportive for the chosen alternative for satisfied DMs than for regretful DMs before the decision process started.

Subject identifications

We found a massive dominance of ego identification, which was found to be the dominating subject identification in 39 out of the 42 coded cases (14 subjects $\times$ 3 time phases). In two cases the DM switched from an ego to an other-oriented perspective. In both cases the subject as a result of unfortunate events in the external world realised that he/she had made an ego-oriented decision that violated another person's interests. As a consequence, he/she saw his or her previous behaviour in a new light and regretted the decision. The third case concerned a person who, before making a decision to divorce his wife, switched from a we-oriented perspective (we = ego + partner) to a pure ego-oriented perspective, implying that the person distanced himself from the partner. Thus, in the three cases where there were shifts in the subject identification there was also a corresponding shift in the evaluation of a to-be-chosen or chosen alternative.

Emotions

The most common types of emotions referred to in the interviews and written protocols taken together are shown in Table 5.3 (negative emotions) and Table 5.4 (positive emotions). The total frequency of negative emotions yielded a number of significant effects, viz. main effects of Time, $F(2,24) = 21.86$, $p < 0.01$, and of Favourability, $F(1,12) < 13.09$, $p < 0.01$, and a Group $\times$ Favourability interaction, $F(1,12) = 7.32$, $p < 0.01$ and a Time $\times$ Favourability interaction, $F(2,24) = 7.32$, $p < 0.01$. These effects may largely be due to two findings. First, satisfied DMs reported a lot of negative emotions in favour of the chosen alternative before the decision process started. That is, these DMs were unhappy with the present situation which they were deciding to leave, but they also felt fear and anxiety with respect to the to-be-chosen alternative. Second, the regretful DMs reported many negative emotions that were not in favour of the chosen alternative after the decision was made. Their most common negative emotions were guilt and regret, as might be expected. By contrast, satisfied DMs reported many positive emotions after the decision (e.g., happiness, love/liking and relief), which, however, to some extent also was true for regretful DMs (see Table 5.4). This pattern is compatible with the significant Time $\times$ Favourability interaction, $F(2,24) = 6.63$, $p < 0.01$ and the significant Favourabilty effect, $F(1,12) = 17.33$ and Time effect,

Table 5.3 The six most frequent negative emotions (percentage of number of coded emotions in interview protocols and written protocols) before, during and after the decision in favour (F) or not (~F) of the chosen alternative for satisfied and regretful DMs

	Before		*During*		*After*		*Total*	
Negative emotion	*F*	*~F*	*F*	*~F*	*F*	*~F*	*F*	*~F*
Unhappiness								
Satisfied	7	1	2	1	0	2	9	4
Regretful	2	0	0	0	0	0	2	0
Fear/Anxiety								
Satisfied	1	4	0	2	0	2	1	8
Regretful	0	0	0	2	0	2	0	4
Regret								
Satisfied	0	0	0	0	0	0	0	0
Regretful	0	0	0	0	0	20	0	20
Ambivalence								
Satisfied	0	0	0	1	0	2	0	3
Regretful	0	3	0	0	0	1	0	4
Hate/Dislike								
Satisfied	1	0	1	0	0	0	2	0
Regretful	0	1	0	3	0	0	0	4
Guilt								
Satisfied	1	0	0	0	0	0	1	0
Regretful	0	0	0	2	0	9	0	11
Total								
Satisfied	10	5	3	4	0	6	13	15
Regretful	2	4	0	7	0	32	2	43
Grand total	12	9	3	11	0	38	15	58

$F(2,24) = 6.88$, $p < 0.01$, that were found for total frequencies of positive emotions.

Considering all emotions together, satisfied DMs reported more emotions (both negative and positive emotions) than regretful DMs before the decision process whereas after the decision the regretful DMs saw themselves as more emotional (mainly negative emotions) than was true for satisfied DMs.

DISCUSSION

The present data show that personal decision making is not only an internal, mental process (the components Beliefs and Preferences), but

Table 5.4 The four most frequent positive emotions (percentage of number of coded emotions in interview protocols and written protocols) before, during and after the decision in favour (F) or not (~F) of the chosen alternative for satisfied and regretful DMs

	Before		*During*		*After*		*Total*	
Positive emotion	*F*	*~F*	*F*	*~F*	*F*	*~F*	*F*	*~F*
Happiness								
Satisfied	2	0	3	1	13	1	18	2
Regretful	0	2	7	0	5	0	12	2
Relief								
Satisfied	0	0	1	1	3	1	4	2
Regretful	0	0	3	0	0	0	3	0
Love/Liking								
Satisfied	0	0	2	0	4	1	6	1
Regretful	0	0	0	0	2	0	2	0
Hope								
Satisfied	1	0	0	0	3	0	4	0
Regretful	0	0	0	0	3	0	3	0
Total								
Satisfied	3	0	6	2	23	3	32	5
Regretful	0	2	10	0	10	0	20	2
Grand total	3	2	16	2	33	3	52	7

also a process in which the individual participates in the external world (Circumstances, Actions), and where also Emotions are important. Our data suggest that in order to understand personal decision making it is necessary to consider both internal and external aspects of the decision process. This picture is supported by two types of qualitative data, viz. protocols written by the subjects and interview data.

As predicted, there was an increasing differentiation between the chosen and non-chosen alternatives from the start of the decision process until the decision was made, although this trend was clear only in the interview data. The increasing differentiation was noticeable for all of the five most common decision components. This uniformity is in line with the assumption that personal decision making may be seen as a negotiation with the environment. When everything is 'right' the decision can be made.

On the other hand, our data showed no consistent signs of consolidation. That is, the overall differentiation between chosen and non-chosen alternatives did not increase after the decision had been made. This was true for both satisfied and regretful DMs. The absence of consolidation contrasts with previous findings (Malmsten, 1996; Svenson, 1992). There are at least two possible explanations of this contrast. First, the previous demonstrations of consolidation involved decision tasks that were defined by the researchers and which did not require an interaction with the environment. Perhaps the need to defend a decision is greater when the DM has fewer possibilities to influence the conditions for the decision. Second, the previous research is typically based on ratings made concurrently with the decision process whereas we used retrospective reports. In retrospect, people may be less anxious to defend their decisions because the possibility of an alternative choice is then less salient.

The extent to which different decision components support or speak against the chosen alternative in different time phases may be seen as being consistent with Montgomery's (1994, 1996) Perspective theory. Montgomery (1996) stressed that the DMs' perspective taking is assisted by their actions (cf. coding category Actions) and by their positive or negative involvement (cf. coding categories Emotions and Preferences) in a focused alternative. When actions and emotional involvement differentiate among alternatives in the same way as is seen from a given perspective (cf. coding categories Circumstances and Beliefs), the perspective is stabilised and the differentiation increases in the sense that it becomes more stable across time.

Most perspective shifts appear to have occurred for regretful DMs after the decision was made. In two cases the subject identification was changed, which in turn was related to changes in the external world. In the other cases, perceived changes in the external situation (Circumstances) and changed Beliefs led to a negative view on the chosen alternative. These results illustrate how the perspective may be changed as a consequence of an interplay between internal and external factors.

Let us now consider how the perspective theory may shed light on differences between satisfied and regretful DMs' pre-decisional processes. In their pre-decisional processes satisfied DMs as compared to regretful DMs expressed more emotional support for the to-be-chosen alternative in the form of more emotional aversion against the non-chosen alternative group. They also reported more Preferences in favour of the to-be-chosen alternative. In contrast, Circumstances relatively speaking were more common among regretful DMs in the coded statements. These results may be interpreted as showing that satisfied DMs viewed their pre-decisional life situation (which always corresponded to the non-chosen alternative) from an outside perspective. They experienced that this situation did not fit their current interests, which in turn gave rise to negative emotions and a wish for something new (= preferences in favour of the to-be-chosen alternative) which could help them out of their dilemma. Although the regretful DMs initially saw negative aspects in the non-chosen alternative (particularly with respect to Beliefs), it appears that this fact did not conflict markedly with their current aspirations. This implies that they initially lacked a clear outside perspective on the non-chosen alternative. Instead the regretful DMs viewed themselves as being guided by external Circumstances, which clearly differentiated between chosen and non-chosen alternative(s) just before the decision was made. It may be noted that in this stage Preferences and Emotions also favoured the to-be-chosen alternative for the regretful DMs. Expressed in terms of perspective theory, regretful DMs may primarily have been guided by an inside perspective on the to-be-chosen alternative rather than on an outside perspective on the non-chosen alternative. This may be an insufficient basis for maintaining a conviction that the right decision has been made in the face of adverse circumstances.

As we see it, the main contribution of the present study is the demonstration that personal decision making is based on a differentiation between different choice alternatives which is facilitated by the DM's interaction with the external world and by his or her emotional reactions. However, we definitely need more knowledge about the role of emotions in personal decision making, which appears to be a neglected area in research on decision making. Moreover, our results appear to be compatible with Montgomery's (1994) Perspective theory, but a closer analysis of the contents of different perspectives and of factors leading to perspectives shifts in personal decision making is necessary in order to validate the theory for such decisions.

ACKNOWLEDGEMENTS

This study was supported by a grant to the second author from the Swedish Council for Research in the Humanities and Social Sciences. The authors are grateful to Darisuh Arai-Ardakani, Maj-Lene Hedenborg, Annika Khan and Robert Lundin for coding protocols, to Per Lindström, Raanan Lipshitz and the editors of this volume for their helpful comments on earlier drafts and to the subjects who made this investigation possible.

REFERENCES

Bagozzi, R.P. (1992) 'The self-regulation of attitudes, intentions, and behaviour', *Social Psychology Quarterly*, 55: 178–204.

Brehmer, B. (1990) 'Strategies in real-time decision making', in R. Hogarth (ed.) *Insights in Decision Making: A Tribute to Hillel J. Einhorn*, Chicago: University of Chicago Press.

Damasio, A.R. (1995). *Descartes' Error: Emotion, Reason and the Human Brain*, New York: Avon Books.

Fischhoff, B. (1996) 'The real world: what good is it?', *Organizational Behavior and Human Decision Processes*, 65: 232–48.

Frijda, N.H. (1986) *The Emotions*, New York: Cambridge University Press.

Gilovich, T. and Husted Medvec, V. (1995) 'The experience of regret: what, when and why', *Psychological Review*, 102: 379–95.

Janis, I.L. and Mann, L. (1977) *Decision Making*, New York: The Free Press.
Karlsson, G. (1988) 'A phenomenological psychological study of decision and choice', *Acta Psychologica*, 68: 7–25.
Klein, G.A. (1993) 'A recognition-primed decision (RPD) model of rapid decision making', in G.A. Klein, J. Orasanu, R. Calderwood and C.E. Zsambok (eds) *Decision Making in Action: Models and Methods*, Norwood, NJ: Ablex.
Klein, G.A., Orasanu, J., Calderwood, R. and Zsambok, C.E. (eds) (1993) *Decision Making in Action: Models and Methods*, Norwood, NJ: Ablex.
Larrick, R. P. (1993) 'Motivational factors in decision theories: the role of self-protection', *Psychological Bulletin*, 113: 440–50.
Lewicka, M. (1990) 'Mood related differences in pre-decisional information search strategies', Paper presented at the 98th Annual Convention of the American Psychological Association, Boston.
Lipshitz, R. and Bar-Ilan, O. (1996) 'How problems are solved: reconsidering the phase theorem', *Organizational Behavior and Human Decision Processes*, 65: 48–60.
Malmsten, N. (1996) 'Studies of post-decision processes', Doctoral thesis, Stockholm University, Department of Psychology.
Montgomery, H. (1983) 'Decision rules and the search for a dominance structure: towards a process model of decision making', in P.C. Humphreys, O. Svenson and A. Vari (eds) *Analyzing and Aiding Decision Processes*, Amsterdam: North-Holland.
Mongomery, H. (1993) 'The search for a dominance structure in decision making: examining the evidence', in G.A. Klein, J. Orasanu, R. Calderwood and C. E. Zsambok (eds) *Decision Making in Action: Models and Methods*, Norwood, NJ: Ablex.
Montgomery, H. (1994) 'Towards a perspective theory of decision making and judgment', *Acta Psychologica*, 87: 155–78.
Montgomery, H. (1996) 'The surrender at Perevolochna: a case study of perspective and action control in decision making under stress', Paper presented at the Decision Making Under Stress Conference, Aberdeen. September.
Montgomery, H. and Svenson, O. (1989) 'A think aloud study of dominance structuring in decision processes', in H. Montgomery and O. Svenson (eds) *Process and Structure in Human Decision Making*, Chichester: Wiley.
Nisbett, R.E. and Wilson, T.D. (1977) 'Telling more than we can know: verbal reports on mental processes', *Psychological Review*, 84: 231–59.
Orasanu, J. and Connolly, T. (1993) 'The reinvention of decision making', in G.A. Klein, J. Orasanu, R. Calderwood and C.E. Zsambok (eds) *Decision Making in Action: Models and Methods*, Norwood, NJ: Ablex.
Ortony, A., Clore, G.L. and Collins, A. (1988) *The Cognitive Structure of Emotions*, New York: Cambridge University Press.
Rasmussen, J. (1993) 'Deciding and doing', in G.A. Klein, J. Orasanu, R. Calderwood and C.E. Zsambok (eds) *Decision Making in Action: Models and Methods*, Norwood, NJ: Ablex.
Rollenhagen, C. (1990) 'On the description of emotion awareness', Doctoral dissertation, Stockholm University, Department of Psychology.
Ross, M. (1989) 'The relation of implicit theories to the construction of personal histories', *Psychological Review*, 96: 341–57.
Sedek, G., Kofta, M. and Tyszka, T. (1993) 'Effects of uncontrollability on subsequent decision making: testing the cognitive exhaustion hypothesis', *Journal of Personality and Social Psychology*, 6: 1270–81.

Shepard, R.N. (1967) 'On subjective optimum selections among multiattribute alternatives', in W. Edwards and A. Tversky (eds) *Decision Making: Selected Readings*, Harmondsworth: Penguin Books.

Sjöberg, L. (1982) 'Beliefs and values as attitude components', in B. Wegener (ed.) *Social Attitudes and Psychophysical Measurement*, Hillsdale, NJ: Erlbaum.

Slovic, P. (1975) 'Choice between equally valued alternatives', *Journal of Experimental Psychology: Human Perception and Performance*, 1: 280–7.

Svenson, O. (1989) 'Eliciting and analyzing verbal protocols in process studies of judgement and decision making', in H. Montgomery and O. Svenson (eds) *Process and Structure in Human Decision Making*, Chichester: Wiley.

Svenson, O. (1992) 'Differentiation and Consolidation theory of decision making: a frame of reference for the study of pre- and post-decision processes', *Acta Psychologica*, 80, 143–68.

Svenson, O. (1996) 'Decision making and the search for fundamental psychological regularities: what can be learned from a process perspective?', *Organizational Behavior and Human Decision Processes*, 65: 252–67.

Toda, M. (1980) 'Emotion and decision making', *Acta Psychologica*, 45: 133–55.

Willén, H. (1994) 'How do couples decide about having their first child? An explorative study', *Göteborg Psychological Reports*, 24: no. 1.

Wolham, B.B. (1982) *Personality Dynamics*, New York: Plenum Press.

Zajonc, R.B. (1980) 'Feeling and thinking: preferences need no inferences', *American Psychologist*, 35: 151–75.

Chapter 6

Is hate wiser than love?

Cognitive and emotional utilities in decision making

Maria Lewicka

According to the classical SEU (Subjective Expected Utility) model of decision making, people should choose the alternative which has the highest sum of the products of estimated subjective probabilities and utilities of its consequences (von Neumann and Morgenstern, 1944; Edwards, 1954; Schoemaker, 1982). This model assumes that probabilities and utilities are two independent but equally important aspects of the representation of a decision problem.

The recent shift from normative to descriptive analyses of decisions, stimulated by observed departures from normative prescriptions, has led researchers to focus more closely on the requirements set by the SEU model by comparing them with real decision behaviour. However, it seems that, of the two components of the SEU equation, subjective probability has attracted relatively more attention than the concept of utility, as evidenced by the disproportionately higher number of theories explaining deviations from the normative prescriptions concerning probability than those concerning utility, and the relatively greater amount of space devoted to the former than the latter in textbooks on judgement and decision making (cf. Plous, 1993). One of the consequences of this asymmetry may be the commonly perceived closer affiliation of decision theory to mathematical psychology or economics rather than to social psychology or the psychology of affect and motivation, i.e., these domains which naturally deal with 'hot' or affect-laden cognitions and hence whose relevance to studies on utility seems obvious.

The present chapter has two purposes. The first is to show how current theories of social cognition can contribute to our understanding of the way in which people ascribe utilities and evaluate decision alternatives. The second purpose is to argue that the way evaluations are made may depend on a number of factors inherent in the decision situation, for instance, how the decision is framed (i.e., whether the decision is to accept or to reject an alternative).

TWO TYPES OF UTILITIES: COGNITIVE VERSUS EMOTIONAL

Are evaluations rooted in descriptions of evaluated objects or are they mere expressions of emotional attitudes? Can they be rationally justified and socially shared, like any other type of descriptive judgement, or are they subjective and thus difficult to communicate? These old philosophical questions (Kołakowski, 1966) are also implicitly present in psychology. In this chapter, I present two arguments related to this issue. My first claim is that the concept of 'utility' (i.e., evaluation of decision alternatives) has shifted its meaning in the literature on decision making from the description of (instrumental) qualities of decision options, present in classical prescriptive models, to an emphasis on its emotional and action-related aspects, more frequent in contemporary, descriptive approaches. My second argument is that this change does not merely represent a shift in the theoretical preferences of the authors, but may reflect real differences between types of utilities. In other words, while the classical normative theories of decision making were focused mostly on 'cognitive', objectively based utilities, the contemporary models, greatly influenced by theoretical contributions coming from other areas of psychology (e.g., social cognition), became interested in 'emotional' utilities. As I shall show later, these two types of utilities can differently influence the overall decision process. I shall also try to show how research in social cognition, particularly research in positive–negative asymmetry in social judgements, may help us meaningfully relate the type of utility, cognitive or emotional, to particular aspects of decision processes.

Cognitive versus emotional roots of social evaluations

Let us first look at how the distinction between emotional and cognitive, applied to evaluations, is handled in other areas of psychology, mostly in research related to social cognition.

Many years ago, Peabody (1967), who was mainly interested in processes of impression formation, introduced a distinction between two types of meaning inherent in trait-adjective concepts: affective and descriptive (cognitive). Affective meaning is an expression of emotional (positive or negative) attitude towards the evaluated property, while descriptive meaning has its anchor in its objective features. Theoretically, these two are uncorrelated. For instance, two trait-adjectives, 'careful' and 'brave', have similar (positive) affective meaning but their descriptive meaning is different, even opposite. Likewise, the two negative adjectives, 'cowardly' and 'risky'. In comparison, 'careful' and 'cowardly', although different in their affective meaning (one positive, the other negative), show considerable descriptive affinity, as both refer to a 'risk-avoidant' attitude. The same set of relations holds for the 'risk-seeking' pair of adjectives, 'brave' and 'risky'.

Most of the terms used to describe personality traits, or the social world in general, have a double meaning, affective and descriptive. According to the studies initiated by Osgood (Osgood *et al.*, 1957), and repeated later many times, most of the concepts which people use to describe the social world are significantly more loaded with affective than with any other meaning (the purely evaluative dimension 'good–bad' explains over 50 per cent of variance of similarity judgements in the majority of cultures studied).

Nevertheless, depending on the cognitive focus of a person, it may happen that, for the same pair of trait adjectives, either the affective or the descriptive relationship between the adjectives will become more salient. This, in turn, will make subjects more sensitive to any inconsistencies between the adjectives on the more salient aspect and thus lead to respective differences in the cognitive representation of the adjective pair.

This distinction stimulated a number of impression formation studies. For instance, Lewicka (1977) investigated the circumstances under which affective or descriptive consistency becomes the prevalent mode of integrating inconsistent information about a hypothetical stranger. She predicted that affective, as compared to descriptive, information processing will occur more often with respect to emotionally involving issues, under time pressure, when fast decisions are required, or when the subject is explicitly asked to evaluate rather than to diagnose a target object (Lewicka, 1979). The reason is that an affectively balanced representation facilitates action and prevents hesitation and future regret. There exists evidence which shows that, for instance, in a situation in which subjects are explicitly asked to make a decision, compared to simple evaluation of the target objects, they prefer affective over descriptive consistency, which leads to cognitively simpler and more polarised representations of compared alternatives (O'Neal and Mills, 1969; Zajonc, 1960).

The dichotomy of affective vs. cognitive processing with clear application to decision situations was taken up by Zajonc (1980) in a seminal paper in which 'preferences' (cues to feel) were set against 'inferences' (cues to understand) and the two were considered the key concepts of two independent modes of information processing. The feeling system (preferences), in contrast to the cognitive system (inferences), was described as primary, instantaneous, irrevocable, not yielding to wilful control, and difficult to change with rational argumentation. This intuitively appealing distinction has been empirically corroborated with the so-called mere exposure effect (Zajonc, 1968), defined as an increase in positive affect towards a stimulus due to a repeated, unreinforced exposure to this stimulus. Mere exposure effects were obtained even though subjects in the experiments were not able to recognise the previously exposed stimuli or to differentiate them from the control, unexposed ones (Zajonc, 1968). Preferences (attitudes) were thus claimed to need no inferences (awareness of distinctive features of the stimuli). According to Zajonc, the majority of important life decisions are made on the basis of preferences, not inferences, hence their emotional, non-cognitive character and their resistance to rational argumentation.

More recently, Epstein (1990) proposed a theory, based on a dichotomy which in a number of ways is strongly reminiscent of Zajonc's distinction, whereby he proposes two qualitatively different conceptual systems, called, respectively, rational and experiential (intuitive). The rational system is 'evolutionarily younger' and 'is a deliberative, verbally mediated, primarily conscious analytical system that functions by a person's understanding of conventionally established rules of logic and evidence' (Denes-Raj and Epstein, 1994: 819). The experiential system, in turn, is evolutionarily older and 'operates in an automatic, holistic, associationistic manner, is intimately associated with the experience of affect, represents events in the form of concrete exemplars and schemas inductively derived from emotionally significant past experience' (ibid.).

In a series of ingenious experiments (Kirkpatrick and Epstein, 1992; Denes-Raj and Epstein, 1994), Epstein demonstrated that prevalence of the experiential system may lead to choices which are suboptimal and non-rational. The paradigm made use of pairs of lotteries where drawing a red ball from an urn would win a prize. Subjects could choose between an urn which consisted of ten balls, in the ratio of one red ball to nine white, and another urn which consisted of 100 balls, with red and white balls in the same proportion (10:90). Even though the odds were exactly the same in both cases, a considerable number of subjects preferred the urn with ten red balls to the one with only one red ball, obviously estimating their chances by the absolute number of (red) balls rather than by their abstract ratio. Subjects who preferred the larger urn were in fact willing to pay an extra sum of money for being allowed to draw from it.

Interestingly, the number of suboptimal choices (willingness to pay for access to the larger urn) depended on whether the situation was phrased in positive or in negative terms (i.e., as wins or losses), and it was significantly higher in the former than in the latter conditions (Kirkpatrick and Epstein, 1992; Denes-Raj and Epstein, 1994). We should perhaps mention that in other areas which made use of the affective–cognitive distinction, there were found significant differences that were due to the valence of the target objects. For instance, Lewicka (1978) found that subjects tended to use more descriptive rules of integrating information when the target was initially described in negative terms than when it was positive (in the latter case affective rules of integrating information predominated). Also mere exposure effects were found to be significantly stronger for initially neutral or mildly positive than for negative stimuli. All this may suggest that valence of the target object may be a significant predictor of which of the two sides of the dichotomy, affective or cognitive, will be activated. This issue will be discussed in more detail in the following sections.

Of other theories currently developed in social cognition, we should mention the distinction between the affective and cognitive origin of attitudes, recently proposed by Aronson *et al.* (1995). Cognitively based attitudes were defined as products of rational argumentation and of the detached weighing of pros and cons of the attitudinal target object, while affective attitudes were either a direct expression of emotions and values or an outcome of often unconscious processes of classical and instrumental conditioning. According to the authors, the origin of an attitude has consequences for whether the attitude will be a good predictor of future behaviour (degree of attitude-behaviour consistency). Wilson (Wilson *et al.* 1989; Wilson *et al.* 1995) demonstrated that reflecting upon the bases of one's own attitudes lowers the attitude-behaviour consistency for affectively but not for cognitively based attitudes.

The above-mentioned approaches, which all make use of the emotional–cognitive distinction, by no means exhaust this large subject. The purpose of this very brief review, however, is not to cover the history of the concept, but to show that research in social cognition has long acknowledged a 'double', emotional and cognitive, origin and nature of human (evaluative) judgements. We want to suggest that this distinction is relevant not only for traditional social issues like impression formation or attitude change, but also for our understanding of how people form evaluative judgements in situations when they have to decide upon a course of action, i.e., in situations of choice.

In the next section, I shall briefly discuss another area of social cognition which seems closely related to the emotional–cognitive distinction in the ascription of utilities: studies in social information integration models.

Prospective vs. diagnostic evaluations

In the late 1940s, Solomon Asch conducted a series of studies concerning the way in which people combine a set of unrelated trait-adjectives into an overall impression of an otherwise unknown person (Asch, 1946). These classical studies initiated a growth of interest in processes of impression formation (e.g., Tagiuri and Petrullo, 1958; Warr and Knapper, 1968). The main controversy which permeated debates at the time dealt with the question of whether people tend to combine single pieces of information in a linear, context-free, way and thus treat each item independently, or whether the combinatory rules are configurational, and the meaning inherent in some pieces of information (usually those presented at the beginning) influences the interpretation of successive items. While Asch (1952) was an adherent of the latter view, others seemed to support the more analytical, linear models (Anderson, 1981).

In subsequent years, the debate between configurationally and more analytically minded researchers continued, and the two points of view were even given labels, becoming known as 'top-down' vs. 'bottom-up', or 'theory-' vs. 'data-driven' forms of information processing. A contemporary reconciliation of the two points of view, applied mostly to research on stereotypes, was made by Fiske (Fiske and Pavelchak, 1986), and is known as the 'categorical' vs. 'piecemeal' model of social perception.

A somewhat different angle on the phenomenon was taken by Lewicka (1988). She suggests that processes of categorisation consist of two, logically opposite, directions of inference, called 'diagnostic' and 'prospective'. Diagnostic inferences infer category membership from specific features of target objects. Prospective inferences, on the other hand, infer features of objects from the information about the category to which the object is known to belong. To take an example: when a person feels ill, she may either engage in diagnostic inferences, and try to identify the disease which has fallen upon her, or in inferences which are prospective and, knowing what the disease probably is, try to predict its development, set up efficient treatment, etc.

Diagnostic inferences are 'data-driven', since a correct diagnosis must rely on accurate identification of relevant symptoms (diagnostic cues). In contrast, prospective inferences are mostly driven by the 'theory', that is, by the content of the relevant categories.

Although good prognosis is dependent on correct diagnosis, and thus theoretically the two directions of inference should be symmetrical and equally important, people nevertheless have been found to prefer prospective over diagnostic inferences (Lewicka, 1993). In somewhat metaphorical terms, we may say that people feel more at ease when predicting the future than when diagnosing the present. 'What follows from X?' or 'What should I do about X?' rather than 'What is it?' or 'Is it really X?' seem the preferred questions.

The two directions of inferences apply also to the formation of evaluative judgements, producing different types of evaluations. I suggest that 'diagnostic' evaluations are evaluations which are built in the 'bottom-up' way, from descriptive cues, and thus their nature is largely cognitive. In contrast, prospective evaluations are products of 'top-down' processing, that is, they are inferences drawn from generalised, global emotional attitudes towards target objects, and their character is largely emotional.

Diagnostic evaluations which are reconstructions of descriptive properties of targets thus have little to do with experienced emotions. When a committee selects suitable candidates for a job, each of the candidates is given a global evaluative score, which manifests his or her 'suitability' on a number of relevant dimensions. This score is not a measure of emotions which the committee may feel towards the candidate, but is a purely descriptive judgement of the candidate's instrumental usefulness for the considered job. Diagnostic evaluations are a form of cognition and this may, or may not, be followed by development of affect. Hence, a woman who reads matrimonial advertisements in newspapers, carefully weighing the pros and cons of each candidate, produces purely diagnostic evaluations of potential partners, but at the same time probably hopes that sooner or later, once a suitable candidate is chosen, her heart will follow the dictates of reason.

Diagnostic evaluations are thus rational: they may be discussed, argued, defended, justified, or changed in the face of convincing argumentation. As we shall see later, the traditional concept of 'utility' has a close affinity to the concept of diagnostic (or 'cognitive') evaluation.

In contrast to diagnostic evaluations, premises of prospective evaluations largely escape rational argumentation. Prolonged exposure to a stimulus, physical proximity of a target, accidentally received information, conditioning, or dissonance-reducing *ex post facto* justifications of previous behaviour towards a target, are different mechanisms which may underlie development of a global, rationally unfounded, positive or negative, emotional attitude. The nursery rhyme 'I do not like you, Mr Fell, the reason why I cannot tell . . .' exemplifies this elusive process.

Once established, the emotional attitude will serve as a global category, producing prospective, 'top-down' inferences. Those may operate through affective consistency, leading to ascription of properties whose evaluative tone is congruent with the global initial attitude (Peabody, 1967; see also above). Sometimes the outcome seems to be a product of the imagination which is scarcely based on objective qualities of the evaluated object. More often, however, the final product of prospective evaluations will be a compromise between affective consistency and descriptive truth. In other words, the final representation will consist of features which support the initial attitude and, at the same time, are not blatantly inconsistent with the target's real nature. For instance, a person, known for his generally risk-avoidant attitude in a variety of situations, may be labelled a 'coward' by somebody who dislikes him, but the same trait in a person who is otherwise liked will be considered a valuable asset ('carefulness', 'wisdom', etc.). The descriptive veridicality hidden behind these evaluations has not been violated: what differentiates the two judgements is merely their evaluative tone (see Peeters, 1989; Kemdal and Montgomery, Chapter 5).

It has been argued elsewhere (Lewicka, 1988) that while diagnostic evaluations ensure realism in our judgements and actions, prospective evaluations may be considered preconditions of commitment. A switch from the 'attribute → category' to the 'category → attribute' inference is thus equivalent to a switch from objective anchoring of a cognitive act (thus open to new information) to anchoring which is subjective, that is, whose roots lie in subject-produced concepts and categories (see also Brickman, 1987; Wojciszke, 1991).

In the next section, I shall argue that, along with the shift from normative to descriptive approaches in the treatment of human decisions, the concept of utility has also shifted its meaning: from cognitive or diagnostic utility to the emotionally based, prospective one.

Cognitive vs. emotional utilities in decision making

'Utility' (from Latin *utilitas*) means 'profitability' or 'usefulness'. *The New Webster Dictionary* (1991) defines utility as 'the quality or state of being useful'. This definition already suggests that utility may have two aspects. On the one hand, it means the evaluation of the target object, the rating of how good or bad it is; on the other hand, its focus is on instrumental qualities. 'To be useful' means to be useful with respect to something. Identification of how instrumental the target is implies recognition and comparison of two sets of descriptive properties: those implied by the goal and those possessed by the target object. The better the match, the higher will be the target's utility. 'Utility' in the meaning of 'instrumentality' is thus a descriptive judgement, although expressed in evaluative terms. The former can easily be translated into the latter and vice versa, if the goal which it serves is known.

The descriptive nature of utilities has always been emphasised in decision theory. For instance, this assumption underlies the notion of 'utility function', which is a mathematical function relating objective intensities of some property to the degree of satisfaction (pleasure–displeasure) experienced in contact with the stimulus. For instance, the money utility function is usually presented as a power function which is concave for gains and convex for losses (Kahneman and Tversky, 1979). Like any descriptive judgement, utility can be discussed, justified, communicated, or modified under the impact of rational argumentation.

Partial utilities (partial evaluations) can be combined into holistic judgements according to a number of integration rules, for instance the averaging rule, elaborated within research in impression formation (Anderson, 1981), or according to a number of 'decision strategies', which are complex recipes of how to weigh, encode and integrate partial evaluations into global utilities of decision alternatives (Svenson, 1979). Instrumental utilities are thus diagnostic; they are inferences from purely descriptive qualities.

The need for radical change in the understanding of utilities in decision processes was first proposed in a seminal paper by March (1978), where he challenged the traditional view that preferences (i.e., criteria for ascribing utilities) must have an extraneous, transitive, stable and choice-independent character. These requirements were for years considered a precondition of rationality of choice. On the one hand, they prevented inconsistencies in choice behaviour; on the other hand, they ensured that the decision taken was indeed the most instrumental with respect to the superordinate goal. The additional advantage was objective justifiability of the decision: choices made according to the stable and socially acknowledged (extraneous) system of preferences could be easily communicated to others and justified with help of rational arguments.

In contrast to this traditional, 'instrumentalist' notion, March (1978) suggested that preferences may have their origin in an active subject, that they may change over the decision process, and thus that they are justifications rather than premises of decisions. Preferences are not given: people tend to modify their values and attitudes throughout their life, and they do it as a consequence, rather than a precondition, of their life choices.

Quite often shifts in preferences take place in the course of the decision process. A 'promising' alternative (Montgomery, 1983) will look even more promising, and may even finally be chosen, if its desirable aspects are bolstered while undesirable aspects appropriately dampened, and/or when the reverse strategy is applied to the competing alternatives (Montgomery, 1983, 1989; Beckmann and Irle, 1985; Lewicka, 1990). This usually involves a number of cognitive manipulations applied to the system of preferences, known as 'wishful thinking', rationalisations, or belief–value correlation (Sjöberg and Biel, 1983). 'Objective' truth disappears behind the fog of subjectivity. Choices can no longer be rationally justified by reference to extraneous criteria, they become private constructions of individual minds. There is no doubt that these cognitive manipulations applied to decision situations would make a classical adherent of rational choice shudder.

This coin, however, has two sides. The other side of these biasing techniques is the emotional consequences of the choice. Rationalisations and *ex post facto* justifications tend to be more resistant to change than a rational estimation of the target's 'objective' value, by definition more open to rational argumentation. Hence, these processes may speed up decisions, promote commitment and emotional involvement, and defend the decision maker against premature abandonment of the chosen option when more attractive alternatives appear (Brickman, 1987). Usually it is the stubborn, irrational side of our nature, our affect and emotional attachments rather than rational argumentation which make us resist the temptation of a better life, and carry the decision through to its very end.

March (1978) was aware of the adaptive consequences of these phenomena. Moreover, he not only defended the emergent character of preferences against the traditional rationalists, but even suggested that the term 'rational' should also be applied to such processes. This, in the opinion of the present author, is going too far, as it obscures rather than clarifies the otherwise well-established meaning of the concept of 'rationality' (see Lewicka, 1993). However, March's attempt shows that, even two decades ago, the concepts of 'utility' and 'preferences' took on a new meaning, showing stronger affinity to 'affect' and 'emotional involvement' than to the previously acknowledged 'instrumentality' (see also Alexander, 1982).

The decision theory which, in the opinion of the present author, departs most from the classical rational approaches, being almost explicitly based on the concept of emotional utility, is the theory of dominance structuring, proposed by Montgomery (1983, 1989). According to this theory, the pre-decisional information search passes through four stages: (1) screening, in which decision options falling short of some important criteria are eliminated; (2) choice of a promising alternative, where the alternative which attracts the temporary attention of the decision maker receives the privileged status of becoming 'promising'; (3) dominance building, in which the promising alternative, due to the application of cognitive manipulations and biasing techniques, is construed as 'dominant'; (4) in case the dominance structuring techniques fail, restructuring of the problem and choice of a new promising option.

According to Montgomery, only the first stage proceeds in an unbiased way: negative candidates are eliminated through a conjunctive decision rule. The second stage is more mysterious. What makes people focus on one and not another candidate? Why should one become more salient than the other? Both theory and relevant empirical research suggest that this process is far from systematic and rational. For instance, Lewicka (1990, 1993) obtained evidence demonstrating that the alternative which becomes promising is simply better known than any other alternative, and that this is independent of whether the information is favourable or unfavourable. This suggests that mere exposure effects may play a crucial role in the formation of initial emotional utilities.

The ensuing stages, which serve to consolidate the evaluative meaning (to ensure that what is promising is also the best), have an equally non-diagnostic character. For instance, once the promising candidate is selected, the decision maker loses interest in other options. In terms of the theoretical distinctions introduced above, we may say that preselection of the promising alternative is followed by a shift from the diagnostic or piecemeal ('attribute → alternative') to the prognostic or category-driven ('alternative → attribute') inference. This would mean a shift from the question 'Which alternative should I choose?' to 'What will happen if I choose alternative X?'.

A large number of studies, both in natural and in experimental settings (Dahlstrand and Montgomery, 1984; Lewicka, 1990, 1993; Bojarska, 1996; Polański, 1996), document the biased distribution of attention paid to different alternatives. As a result, subjects tend to make their decisions on the basis of considerably richer knowledge about the finally selected candidate than about those which have not been chosen.

Other biasing techniques include evaluative manipulations: differential weighing of evaluative criteria, employment of affective inferences and perspective shifts, etc., which all produce emotionally homogeneous (positive) representations of the preselected alternative (Kemdal and Montgomery, Chapter 5). As a consequence, the alternative which is finally chosen is most often the one that appeared promising in the very beginning.

POSITIVE–NEGATIVE ASYMMETRY IN EVALUATIONS AND DECISION MAKING

Are all utilities emotional and category-driven? From what we have written so far, should we conclude that the rational approach is no longer applicable to real processes of decision making, and that its function is purely prescriptive? By no means. In the preceding sections, we mentioned the possibility that both cognitive and emotional utilities may be present in every decision process. However, which of the two will prevail may depend on a number of factors.

This section summarises a set of findings collected mainly within research on social cognition, known as 'positive–negative asymmetry', which suggest that the 'emotional–cognitive' dichotomy may be related to the target's valence. In this section I argue that positive utilities may have a more 'emotional' character than negative utilities, which are more often 'cognitive'.

The concept 'positive–negative asymmetry' (PNA) refers to the asymmetrical way in which people encode, process and react to positive and negative stimuli (Peeters, 1971; Peeters and Czapiński, 1990; Lewicka *et al.,* 1992). Its diverse manifestations include 'positivity bias', that is, the tendency to assume that what is unknown is benevolent rather than dangerous (an optimistic view of the world), and the 'negativity effect', a stronger reaction to negative stimuli than to equally intense, positive ones.

In decision situations, PNA is manifested through both aspects but the negativity effect appears to have drawn more attention from decision researchers. For instance, the utility function is known to be steeper for losses than for gains, demonstrating that people experience greater dissatisfaction with the loss of a certain amount of money than satisfaction with a gain of the same amount. The status-quo bias (preferring the known to the unknown) and risk aversion in lotteries can be explained by more weight being attached to negative than to positive consequences of one's actions. A negativity effect is also manifested in the screening stage of a decision process: decision makers give priority to the elimination of negative alternatives over the choice of a positive one (Beach and Strom, 1990; Beach, 1993; Rodin, 1978). Negative information also plays a decisive role in further stages of the decision process. For instance, in a series of experiments, Beach and Strom (1990) demonstrated that the final outcome of a decision is influenced more by negative than by positive information.

Apart from the asymmetrical emotional consequences, labelled 'affective negativity effect' (Peeters and Czapiński, 1990), negative evaluations are known to influence our judgements through cognitive aspects. They have been found to be more diagnostic than positive evaluations, as evidenced for instance by the fact that it is easier to identify a person described in negative than in positive terms (Czapiński, 1986). This may be due to the different linguistic structure of negative and positive terms. Negative words were found to be narrower and to have more precise meanings than positive words (Claeys and Timmers, 1993).

Negative phenomena attract more attention (Fiske, 1980), stimulate more attributional questions (Wong and Weiner, 1981), more often trigger counterfactual thought (Gleicher *et al.*, 1990), and more frequently stimulate the curiosity of scientists (Czapiński, 1985) than positive phenomena. Negative events also lead to more interpersonal consensus than positive events, that is, people agree more on what is undesirable than on what is desirable (Peeters and Czapiński, 1990) and criteria of negative preferences are more consistent across different individuals than criteria of positive preferences (Beach, 1993). These phenomena became known as manifestations of the 'informational negativity effect', defined as the higher informational value of negative compared to positive evaluations (Peeters and Czapiński, 1990).

Affective and informational negativity effects have a clearly adaptive function. The former sensitises an organism to imminent danger and triggers immediate protective reactions (escape, avoidance). The latter is responsible for veridical perception of the nature and causes of the threatening event and thus for the knowledge which may be used in elaboration of future programmes of preventive action. Together, the two manifestations of the negativity effect testify to the human ability to assess realistically dangers and unforeseen obstacles.

Since correct recognition of a danger is adaptively more important than veridical perception of a beneficial event, we predict that negative targets should instigate data-based inferences more often than positive targets. This should imply a relatively more emotional character for positive utilities and a relatively more cognitive character for negative ones. Metaphorically, we might say that reasons to hate may be cognitively easier to grasp than reasons to love.

Do we find grounds for these claims in decision research? Do ascriptions of negative and positive utilities in situations of choice conform to different principles? Existent data, although unsystematic, provide preliminary evidence corroborating the above claim. Relevant evidence comes mostly from those studies where choice situations were framed in either positive terms (decisions to 'accept') or in negative terms (decisions to 'reject'). This explicit framing led subjects either to attribute positive utility to the finally chosen alternative or negative utility to the finally rejected alternative.

In a series of decision tasks simulating a publication review procedure, Westenberg and Koele (1989) asked subjects either to choose manuscripts which they considered suitable for publication or to reject manuscripts which were unsuitable. Decisions to reject involved a significantly more attribute-wise search than decisions to accept, which used more alternative-wise search. In other words, subjects who were asked to choose tended to pick out one alternative and check its position on consecutive attributes, whereas subjects who were asked to reject preferred to compare consecutive alternatives on one attribute.

An analogous pattern of data was obtained by Wojcik (cf. Lewicka, 1993) in a study in which participants collected information with the goal of either accepting or rejecting one out of five potential co-workers on a future task. Rejecting subjects asked significantly more questions about attributes and significantly less questions about candidates than did accepting subjects.

The findings are interpretable within the presented framework. Attribute-wise search involves focusing attention on 'objective' comparison criteria (attributes) and hence it is unbiased with respect to any tentative hypothesis which the subject may foster about a particular alternative. The overall utility of each alternative within this type of search is built from its partial evaluations on successive attributes and thus has a data-driven character. In contrast, alternative-wise search involves focusing on a specific alternative, and since it is often triggered by a biased emotional or cognitive precommitment to this alternative, it is theory- or category-driven (Lewicka, 1990).

A series of five further studies (Lewicka, 1993) corroborated the claim about less partial pre-decisional information processing under reject than accept instruction. The same framing procedure as before was employed (to reject or to accept a candidate) but the tasks varied on a number of additional dimensions: (1) number of available alternatives to select from (three to nine); (2) ratio of positive to negative traits on each alternative (i.e., the overall evaluation of the candidates – positive, ambivalent, negative alternatives); (3) how different the alternatives were from each other on general attractiveness (matched vs. differentiated on overall attractiveness); and (4) ways of collecting information about the alternatives (attribute-wise vs. alternative-wise vs. mixed). Framing of the instruction (accept vs. reject) significantly influenced pre-decisional information search. In all five experiments, independent of additional variables, the rejecting subjects manifested significantly more careful behaviour by spreading their attention more evenly over different candidates and displaying less biased information search than they did in the 'accept' condition (Lewicka, 1993). In turn, the accepting subjects devoted disproportionate attention to their first choices which they finally selected, thus conforming more to dominance structuring processes (Montgomery, 1983). The ensuing, more balanced picture of the candidates when their drawbacks rather than their merits were scrutinised may be viewed as another manifestation of the informational negativity effect.

CONCLUDING REMARKS

The classical models of rational decision making emphasised the reconstructive, data-driven process of ascribing utilities to decision alternatives. In contrast, social cognition research frequently demonstrated that forming evaluations of social objects is a process which is mostly constructive and category-driven. This chapter makes an attempt to reconcile the two views by postulating that utilities may have either a cognitive (diagnostic, data-driven) or an emotional (prognostic, category-driven) character and that the type of ascribed utility may have profound consequences for the nature of the decision process.

An obvious question which must arise is 'When do people choose which type of utility?' The last section of the chapter reviews evidence which suggests that evaluative valence of a target option (whether it is a target of the decision to accept or to reject) may play a crucial role here.

Is hate then wiser than love? Are negative decisions more impartial and rational than positive decisions? Although these questions may sound paradoxical, they are not unfounded in the light of the presented data.

Altogether, the reviewed evidence suggests that a human decision maker may be endowed with considerable flexibility in ascribing utilities to decision targets. The ability to realistically assess negative decision targets (ascription of cognitive utilities), combined with a tendency to construct positive targets (emotional utilities), suggest a picture of a decision maker who is both rational and capable of emotional commitment. We believe that this picture avoids either of the two pitfalls present in decision literature: of the overly optimistic and overly pessimistic view on human skills to take rational decisions.

ACKNOWLEDGEMENT

This chapter was financed from the research grant no. 835/H01/96/10, given by the Committee of Scientific Research to the author.

REFERENCES

Alexander, J.C. (1982) *Positivism, Presuppositions, and Current Controversies*, Berkeley and Los Angeles: University of California Press.

Anderson, N.H. (1981) *Foundations of Information Integration Theory*, New York: Academic Press.

Aronson, E., Wilson, T.D. and Akert, R.M. (1995) *Social Psychology: The Heart and the Mind.* New York: HarperCollins.
Asch, S.E. (1946) 'Forming impressions of personality', *Journal of Abnormal and Social Psychology*, 41: 258–90.
Asch, S.E. (1952) *Social Psychology,* Englewood Cliffs, NJ: Prentice Hall.
Beach, L.R. (1993) 'Broadening the definition of decision making: the role of prechoice screening of options', *Psychological Science*, 4: 215–20.
Beach, L.R. and Strom, E. (1990) 'A toadstool among the mushrooms: screening decisions and image theory's compatibility test', *Acta Psychologica*, 72: 1–12.
Beckmann, J. and Irle, M. (1985) 'Dissonance and action control', in J. Kuhl and J. Beckman (eds) *Action Control: From Cognition to Behavior*, Berlin: Springer-Verlag, 129–50.
Bojarska, K. (1996) 'Podejmowanie decyzji przez osoby depresyjne i niedepresyjne' (Decision taking by depressed and non-depressed persons), Unpublished MA thesis, University of Warsaw.
Brickman, P. (1987) *Commitment, Conflict, and Caring,* Englewood Cliffs, NJ: Prentice Hall.
Claeys, W. and Timmers, L. (1993) 'Some instantiations of the informational negativity effect: positive–negative asymmetry in category breadth and in estimated meaning similarity of trait adjectives', *European Journal of Social Psychology*, 23: 111–29.
Czapiński, J. (1985) 'Negatywizm w psychologii. Analiza polskich publikacji' (Negativity in psychology. Analysis of Polish publications), *Studia Psychologiczne*, 22: 25–53.
Czapiński, J. (1986) 'Informativeness of evaluations in interpersonal communication: effects of valence, extremity of evaluations, and ego-involvement of evaluator', *Polish Psychological Bulletin*, 17: 155–64.
Dahlstrand, U. and Montgomery, H. (1984) 'Information search and evaluative processes in decision making: a computer based process tracing study', Unpublished manuscript, University of Göteborg.
Denes-Raj, V. and Epstein, S. (1994) 'Conflict between intuitive and rational processing: when people behave against their better judgment', *Journal of Personality and Social Psychology*, 66: 819–29.
Edwards, W. (1954) 'The theory of decision making', *Psychological Bulletin*, 51: 380–417.
Epstein, S. (1990) 'Cognitive experiential self theory', in L. Pervin (ed.) *Handbook of Personality: Theory and Research*, New York: Guilford Press, 165–92.
Fiske, S.T. (1980) 'Attention and weight in person perception: the impact of negative and extreme behavior', *Journal of Personality and Social Psychology*, 38: 889–906.
Fiske, S.T. and Pavelchak, M. (1986) 'Category-based versus piecemeal-based affective responses: development in schema-triggered affect', in R.M. Sorrentino and E.T. Higgins (eds) *Handbook of Motivation and Cognition: Foundations of Social Behavior*, vol. 1, New York: Guilford Press, 167–202.
Gleicher, F., Kost, K.A., Baker, S.M., Strathman, A.J., Richman, S.A. and Sherman, S.J. (1990) 'The role of counterfactual thinking in judgements of affect', *Personality and Social Psychology Bulletin*, 16: 284–95.
Kahneman, D. and Tversky, A. (1979) 'Prospect theory: an analysis of decision under risk', *Econometrica*, 47: 263–91.
Kirkpatrick, L.A. and Epstein, S. (1992) 'Cognitive–experiential self-theory and subjective probability: further evidence for two conceptual systems', *Journal of Personality and Social Psychology*, 63: 534–44.

Kołakowski, L. (1966) *Filozofia pozytywistyczna. Od Hume'a do Koôa Wiedeńskiego* (Philosophy of positivism. From Hume to Vienna Circle). Warsaw: PWN.

Lewicka, M. (1977) 'Evaluative and descriptive aspects of organization of cognitive structures', *Polish Psychological Bulletin*, 8: 3–12.

Lewicka, M. (1978) 'Zjawisko Pollyanny' (Pollyanna phenomenon), *Przegład Psychologiczny*, 3: 445–66.

Lewicka, M. (1979) 'Effect of cognitive set: to diagnose or to evaluate upon impression formation and change', *Polish Psychological Bulletin*, 10: 21–30.

Lewicka, M. (1988) 'On subjective and objective anchoring of cognitive acts. How behavioral valence modifies reasoning schemata', in W.J. Baker, L.P. Mos, H.V. Rappard and H.J. Stam (eds) *Recent Trends in Theoretical Psychology*, New York: Springer-Verlag, 285–301.

Lewicka, M. (1990) 'Rational or uncommitted? Depression and indecisiveness in interpersonal decision making'. Unpublished manuscript.

Lewicka, M. (1993) *Aktor czy obserwator? Psychologiczne mechanizmy odchyleń od racjonalności w rozumowaniu potocznym* (Actor or observer? Psychological mechanisms of departures from rationality in lay thinking), Warszawa-Olsztyn: PTP.

Lewicka, M., Czapiński, J. and Peeters, G. (1992) 'Positive–negative asymmetry or "when the heart needs a reason"', *European Journal of Social Psychology*, 22: 425–35.

March, J.G. (1978) 'Bounded rationality, ambiguity, and the engineering of choice', *Bell Journal of Economics*, 9: 587–608.

Montgomery, H. (1983) 'Decision rules and the search for a dominance structure: towards a process model of decision making', in P. Humphreys, O. Svenson and A. Vari (eds) *Analyzing and Aiding Decision Processes*, Amsterdam: North-Holland, 343–69.

Montgomery, H. (1989) 'From cognition to action: the search for dominance in decision making', in H. Montgomery and O. Svenson (eds) *Process and Structure in Human Decision Making*, Chichester: Wiley.

New Webster Dictionary and Thesaurus of the English Language (1991) New York: Lexicon Publications, Inc.

O'Neal, E. and Mills, J. (1969) 'The influence of anticipated choice on the halo effect', *Journal of Experimental Social Psychology*, 5: 347–51.

Osgood, C.E., Suci, G.J. and Tannebaum, P.H. (1957) *The Measurement of Meaning*, Urbana, IL: University of Illinois Press.

Peabody, D. (1967) 'Trait inferences: evaluative and descriptive aspects', *Journal of Personality and Social Psychology*, Monograph, 7 (4, Pt. 2).

Peeters, G. (1971) 'The positive–negative asymmetry: on cognitive consistency and positivity bias', *European Journal of Social Psychology*, 1: 455–74.

Peeters, G. (1989) 'National stereotypes', Paper presented at the conference Affect and Cognition, June, Sopot, Poland.

Peeters, G. and Czapiński, J. (1990) 'Positive–negative asymmetry in evaluations: the distinction between affective and informational effects', in W. Stroebe and M. Hewstone (eds) *European Review of Social Psychology*, vol. 1, Chichester: Wiley, 33–60.

Plous, S. (1993) *The Psychology of Judgement and Decision Making*, New York: McGraw-Hill.

Polański, P. (1996) 'Trudności w podejmowaniu decyzji' (Difficulties in decision making), Unpublished MA thesis, University of Warsaw.

Rodin, M.J. (1978) 'Liking and disliking: sketch on an alternative view', *Personality and Social Psychology Bulletin*, 4: 473–8.

Schoemaker, P.J. (1982) 'The Expected Utility model: its variants, purposes, evidence and limitations', *Journal of Economic Literature*, 20: 529–63.

Sjöberg, L. and Biel, A. (1983) 'Mood and belief-value correlation', *Acta Psychologica*, 53: 253–70.

Svenson, O. (1979) 'Process descriptions of decision making', *Organizational Behavior and Human Performance*, 23: 86–112.

Tagiuri, R. and Petrullo, L. (1958) *Person Perception and Interpersonal Behavior*, Stanford, CA: Stanford University Press.

Von Neumann, J. and Morgenstern, O. (1944) *Theory of Games and Economic Behavior,* Princeton, NJ: Princeton University Press.

Warr, P.B. and Knapper, C. (1968) *The Perception of People and Events*, New York: Wiley.

Westenberg, M.R.M. and Koele, P. (1989) 'Response modes and decision strategies', in K. Borcherding, O.I. Larichev and D.M. Messick (eds) *Contemporary Issues in Decision Making*, Amsterdam: North-Holland.

Wilson, T.D., Dunn, D.S., Kraft, D. and Lisle, D.J. (1989) 'Introspection, attitude change, and attitude–behaviour consistency: the disruptive effects of explaining why we feel the way we do', in L. Berkowitz (ed.) *Advances in Experimental Social Psychology*, vol. 22, New York: Academic Press, 287–343.

Wilson, T.D., Lisle, D.J., Schooler, J.W., Hidges, S.D., Klaaren, K.J. and LaFleur, S.J. (1995) 'Introspecting about reasons can reduce post-choice satisfaction', *Personality and Social Psychology Bulletin*, 19: 331–39.

Wojciszke, B. (1991) *Procesy oceniania ludzi,* Poznań: Nakom.

Wong, P.T.P. and Weiner, B. (1981) 'When do people ask "why" questions, and the heuristics of attributional search', *Journal of Personality and Social Psychology*, 40: 650–63.

Zajonc, R.B. (1960) 'The process of cognitive tuning in communication', *Journal of Abnormal and Social Psychology*, 61: 159–67.

Zajonc, R.B. (1968) 'Attitudinal effects of mere exposure', *Journal of Personality and Social Psychology Monograph*, 9: 1–28.

Zajonc, R.B. (1980) 'Feeling and thinking: preferences need no inferences', *American Psychologist*, 35: 151–75.

Part III

The risk dimension

Introduction to Part III

In decision research, the formal language of risk and uncertainty is somewhat confusing. Traditionally the two terms have been differentiated according to whether or not precise probabilities can be attached to events. Edwards (1954) gave tossing a coin as an example of an event involving risk and the proposition 'Will you drink a glass of beer immediately after reading this paper?' as an example of uncertainty. In the latter case, he suggested, there are no generally accepted rules for assigning a precise probability to the event, whereas most people accept that the probability of the coin landing 'heads' is precisely 0.5. To complicate matters, risky and uncertain events (as defined above) which may result in *negative* consequences are both termed risks in everyday language. The less confusing terms *well-defined* and *ill-defined* risks might better distinguish risk and uncertainty in Edwards' sense. Much early research focused on well-defined risks and used simple gamble tasks to test alternative theories. Such lotteries provide precise probability information, but apart from notable exceptions such as the National Lottery and the gambling casino, most real-life risks are ill-defined. That is, the probabilities of uncertain events which may follow a decision are imprecise, vague or ambiguous, and are essentially subjective. Researchers questioning the idea that lotteries display the essential characteristics of real-world risks have begun to focus on alternative tasks. For example, Tversky and Kahneman have departed from the standard lottery in developing Cumulative and Generic Prospect Theory.

The following three chapters make distinctive and complementary contributions to the study of real-life, ill-defined risk decisions. In Chapter 7, Teigen and Brun examine the nature and role of risk appraisal processes in decision making. They question one of the central assumptions of traditional theories, that when people are facing risks they judge and take into account the subjective probabilities of success or failure associated with various options. They argue that, mathematically, these probabilities should be complementary, but psychologically they require a change of focus, or even a different motivational attitude. In both cases, what is being appraised should perhaps not be conceived of as probabilities, but rather as a product of expectations, reservations, and more or less life-like images of the outcome in focus.

In the first part of their chapter, Teigen and Brun point to four different foci in the appraisal of uncertain events. First, one may attend to either the possible occurrence or the non-occurrence of a positive outcome (success, goal attainment). Attention to its occurrence defines the focus, 'opportunity orientation' (what can be gained), which is distinguished from 'uncertainty orientation', the focus on a positive outcome not happening. Similarly, they distinguish between 'risk orientation' (what can go wrong), a focus on the occurrence of negative outcomes (accidents and failures), and a 'safety orientation' if the focus is on how the negative outcome can be prevented or counteracted.

In the second part of their chapter, the authors discuss how future outcomes in general, and negative outcomes in particular, are appraised. They suggest that risks are weighted or anticipated according to their *reality character* rather than by their probabilities, as this term is usually understood. They go on to present an analysis of risk appraisal based on two processes for assessing the reality character of risks that they term 'reality by appearance' and 'reality by extension'. Teigen and Brun's framework offers both a stimulating challenge to traditional approaches and an important agenda for future research.

A related area of contemporary research aimed at understanding real-life, ill-defined risks is reviewed by Kühberger in Chapter 8. Kühberger examines the framing effect, the finding that a preference reversal can be induced by wording a risk problem in terms of negative rather than positive outcomes. Clearly, this is related to Teigen and Brun's analysis of the implications of focusing on positive or negative outcomes in risk appraisal. The dominant interpretation of the framing effect is in terms of prospect theory's weight and value functions. This assumes that probabilities are thought of as precise and well defined. However, consider Tversky and Kahneman's well-known 'Asian Disease' problem, where in one version subjects are asked to consider a treatment which has a one-third chance of saving 200 lives. Although precise probability information is presented in such problems, it is ill defined in that stated values seem to be subjective, and not backed up by logical or frequency arguments. Kühberger reviews a considerable number of alternative explanations of how people process such decision problems. He argues that several offer the potential for a richer and deeper psychological analysis in terms of underlying motives and cognitions. He observes that cognitive theories highlight the important notions that framing is content-specific and that it is dependent on elaboration processes, while motivational theories emphasise the importance of understanding the role played by hopes, wishes and fears.

In Chapter 9, Huber argues that a more detailed examination of real-world, ill-defined risks should be a major priority for process-tracing research. He points out that the traditional process-tracing methods, discussed by Harte and Koele in Chapter 2, are of limited value for the study of real-life problems. Huber describes a new technique he and his colleagues have recently developed as an alternative to the information board procedure. This is the very productive 'Active Information Search' (AIS) technique for the study of patterns of pre-decision information seeking. The AIS method uses a very well-briefed researcher who provides information requested in an informal, face-to-face setting.

A number of researchers are currently investigating the extent to which people think about ill-defined risks probabilistically. Huber argues that compensatory, probabilistic thinking does not necessarily dominate decision making with ill-defined risks. He presents evidence that people seek to reduce or even eliminate uncertainty via the application of *defusing operations*. For example, they may search for the means of controlling relevant variables to reduce uncertainty below a threshold; or they may construct alternative courses of action to avoid the uncertainty altogether; or they may construct worst-case scenarios in which the impact of a possible negative outcome is minimised. These defusing operations can be seen as that part of the decision process which can lead to the construction of essentially *riskless* representations of ill-defined risks. Huber summarises two studies he and his colleagues have recently carried out which have produced interesting evidence concerning the role of defusing operations. He also presents a new process model of risk management in decision making.

To summarise, the chapters of Part III each contribute towards a deeper understanding of the psychological processes that are brought to bear on decisions involving ill-defined risks. Teigen and Brun underline the importance of the process of appraising the reality character of ill-defined risks; Kühberger shows how risk domain, elaboration processes and motivational factors all need to be taken into account for a full explanation of how ill-defined risks are framed; and Huber describes how defusing operations are used to manage risks in everyday decision making.

REFERENCE

Edwards, W. (1954) 'The theory of decision making', *Psychological Bulletin*, 51: 380–417.

Chapter 7

Anticipating the future

Appraising risk and uncertainty

Karl Halvor Teigen and Wibecke Brun

> A windy day, Winnie-the-Pooh and his friend Piglet were walking through the woods, . . . listening a little nervously to the roaring of the gale among the tree-tops.
> – 'Supposing a tree fell down, Pooh, when we were underneath it?'
> – 'Supposing it didn't,' said Pooh, after careful thought. Piglet was comforted by this.
>
> (Milne, 1928/1974: 130)

The dialogue between Pooh and Piglet is obviously about risk. Risks, as currently defined, are situations where negative or adverse outcomes, like losses, accidents, health injuries, or deaths cannot be ruled out. We don't *know* that they will happen, but neither can we guarantee that they will not. What we can do is, like Pooh and Piglet, to suppose.

Inspired by risk analysts and formal decision making models, we often hope to go a step further and estimate the *probabilities* of the adverse outcome. In fact, some decision theorists distinguish between risky prospects, where the probabilities associated with the possible outcomes are assumed to be known, and uncertain prospects, where the probabilities are not established (Knight, 1921/1965; Tversky and Fox, 1995).

The idea of linking degree of riskiness to degree of loss likelihood is an appealing one, for at least two reasons: (1) It connects the concept of risk to the well-known mathematical concept of probability, which offers a standard to which subjective estimates of risk may be compared. (2) It also seems to reflect an important psychological component of the risk concept (cf. Brun, 1994; Drottz-Sjöberg, 1991; Yates and Stone, 1992). Most people would agree that it is more risky to play Russian roulette with a revolver charged with two bullets rather than just one, as the chances of being shot increase from 1/6 to 2/6. Piglet may think it is more risky to walk in the woods on a windy than on a calm day, as the probability of trees falling down is greater the stronger the wind.

Yet, there are two aspects of the conversation in the woods not adequately captured by the concept of subjective probability. One is the term 'supposing'. Supposing is both less and more than performing a probability estimation. It does not say much about degrees of likelihood, but requires instead an act of the imagination. One is asked to pretend that something presently non-existent is, in fact, real or – to use a more modern term – to perform 'a mental simulation'. According to the 'simulation heuristic' (Kahneman and Tversky, 1982), the ease of this operation may, in turn, be used as evidence for the probability of the outcome in question, but it may alternatively (and perhaps more directly) be conceived as a test of its reality-character. According to Taylor and Pham, 'research suggesting that mental simulations make events seem true is voluminous' (1996: 220).

The second noteworthy feature of the little dialogue is that one 'supposing' can be met (and neutralised) by another. The two suppositions are not probabilities between 0 and 1. If they were, the first one would already imply the second one, like $p = 0.20$ for being hit over the head by a falling tree implies $p = 0.80$ for not being hit, the second statement being redundant. But in our example, the two suppositions do not add up to 1; rather, the first is alarming and the second reassuring, not only by their strength but by their mere articulation.

The adult reader may of course not feel very impressed by this example, not being so easily alarmed and comforted as Piglet, yet the thesis of the present chapter is that we are able to enjoy this fictitious dialogue precisely because there is a grain of truth in it. In the rest of the chapter we will try to expand this grain into a theoretical framework for understanding perception of risk (see also Teigen and Brun, 1995a).

FOUR FOCI IN THE PERCEPTION OF UNCERTAIN EVENTS

When people are explicitly asked to estimate the chances or frequencies of various adverse events, like diseases and accidents, they often seem to *overestimate* the dangers. This is especially the case with rare but dramatic disasters, like fires, floods, aircraft accidents, nuclear catastrophes, AIDS and violent assaults (Slovic *et al.*, 1979). For instance, in a sample of Dutch psychology students the estimated probability of becoming the victim of mugging averaged about 25 per cent (Otten, 1995), clearly higher than the population frequencies. A Norwegian student sample estimated a woman's probability of contracting HIV after one unprotected heterosexual intercourse with an HIV+ partner to be about 75 per cent (Andenæs and Røsshag, 1995), whereas the true statistical estimates are closer to 0.2 per cent (Hearst and Hulley, 1988). Yet public health authorities often claim that people should be made more 'risk conscious', as they seem to neglect safety measures and expose themselves to risks that could easily have been avoided. However, when such 'risk taking' behaviour is more closely studied, it often appears that it is not based on risk evaluations at all, so it may be more appropriate to say that people are *running* risks rather than intentionally *taking* them (Pitz, 1992; Wagenaar, 1992).

This apparent discrepancy between risk evaluation and risk behaviour may be explained by the fact that people facing a risk questionnaire and people considering a particular action are not focusing on the same event. In the first case, they are instructed to attend to possible harms and losses. In the second, they are typically set on attaining a goal, which implies the contemplation of a positive rather than a negative outcome. The drugged driver, or the couple engaged in unprotected sex, are probably more focused on the positive aspects of these behaviours, i.e., what can be attained by them, than upon the dangers they imply. After all one doesn't drive to be safe, but to get from one place to another, and sex may be regarded as a source of excitement and pleasure rather than a kind of health behaviour.

Several investigators of risk, particularly in the economic domain, have noticed the figure/ground relationship between the positive and negative outcomes of a risky event. It is difficult to focus on both at the same time. When we pay attention to the positive outcome, the negative recedes into the background. When we focus on the negative, it becomes more urgent to engage in preventive behaviour than to exploit the opportunities.

Focus may be determined by something as simple as question wording, often called 'framing' (Tversky and Kahneman, 1981). A venture with 75 per cent probability of success has more appeal than the same venture described as having a 25 per cent chance of failure.

It may also be determined by personality disposition. Lopes (1987, 1993) has suggested a typology based on habitual loss-focused vs. gain-dominated behaviour, distinguishing between risk-averse 'security-mindedness' on one hand, and risk-seeking 'potential-mindedness' on the other. In their review of adolescent risk taking, Furby and Beyth-Marom (1992) suggest that adolescents focus more on the opportunity for gain (potential), i.e., what they can achieve by engaging in various forms of risky behaviour, and less on the possibility of loss, as opposed to parents and other adult authorities who more often assume a security-minded stance.

Finally, focus may be determined by situational characteristics. March and Shapira (1992) have suggested that people become more 'survival oriented', focusing on losses, when their resources are threatened by depletion, otherwise their perceptions and behaviours may be more 'aspiration oriented', focused on positive goal attainment.

But even among people considering the same outcome, for instance the negative one, two different orientations are possible. Like Piglet, one may focus on the possibility that this particular outcome will occur, or, like Pooh, on the hope that it may not. In a study of so-called verbal probabilities, i.e. phrases expressing different levels and varieties of probability and uncertainty (like 'perhaps', 'possible', 'doubtful' and 'not certain'), it was found that these linguistic expressions could be divided into two distinct categories, namely, those referring to the occurrence and those referring to the non-occurrence of a target outcome (Teigen and Brun, 1995b). For instance, 'probable' and 'possible' are in a sense affirmations, in that they refer to the potential occurrence of a particular event, whereas 'doubtful' and 'uncertain' are negations, drawing attention to the alternative, namely, the fact that the event may *not* occur. This linguistic directionality is not equivalent to degree of probability; for instance 'a slight possibility' may be thought of as positive, despite its smallness, whereas 'not completely sure' is negative, even when referring to a probability close to 1.0. The same reasoning can readily be applied to risk evaluations.

Table 7.1 summarises four possible orientations or foci in the consideration of a risky event. One may focus on the negative outcomes – accidents, failures, losses – or, alternatively, on the positive side of the coin – potential successes, goal attainments, or gains. In both cases, attention can be directed either towards the occurrence or towards the non-occurrence of the target outcome. For instance, the idea of a feared event can activate thoughts about everything that can go wrong, or about how it can be prevented or avoided. The first mode of thinking may be termed *risk orientation* and the second *safety* (or security) *orientation.*

Correspondingly, thoughts about a positive outcome may be expressed as images of its attainment, i.e., of the opportunity or positive potential inherent in the situation, which may be called an *opportunity* (or potentiality) *orientation.* Alternatively, they may be reflected in doubts that the positive outcome may not be realised at all, that important conditions are absent, or that knowledge about how the goal can be achieved is missing. Concern about this lack of reassurance may be described as an *uncertainty orientation.*

The two dimensions described in Table 7.1 may be helpful in solving an apparent contradiction between predictions from prospect theory (Kahneman and Tversky, 1979) and findings reported in the literature on

Table 7.1 Four foci in the appraisal of uncertain events

Type of outcome	*Occurrence*	*Non-occurrence*
Negative (losses, accidents, failures)	RISK ORIENTATION What can go wrong?	SAFETY ORIENTATION How can it be counteracted or prevented?
Positive (gains, successes, goal attainments)	OPPORTUNITY ORIENTATION What can be gained? How promising is it?	UNCERTAINTY ORIENTATION What is missing?

decisions in organisations under threat, as discussed by e.g. Highouse and Yüce (1996). According to prospect theory, people tend to be risk averse in situations involving gains, but risk seeking when the same situation is framed in terms of losses. But other observations suggest that people – and organisations – tend to become very conservative and take few chances when confronted with a serious threat (Staw *et al.*, 1981). Highouse and Yüce (1996) explain this by distinguishing between a loss frame and the threat of losing. According to these authors, people in a loss frame are typically concerned about the possibility of *avoiding* the loss so, in a sense, their primary motivation is hope rather than fear. In the present terminology, we would say that they are focused upon the non-occurrence of the negative outcome. Similarly, so-called 'risk averse' subjects in a gain frame appear to be primarily concerned about missing out on the gain, in other words about its possible non-occurrence. The point stressed by the present framework is that different foci may lead to different behaviours. Whether this behaviour is characterised by 'risk taking' (in the sense of choosing an uncertain rather than a certain option) will depend upon what it takes to achieve the aim in question.

In the remainder of this chapter, we will zoom in on the risk cell and ask what makes a risk – defined as the potential occurrence of a negative outcome – loom large or small. In principle, similar analyses can be performed within each of the other cells.

THE REALITY OF THE FUTURE

The events in focus, negative or positive, belong to the future. As such, they possess a peculiar status of half-baked reality. They are not factual in the sense that they can be touched, tasted, or smelled in the present. Neither are they regular counterfactuals or alternatives to reality, as their full and decisive presence may be only seconds, hours or days away. And with uncertain events, we do not know which outcomes will end up as factuals and which ones will eventually belong to the counterfactual category.

Appraising a risk means accordingly to try to discern this particular outcome's reality status when it still lingers, so to speak, on the horizon. How successfully can we 'suppose' its reality? The position taken in the present chapter is that such judgements are mediated by whatever makes the event appear lifelike, substantial, or psychologically real. The logic behind this supposition is a simple one: what concerns us most in the present is, almost by definition, the parts of our environment that we consider to be real. By implication, our most important future concerns are those outcomes that look as though they *may become real.* It is natural to assume that these are the ones that already have a reality-like character, or display some lifelike features.

In the risk and decision making literature, such possibilities are traditionally described as being more or less *likely* or, more precisely, as having a certain *subjective probability value*. Our suggestion is that it may be more accurate and perhaps more theoretically fruitful to speak about their *psychological reality* than about their subjective *p* values, even if these two concepts may turn out to be highly correlated. After all, the concept of probability translates in many European languages as 'truth-likeness' or 'verisimilitude' (e.g. French *vraisemblance*, German *Wahrscheinlichkeit*, Swedish *sannolikhet*, and Polish *prawdopodobieństwo*). Still, speaking about truth- or reality-likenesses rather than probabilities may serve a purpose: (1) by uncoupling the psychological risk concept from the normative doctrine of probabilities, making some biases and discrepancies in the risk perception literature appear less anomalous and puzzling; (2) by providing a heuristic device for isolating potential risk determinants. For instance, if reality-likeness is more essential than probability judgements for risk perception, it comes as no surprise that people may become more alarmed by a single-case story than by a statistical overview (Borgida and Nisbett, 1977), and that certain types of accidents may evoke a feeling of risk and be interpreted as 'warning signals' even when the actual fatality rates for the same hazards are not overwhelming (Slovic *et al.*, 1984; Slovic, 1992).

So how do we tell the reality character of a future event? Two strategies seem possible.

1 We can contemplate the future target event, looking for potential 'reality-cues'. Does the target outcome carry the characteristics usually associated with a real event? Does it look plausible?
2 Alternatively, we can contemplate the past and the present, in other words those parts of our life space already *known* to be real, and ask whether the target outcome appears to *follow* from these, by a kind of extension or extrapolation.

The relation between the present and the future can be visualised as an analogy to a half-completed jigsaw puzzle (see Figure 7.1). The completed part (top) consists of those events we acknowledge as factual and real, by virtue of their having already happened. The future target outcome (bottom) corresponds to a piece we still don't know where to place. Does it belong to the puzzle at all, and if it does, is it next in line or does it have to wait until later? To place the pieces correctly, one may start by inspecting those already on the board. What do they represent? If it is obvious that they make up the body and neck of a giraffe, we have to look for the giraffe's head. If they look like the antecedents of a disastrous event, with ominous clouds gathering on the horizon, the scene seems prepared for a shipwreck. Alternatively, one may pick up a piece and examine it to decide whether it is a good candidate for a place in the puzzle. Does it have the shape, the colours and the substantiality characterising the true pieces of this puzzle? The first strategy may be called reality anticipation *by extension*, or how well a focused outcome *fits*, the second reality anticipation *by appearance*, or how convincing the target outcome *looks*.

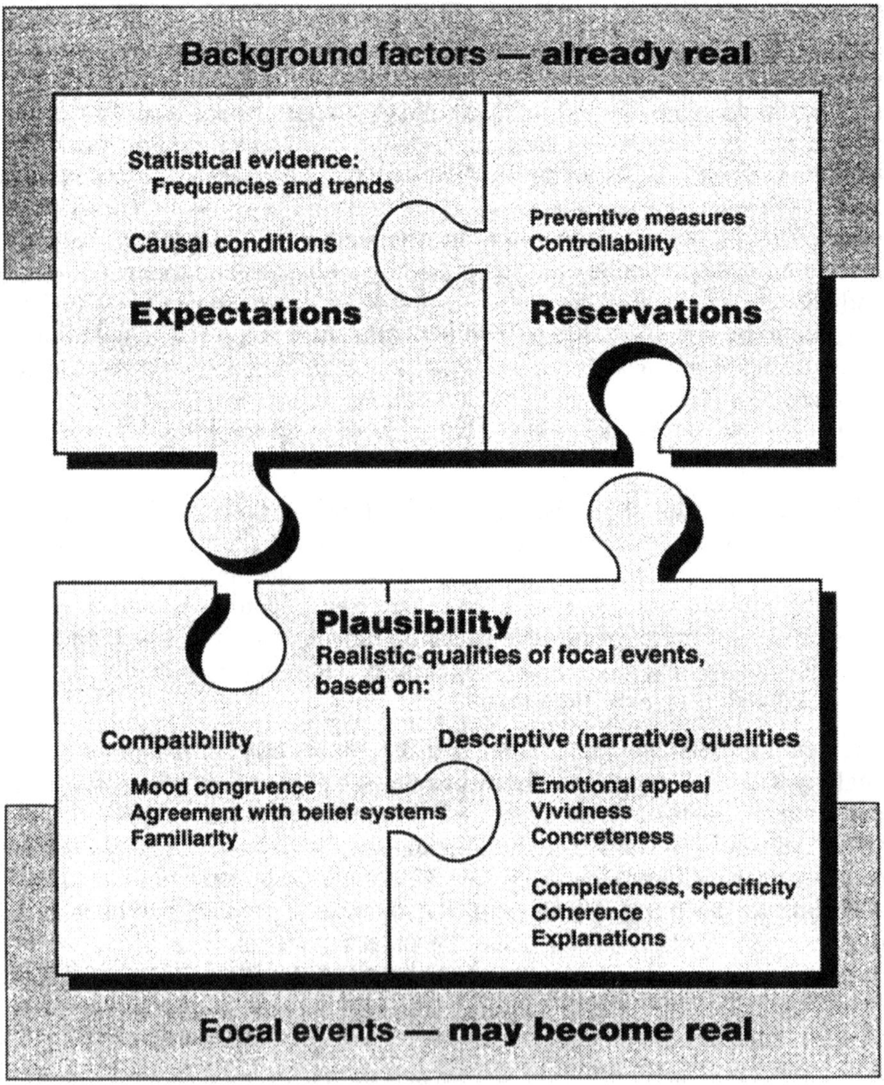

Figure 7.1 The 'puzzle' model for perceived realism of a future event

PSYCHOLOGICAL REALITY BY EXTENSION: THE ROLE OF BACKGROUND FACTORS

The present and the past contain a number of indicators making a particular future event – in this case a loss or an accident – look more or less imminent or expected. Experience, aided by inductive inference, tells us what regularly *does* go wrong, what *tends* to go wrong, and what hypothetically *can* go wrong; it also informs us about what can *prevent* a negative sequence from unfolding. For our purposes, it may be helpful to distinguish between expectations built upon purely *empirical/statistical* considerations and those based on a *causal* analysis. Similarly, we can hold statistically or causally based *reservations* or reasons for why the negative target outcome may not occur after all. A schematic overview of these factors is shown in the upper half of Figure 7.1.

Statistical evidence

To the risk expert, risks are primarily a matter of accident *frequencies*. An activity or technology that leads to a number of injuries, or casualties, is by definition a risky one, the more risky the higher the accident percentage. To lay people, this is not the only (and maybe not even the most decisive) determinant of risk (Slovic *et al.*, 1985), but it is nevertheless an important one. One's opinions about the riskiness of, say, downhill skiing are certainly influenced by information about the injury rate.

But even when perceived riskiness is *based* on injury rates, it may not be thought about as *identical* to these rates. Recent research on concept formation has stressed the human tendency to go behind appearances and think of features as expressing rather than defining an object's identity. According to the 'essentialist' view (Medin, 1989), people may not only think of a tree as a plant because it can grow, but also – or rather – that it can grow because it is a plant. Similarly, it may be true that downhill skiing is risky because it leads to injuries, but it may sound equally convincing that it leads to injuries because it is risky. Number of fatalities therefore *indicates* rather than *defines* a particular hazard's degree of riskiness.

Statistical information can also tell about *trends*. Life in large cities is often perceived to be more risky nowadays than it used to be because of the rise in crime rates. In such cases it is particularly easy to see that the perceived riskiness is not identical to the present rate, but rather a projection or extrapolation from the increasing trend. Even objectively small risks can under such circumstances be perceived as threatening, since they may be taken as a 'danger signal' or a warning that something is wrong (Slovic *et al.*, 1980, 1985). This psychological use of statistical trends again suggests that the empirical data are not taken at face value, but interpreted as 'signs' of the underlying 'essences'.

Causal inferences

Past experience and present conditions can inform us about more than accident frequencies. They also create expectations about future outcomes by indicating the presence of *causal conditions* for such accidents. An old and decrepit bridge does not have to collapse a certain number of times to be considered risky. It is enough to notice cracks in the construction, corroded bolts and rotten planks, to be convinced that at least some of the conditions for a breakdown are already present.

An analysis of the causal conditions for failure is especially central for risk judgements of unique events, where frequencies are irrelevant or unavailable. For instance, Hendrickx and colleagues have found subjects to be more sensitive to causal process information when evaluating small-scale, personally controllable risks, whereas frequentistic information was more important for large-scale and uncontrollable risks (Hendrickx *et al.*, 1989; Hendrickx *et al.*, 1992). The distinction between unique and repeated events is, however, a fuzzy one. Two situations rarely duplicate each other in all possible respects. Even in situations where it is possible to build upon extensive statistical material, for instance in judging the riskiness of smoking, motorcycle riding, or aviation, people may prefer to think in terms of causes operating on the particular case rather than in terms of accident frequencies.

In situations where it is obvious that important conditions for an adverse outcome are present, or that 'many things can go wrong', the causal analysis may paint a more threatening picture than do the statistics. For instance, anything high up (including aeroplanes) may appear risky, since by its position it satisfies one important condition for falling down. Accident frequencies may tell a more reassuring story.

In other cases, the causal simulation may miss the point and be more hopeful than the statistical picture. The naïve tourist may see no reason why she should be cautious about accepting an 'innocent' invitation from a stranger, in stark contrast to the accumulated wisdom of the local police records.

Reservations

An intuitive analysis of the situation, causally as well as statistically, can also disclose factors that make an otherwise hazardous activity appear *less* risky after all. Statistically, frequencies may be small enough to appear negligible, and trends may be comfortingly decreasing. Causally (and perhaps more importantly) there may be preventive measures available, forming a second line of defence. In case of an emergency, is there something that can be done? Studies of risk perception (Brun, 1992; Hendrickx and Vlek, 1991) have pointed to the importance of perceived *control.*

Perceived control is held by some authors to be at least partly responsible for the phenomenon of 'unrealistic optimism' (Weinstein, 1980, 1984; Zakay, 1984). Unrealistic optimism seems to be especially relevant when people engage in activities under personal control. For instance, it has been shown that car drivers generally perceive themselves as more skilful and less likely to become involved in a road accident than other drivers (Svenson, 1981; Svenson *et al.*, 1985). But as passengers, they do not think of themselves as more safe compared to other passengers (McKenna, 1993). The difference seems to be that, as a driver, one has control and is able to prevent accidents, which passengers are not in a position of doing. According to Hoorens and Buunk (1993), high scorers on an internal locus of control scale tend also to be more optimistic about health risks.

Another type of reservation, also claimed to be a factor in studies of unrealistic optimism, is the existence of more extreme groups at risk. One may for instance feel relatively safe from contracting HIV, knowing that one does not belong to any of the known 'risk' groups, like drug addicts and homosexuals.

An *absence* of preventive measures and known risk groups may, on the other hand, make an otherwise not very likely loss appear more threatening. People do not feel comfortable about a situation where there is 'nothing to prevent' an accident from occurring. No obstacles mean easy access and a high degree of perceived reality. This phenomenon may be akin to the 'equiprobability effect' (Teigen, 1988). When several outcomes are *equally* probable they are often described as *highly* probable, even if the individual probabilities for each out of n outcomes cannot exceed $1/n$. Risks that 'strike out of the blue' are often perceived as more frightening than more frequent, but apparently more predictable or controllable hazards. See, for example, the newspaper headline: 'What is horrible about the TWAR-bacteria is that it can hit anybody' (quoted in Brun, 1994).

PSYCHOLOGICAL REALITY BY APPEARANCE: QUALITIES OF THE FOCAL EVENT

Sometimes, an outcome may look alarmingly real regardless of how well or poorly it 'fits' the actual situation. A tropical disease may be described so vividly as to alarm even a reader in the Arctic. There is nothing here to warrant its reality by extension, as it does not 'follow' from the actual situation at hand. But it may still arouse the imagination in a way that makes it look plausible.

Conversely, there are cases in which imminent, expected dangers are played down or neglected because they are difficult to picture. Looking over the peaceful landscape, people find it hard to believe that, in a few days, it will in all probability be wrecked by a flood which is already creating havoc 100 miles upstream. In this case, the disaster may only become psychologically real by an act of extrapolation, rather than by an act of the imagination.

The plausibility, or reality character, of an isolated target event may be dependent upon two main sources, one being inherent in the way the risky target event is described, the other in the event's compatibility with schemata and attitudes already in the mind of the perceiver. A tentative overview of such factors is presented in the lower half of Figure 7.1.

Compatibility

A target event may not only be judged by how well it fits various background conditions, but also by how well it fits and completes the perceiver's knowledge structures and his or her state of mind.

A dangerous outcome seems more real to an already frightened person, by the principle of *mood congruity* (Gilligan and Bower, 1984). It also seems more real if it is compatible with one's *belief systems*. It is, for instance, easier to imagine an ultimate catastrophic outcome for somebody who has learned to believe that undeserved success is not an occasion for pride (hubris), but will sooner or later bring its own punishment.

Outcomes become real also by virtue of their *familiarity*. A person who has no previous experience with failure will find it hard to believe that something can go wrong, even if the present situation is completely different from the ones that formed the basis for earlier successes, whereas someone who knows of or has experienced accidents and failures before may be more inclined to see a situation as risky. *Novelty* has also proved to contribute to perceived riskiness (Slovic *et al.*, 1985), perhaps by an association between the new and the unknown.

Descriptive qualities

Outcomes also tend to become more real when they are convincingly described, for instance by being embedded in a story showing appropriate *narrative* qualities (see Bruner, 1986, 1990). According to Bruner, the narrative (as opposed to the scientific or 'paradigmatic') way of knowing works by creating lifelikeness rather than establishing and proving truths. In a recent chapter on 'variants of probability' (Teigen, 1994), some speculations were offered about people's willingness to discuss the probabilities of clearly fictional events. We say, for instance, that a movie character, or the plot in a novel, appears to be 'probable' or 'improbable'. In such cases we are apparently able to judge a situation or event's truth-likeness independent of its actual occurrence. Writers and artists have always been aware that 'truth is not always probable' and, consequently, that realism is not always best achieved by a literal chronicle of the facts (Maupassant, 1888/1984). Literary critics like Barthes (1984) and Eco

(1994) have offered valuable insights into textual characteristics conducive to creating a 'reality effect'.

Most people would agree that a more *vivid* description of an event makes it (regardless of its improbability) appear more real, although the concept of vividness is in itself in need of a closer analysis (Nisbett and Ross, 1980; Taylor and Thompson, 1982). Vividness has variously been conceptualised as *picture-like* (calling upon visual imagery), including *concrete* features, and easily *memorable* and *recallable* (hence related to the well-known 'availability heuristic' (Tversky and Kahneman, 1973)).

Vividness has further been identified with stimuli that are *emotionally engaging*. From the risk perception literature, it is well known that degree of riskiness is related to the hazard's 'dread' potential, defined as 'a risk ... that people have great dread for – on the level of a gut reaction' (Fischhoff *et al.*, 1978; Slovic, 1992).

Nisbett and Ross (1980) add that information also seems vivid in proportion to one's temporal, spatial and sensory *proximity* to it. 'The news that a bank in one's neighbourhood has been robbed just an hour ago is more vivid than the news that a bank on the other side of the town was robbed last week' (1980: 49). It is natural to assume that the close and recent robbery will also contribute more to increase the perceived risk of bank robberies.

It is hard to say whether factors like proximity, emotionality, concreteness, memorability and imaginability work through their contributions to 'vividness', or whether it is better to regard vividness as a handy but not very precise term summarising the impact of these and other 'reality-creating' characteristics. One advantage of thinking in terms of reality-likeness, or plausibility, rather than vividness, is that the former concepts suggest a greater range of possible determinants.

For instance, a *completely* described event will look more truth-like than one that is only partly known. A summary usually appears less credible than the full story. And *specific* information makes a statement sound more convincing than the use of general estimates, even if the latter are more inclusive and accordingly have a better chance of capturing the true values (Teigen, 1990).

But all parts of a scenario do not have to be spelled out to the same extent. A few concrete, even irrelevant, details may serve as highlights, lending a 'reality effect' to the complete scene (Barthes, 1984). Parts not explicitly mentioned, which have to be added or inferred by an act of presupposition, may actually enhance the lifelikeness of the complete story (Bruner, 1986).

Regardless of the level of completeness and the use of details, the different parts of a story or a risk scenario have to form a *coherent* pattern. Reality is believed to form a coherent story, with a minimum of internal contradictions and unmotivated leaps.

Perhaps the best way of creating coherence is to include both causes and effects. A description of a loss or an accident becomes more convincing when it contains *explanations* as well as results, i.e., underlying reasons, how events may develop and why they can go wrong. In their classical study of the 'Conjunction fallacy', Tversky and Kahneman (1983) showed the prospect of 'a massive flood somewhere in North America in 1983, in which more than 1000 people drown' appeared less likely than the more specific causal scenario: 'An earthquake in California sometime in 1983, causing a flood in which more than 1000 people drown'.

Causal considerations are appealing because they ensure coherence. They also provide a kind of depth dimension, by going beneath the surface flow of events. Causally anchored outcomes will almost by necessity appear more real than 'uprooted', superficially described ones. Finally, causes may forge the links between the future focal event and the 'already real' past and present parts of the puzzle, thus contributing to what we have termed 'reality by extension' as well as to 'reality by appearance'.

ANTICIPATIONS AND DECISIONS

Psychological studies of perceived risk have occasionally been criticised for being predominantly exploratory, descriptive, and lacking an integrated theoretical basis (see Hendrickx, 1991; Brun, 1994). In the present chapter, an attempt has been made to point to links between risk perception and a more general framework for how people relate to future events, according to (a) the outcome in focus and (b) the perceived realism of this outcome. The assumptions are that the same outcome will appear more or less real according to (1) whether it is focused upon or not, (2) how well it fits our past and present reality, and also (3) how convincingly it is described or presented when focused upon. It follows that statistical evidence, the risk analyst's major tool for assessing riskiness, can play only a relatively minor part in everyday risk appraisal.

Perceived realism is, in turn, believed to determine decisions under risk and uncertainty. It has been shown that people who are asked to consider a particular course of events 'as real' will subsequently behave differently from those who are given only arguments supporting a particular course of action (Gregory *et al.*, 1982). Richard *et al.* (1996) found that people who were asked to imagine how they would feel after a particular action (sex without the use of condoms) were likely to change their sexual practices later on. In these cases people seem to be affected by generating *prefactuals*, i.e., thoughts about 'what may be' (Boninger *et al.*, 1994).

The lifelikeness, or reality character, of an anticipated outcome will not only influence perceptions and decisions under risk. A similar analysis could also be applied to positive outcomes, like hopes and goals. Beach (1990) has presented an 'Image theory' of decision making, in which *goal images* (also called 'trajectory images') play a central part. Contrasting images with verbal descriptions, Beach observes that 'the striking things about images is that they are so striking' (1990: 17). This could bring one to assume that the theory is indeed concerned about how *striking* (vivid, lifelike) goals are pictured. But despite its suggestive label, Image theory has very little to say about imagination, or the process by which images are created and nourished. From the present analysis of the lifelikeness of outcomes, we would guess that the lifelikeness of a goal candidate will increase its likelihood of being adopted by the decision maker. Further, that changes in the lifelikeness of an already adopted goal will strongly affect the decision maker's initiatives, efforts and persistence of goal-directed behaviour.

REFERENCES

Andenæs, G. and Røsshag, E. (1995) 'Risikovurderinger av HIV/AIDS belyst ved to komplementære tilnærminger', Unpublished Master's thesis, University of Tromsø, Norway.

Barthes, R. (1984) 'L'effet de réel', in *Essais critiques IV: le bruissement de la langue*, Paris: Seuil.

Beach, L.R. (1990) *Image Theory: Decision Making in Personal and Organizational Contexts*, Chichester: Wiley.

Boninger, D.S., Gleicher, F. and Strathman, A. (1994) 'Counterfactual thinking: from what might have been to what may be', *Journal of Personality and Social Psychology*, 67: 297–307.

Borgida, E. and Nisbett, R.E. (1977) 'The differential impact of abstract vs. concrete information on decision behaviour', *Journal of Applied Social Psychology*, 7: 258–71.

Brun, W. (1992) 'Cognitive components in risk perception: natural versus manmade risks', *Journal of Behavioral Decision Making*, 5: 117–32.

Brun, W. (1994) 'Risk perception: main issues, approaches and findings', in G. Wright and P. Ayton (eds) *Subjective Probability*, London: Wiley, 295–320,

Bruner, J. (1986) *Actual Minds, Possible Worlds*, Cambridge, MA: Harvard University Press.

Bruner, J. (1990) *Acts of Meaning*, Cambridge, MA: Harvard University Press.

Drottz-Sjöberg, B.M. (1991) *Perceptions of Risk: Studies of Risk Attitudes, Perceptions, and Definitions*, Stockholm: Risk Research.

Eco, U. (1994) *Six Walks in the Fictional Woods*, Cambridge, MA: Harvard University Press.

Fischhoff, B., Slovic, P., Lichtenstein, S., Read, S. and Combs, B. (1978) 'How safe is safe enough? A psychometric study of attitudes towards technological risks and benefits', *Policy Sciences*, 9: 127–52.

Furby, L. and Beyth-Marom, R. (1992) 'Risk taking in adolescence: a decision-making perspective', *Developmental Review*, 12: 1–44.

Gilligan, S.G. and Bower, G.H. (1984) 'Cognitive consequences of emotional arousal', in C. Izard, J. Kagan and R. Zajonc (eds) *Emotions, Cognition, and Behavior*, New York: Cambridge University Press.

Gregory, L.W., Cialdini, R.B. and Carpenter, K.M. (1982) 'Self-relevant scenarios as mediator of likelihood estimates and compliance: does imagining make it so?', *Journal of Personality and Social Psychology*, 43: 89–99.

Hearst, N. and Hulley, S.B. (1988) 'Preventing the heterosexual spread of AIDS', *Journal of the American Medical Association*, 259: 2428–32.
Hendrickx, L. (1991) 'How versus how often: the role of scenario information and frequency information in risk judgment and risky decision making', Ph.D. thesis, University of Groningen, The Netherlands.
Hendrickx, L. and Vlek, C. (1991) 'Perceived control, nature of risk information and risk taking: an experimental test of a simple taxonomy of uncertainty', *Journal of Behavioral Decision Making*, 4: 235–47.
Hendrickx, L., Vlek, C. and Caljé, H. (1992) 'Effects of frequency and scenario information on the evaluation of large scale risks', *Organizational Behaviour and Human Decision Processes*, 52: 256–75.
Hendrickx, L., Vlek, C. and Oppeval, H. (1989) 'Relative importance of scenario information and frequency information in the judgment of risk', *Acta Psychologica*, 72: 41–63.
Highouse, S. and Yüce, P. (1996) 'Perspectives, perceptions, and risk-taking behavior', *Organizational Behavior and Human Decision Processes*, 65: 159–67.
Hoorens, V. and Buunk, B.P. (1993) 'Social comparison of health risks: locus of control, the person-positivity bias, and unrealistic optimism', *Journal of Applied Social Psychology*, 23: 291–302.
Kahneman, D. and Tversky, A. (1979) 'Prospect theory: an analysis of decision making under risk', *Econometrica*, 47: 263–91.
Kahneman, D. and Tversky, A. (1982) 'The simulation heuristic', in D. Kahneman, P. Slovic and A. Tversky (eds) *Judgment under Uncertainty: Heuristics and Biases*, Cambridge: Cambridge University Press, 201–8.
Knight, F. (1965) *Risk, Uncertainty, and Profit*, New York: Harper and Row (first published 1921).
Lopes, L.L. (1987) 'Between hope and fear: the psychology of risk', *Advances in Experimental Social Psychology*, 20: 255–95.
Lopes, L.L. (1993) 'Reasons and resources: the human side of risk taking', in N.J. Bell and R.W. Bell (eds) *Adolescent Risk Taking*, Newbury Park: Sage, 29–54.
McKenna, F.P. (1993) 'It won't happen to me: unrealistic optimism or illusion of control?', *British Journal of Psychology*, 84: 39–50.
March, J.G. and Shapira, Z. (1992) 'Variable risk preferences and the focus of attention', *Psychological Review*, 99: 183–92.
Maupassant, G. de (1984) 'Le roman'. Introduction to *Pierre et Jean*, Paris: Albin-Michel (first published in 1888).
Medin, D.L. (1989) 'Concepts and conceptual structure', *American Psychologist*, 44: 1469–81.
Milne, A.A. (1974) *The House at Pooh Corner*, London: Methuen (first published 1928).
Nisbett, R. and Ross, L. (1980) *Human Inference: Strategies and Shortcomings of Social Judgement*, Englewood Cliffs, NJ: Prentice-Hall.
Otten, W. (1995) *Optimism*, Amsterdam: University of Amsterdam.
Pitz, G.F. (1992) 'Risk taking, design, and training', in J.F. Yates (ed.) *Risk-Taking Behavior*, London: Wiley, 49–86.
Richard, R., van der Pligt, J. and de Vries, N.K. (1996) 'Anticipated regret and time perspective: changing sexual risk-taking behaviour', *Journal of Behavioral Decision Making*, 9: 185–200.
Slovic, P. (1992) 'Perception of risk: reflections on the psychometric paradigm', in S. Krimsky and D. Golding (eds) *Social Theories of Risk*, Westport, CT: Praeger, 117–52.
Slovic, P., Fischhoff, B. and Lichtenstein, S. (1979) 'Rating the risks', *Environment*, 21: 14–20, 36–9.

Slovic, P., Fischhoff, B. and Lichtenstein, S. (1980) 'Facts and fears', in R.C. Schwing and W.A. Albers (eds) *Societal Risk Assessment: How Safe is Safe Enough?*, 181–216, New York: Plenum Press.

Slovic, P., Fischhoff, B. and Lichtenstein, S. (1985) 'Characterising perceived risk', in R.W. Kates, C. Hoenhemser and J.X. Kasperson (eds) *Perilous Progress: Managing the Hazards of Technology*, Boulder, CO: Westview, 91–125.

Slovic, P., Lichtenstein, S. and Fischhoff, B. (1984) 'Modeling the societal impact of fatal accidents', *Management Science*, 30: 464–73.

Staw, B.M., Sandelands, L. and Dutton, J.E. (1981) 'Threat-rigidity cycles in organizational behaviour: a multi-level analysis', *Administrative Science Quarterly*, 26: 501–24.

Svenson, O. (1981) 'Are we all less risky and more skilful than our fellow drivers?', *Acta Psychologica*, 47: 143–8.

Svenson, O., Fischhoff, B. and MacGregor, D. (1985) 'Perceived driving safety and seatbelt usage', *Accident Analysis and Prevention*, 17: 119–33.

Taylor, S.E. and Pham, L.B. (1996) 'Mental simulation, motivation, and action', in P.M. Gollwitzer and J.A. Bargh (eds) *The Psychology of Action*, New York: The Guilford Press, 219–35.

Taylor, S.E. and Thompson, S.C. (1982) 'Stalking the elusive "vividness" effect', *Psychological Review*, 89: 155–81.

Teigen, K.H. (1988) 'When are low-probability events judged to be "probable"? Effects of outcome-set characteristics on verbal probability judgements', *Acta Psychologica*, 67: 157–74.

Teigen, K.H. (1990) 'To be convincing or to be right: a question of preciseness', in K. Gilhooly, M. Keane, R. Logan and G. Erdos (eds) *Lines of Thinking: Reflections on the Psychology of Thought*, Chichester: Wiley, 299–314.

Teigen, K.H. (1994) 'Variants of subjective probabilities: concepts, norms, and biases', in G. Wright and P. Ayton (eds) *Subjective Probability*, London: Wiley, 211–38.

Teigen, K.H. and Brun, W. (1995a) 'Risk perception: a problem solving perspective', in G. Kaufmann, T. Helstrup and K.H. Teigen (eds) *Problem Solving and Cognitive Processes: A Festschrift in Honour of Kjell Raaheim*, Bergen: Fagbokforlaget, 249–64.

Teigen, K.H. and Brun, W. (1995b) 'Yes, but it is uncertain: direction and communicative intention of verbal probabilistic terms', *Acta Psychologica*, 88: 233–58.

Tversky, A. and Fox, C.R. (1995) 'Weighting risk and uncertainty', *Psychological Review*, 102: 269–83.

Tversky, A. and Kahneman, D. (1973) 'Availability: a heuristic for judging frequency and probability', *Cognitive Psychology*, 4: 207–32.

Tversky, A. and Kahneman, D. (1981) 'The framing of decisions and the psychology of choice', *Science*, 211: 1124–30.

Tversky, A. and Kahneman, D. (1983) 'Extensional versus intuitive reasoning: the conjunction fallacy in probability judgment', *Psychological Review*, 90: 293–315.

Wagenaar, W.A. (1992) 'Risk taking and accident causation', in J.F. Yates (ed.) *Risk-Taking Behaviour*, London: Wiley, 257–82.

Weinstein, N.D. (1980) 'Unrealistic optimism about future life events', *Journal of Personality and Social Psychology*, 39: 806–20.

Weinstein, N.D. (1984) 'Why it won't happen to me: perceptions of risk factors and susceptibility', *Health Psychology*, 3: 431–57.

Yates, J.F. and Stone, E.R. (1992) 'Risk appraisal', in J.F. Yates (ed.) *Risk-Taking Behaviour*, London: Wiley, 49–86.

Zakay, D. (1984) 'The influence of perceived event's controllability on its subjective occurrence probability', *Psychological Record*, 34: 233–40.

Chapter 8

Theoretical conceptions of framing effects in risky decisions

Anton Kühberger

Risky decision making is full of so-called biases, that is, deviations of actual behaviour from normative models. One of the most influential biases in decision making is the preference reversal phenomenon, which refers to the finding that preferences are not invariant with regard to either the procedures that are used to elicit them or to alternative problem descriptions. The framing effect is one such bias. In framing experiments, the description of formally identical problems is varied, thus highlighting different aspects of them. Typically, valued objects are used and are presented so as to highlight either their gains or losses. Tversky and Kahneman (1981: 453) were the first researchers to raise these issues in their famous Asian disease problem, which is given below:

> Imagine that the U.S. is preparing for the outbreak of an unusual Asian disease, which is expected to kill 600 people. Two alternative programs to combat the disease have been proposed. Assume that the exact scientific estimate of the consequences of the programs are as follows:
>
> If Program A is adopted, 200 people will be saved.
> If Program B is adopted, there is 1/3 probability that 600 people will be saved and 2/3 probability that no people will be saved. Which of the two programs would you favour?

This represents the positively framed version of the Asian disease story, since the options are described as if they were gains. Tversky and Kahneman varied the framing of the story by presenting also a negatively framed version. In the negative frame the options are described as if they were losses:

> If Program C is adopted, 400 people will die.
> If Program D is adopted, there is 1/3 probability that nobody will die and 2/3 probability that 600 people will die.

Formally the two versions do not differ from each other: a program that saves 200 people out of 600 that otherwise will die is formally identical to a program that condemns 400 people out of 600 to death.

Psychologically, however, the presentation of the options make a difference. In Tversky and Kahneman's original research, a clear majority of respondents preferred saving 200 lives for sure (72 per cent), i.e., they preferred the risk averse option over the risky option in the positively framed version. In the negatively framed version, however, most people preferred 1/3 probability that nobody would die and 2/3 probability that 600 people would die (78 per cent), i.e., they preferred the risky option over the risk averse option.

THE FRAMING EFFECT

Framing the options of formally identical problems as gains or as losses has formed the basis of an impressive and important research endeavour. In the domain of risky decision making nearly 130 empirical articles and 80 theoretical treatments were published from 1981 until the end of 1994 (Kühberger, 1996). The usual finding, the framing effect, is risk averse choices with gains (choosing a riskless gain over a risky gain with identical expected value) and risk seeking with losses (choosing a risky loss over a riskless loss). The effectiveness of the framing manipulation seems to vary between different research paradigms, but, overall, a conservative estimate of the framing effect size is considerable ($d = 0.37$; Kühberger, 1996). Thus, there is ample evidence for a framing effect. There is negative evidence too, however (e.g., Bateman and Zeithaml, 1989; Urbany and Dickson, 1990), and there are some groups of experiments where the evidence is generally equivocal. These are experiments on (1) social dilemma situations, (2) the escalation of commitment, (3) message compliance, and (4) some health-related problems.

In social dilemma situations, framing is manipulated by presenting identical choices as either 'give-some' or 'take-some' situations. Co-operation is often found to be uncorrelated or only loosely correlated with framing (e.g., Komorita and Carnevale, 1992), and other players' frames are found to interact with one's own frame (e.g., De Dreu *et al.*, 1992).

The escalation of commitment literature, where framing is manipulated via capitalising on the money saved (by not investing further) or on the money lost (by staying committed to an initial investment) often reports interactions of framing with responsibility (e.g., Barton *et al.*, 1989).

In the message compliance paradigm the effectiveness of positively vs. negatively framed messages is found to be influenced by many different factors, but often not by framing (e.g., Lerman *et al.*, 1992). Finally, the results of some health-related studies are inconclusive (e.g., Christensen *et al.*, 1991).

In Kühberger's (1996) meta-analysis, out of 129 results, 36 (28 per cent) were not significant, and 9 (7 per cent) were significant in the direction opposite to that of the usual framing effect. Most of the studies that report inconclusive results do not present a decision between a sure and a risky option, however. Instead, they present options differing in riskiness (for the relevance of this distinction, see Kühberger, 1996). In such situations it may be unclear what constitutes the more and the less risky option.

With the Asian disease paradigm, the framing effect could also be made to disappear or even to be reversed (Kühberger, 1995), by the highlighting of information omitted in the standard version. For instance, if 600 people are at stake and you save 200, then this means that 400 will not be saved. Kühberger (1995) varied the information presented in the sure alternative by presenting a version which highlighted the missing aspect (e.g., *400 people will not be saved*). This led to a reversal of the standard framing effect.

In summary, the framing effect depends on the methodology used. But this does not come as a big surprise: if a phenomenon gets so much attention in such different areas and is researched within so many different approaches, it is not surprising that some of them are ineffective in some areas. The important question is why. The theoretical accounts for framing effects given in the remainder of this chapter may give some answers.

MODELS OF FRAMING

Theories of framing can be grouped as follows: (i) *Formal models* concentrate on values and weights and use different value and weighting functions dependent on the domain for the prediction of judgements and choices. In essence they view the framing phenomenon as a cognitive illusion, very similar to a perceptual illusion. The structure of the problem is of greatest relevance. (ii) *Cognitive models* are interested in identifying the details of information processing that occur between stimulus and response. The structure of the processing system is mainly relevant. Some cognitive models are not purely cognitive, but often use cognitive in addition to formal concepts. Thus they may be labelled more accurately as hybrid formal-cognitive models. (iii) *Motivational models* see the framing effect as a consequence of motivational forces such as wishes and fears within the individual. The content of the system is relevant. Again, some of these are more accurately termed hybrid formal-motivational. (iv) *Metaphorical models* of framing use concepts which stem from a different scientific background.

Formal modelling: values and weights

In formal models it is the structure that is relevant, not the content or the purpose. This idea is translated in formal models as differences in value or weighting functions for gains and losses, which do not depend on the surface structure of a problem, but depend on a deep structure, which is assumed to have the syntax of a gamble. Pure formal models give an account of framing in terms of a set of psychophysical functions, whose forms may vary. Highlighting either gain or loss aspects of a problem brings different psychophysical functions to bear on the presented information. Some of the more influential formal models are presented below.

Prospect theory

Framing research is heavily dominated by Prospect theory (Kahneman and Tversky, 1979), which distinguishes three phases in decision making. In the translation phase, outcomes are coded relative to a reference point and are assigned a subjective value, and probabilities are translated into decision weights. In the combination phase, subjective values and decision weights are combined. Finally, in the decision phase, the prospect value is evaluated or a prospect is chosen. Prospect theory's essential point for framing lies in the subjective value function, which has three noteworthy characteristics: (1) The value function has a reference point, which is the focal level of the pertinent outcome such that lower values are perceived as losses and higher values are perceived as gains. (2) The shape of the value function changes markedly at the reference point: above the reference point, in the domain of gains, the value function is concave, showing diminishing marginal value. Below the reference point in the domain of losses, however, the value function is convex. (3) The slope of the value function is steeper for losses than for gains, which means that reaction to losses is more profound than reaction to gains.

For the Asian disease problem, Prospect theory predicts the results by the following logic: the positive framing induces an adoption of the reference point so that the disease is allowed to take its toll of 600 lives. Thus the outcomes of the two options are perceived as possible gains. Therefore saving 200 people with probability 1 is more attractive than saving 600 people with probability 1/3, since 600 is subjectively less than 3 times 200 at the convex value function for gains. In the negatively framed version, the reference point is zero people dying, and the outcomes thus are perceived as possible losses. Therefore having 400 people dying with probability 1 is less attractive than having 600 people dying with probability 2/3, since 600 is subjectively more than 3/2 times 400 at the concave value function for losses. Thus, we see risk aversion in the domain of gains, and risk seeking in the domain of losses.

Cumulative prospect theory

In 1992, Tversky and Kahneman presented Cumulative prospect theory, a refined version of Prospect theory. The refinements mainly deal with the weighting function: the weights are cumulative rather than separable, thus allowing different weighting functions for gains and for losses. Cumulative prospect theory leads to the interesting prediction of 'a distinctive fourfold pattern of risk attitudes: risk aversion for gains and risk seeking for losses of high probability; risk seeking for gains and risk aversion for losses of low probability' (Tversky and Kahneman, 1992: 297). According to Cumulative prospect theory, risk attitudes do not depend solely on the value function, but are determined jointly by the value function and the cumulative weighting functions.

Prospect theory as well as Cumulative prospect theory are not pure formal models, but rather are hybrid models since they incorporate two stages: an initial framing stage and a subsequent stage of valuation. The framing stage is cognitively modelled, and incorporates coding and simplification operations whereas the valuation stage is formally modelled. Interestingly, it is the valuation phase and not the framing phase, however, which is applied to framing. These models are therefore treated under the heading of formal models.

Markowitz's utility theory

Markowitz's utility theory has a value function which is defined over gains and losses. It has one inflection point at the reference point, and two further inflection points in the domains of gains and losses, respectively. It is assumed to be convex for large losses and small gains, and concave for small losses and large gains. Thus, risk seeking and risk aversion are possible in both domains, risk seeking being predominant for large losses and small gains, and risk-aversion being predominant for small losses and large gains.

Venture theory

Hogarth and Einhorn (1990) presented a model that translates probabilities into decision weights. In Venture theory, framing effects result from the probability weighting function.

The Advantage model

The Advantage model (Shafir *et al.*, 1993) has both absolute aspects (a lottery's attractiveness depends solely on the lottery itself) and comparative aspects (the attractiveness of a lottery depends on the options against which it is compared). The absolute part captures a lottery's size and the comparative part evaluates the relative difference in payoff and probability. This is done separately for gains and for losses. In the Advantage model it is a person's relative weight of payoffs to probabilities that differs when the payoffs represent gains as opposed to losses.

Table 8.1 summarises these formal models, with their relevant concepts and predictions.

Cognitive modelling: levels of processing

Cognitive models assume that the level of cognitive processing is determined by the content and importance of the problem and that thinking is dependent on the problem domain.

Fuzzy-trace theory

Fuzzy-trace theory holds that framing effects are the result of information processing strategies that operate on a superficial, simplified level.

Table 8.1 Prominent concepts and predictions for formal models

Theory	*Prominent concepts*	*Predictions*
Prospect theory	Reference point Value function	Risk aversion for gains Risk seeking for losses
Cumulative prospect theory	Reference point Value function Weighting function	High probabilities: risk aversion for gains; risk seeking for losses Low probabilities: risk seeking for gains; risk aversion for losses
Markowitz's utility theory	Reference point Value function Magnitude of payoff	Large payoffs: risk aversion for gains; risk seeking for losses Small payoffs: risk seeking for gains; risk aversion for losses
Venture theory	Reference point Magnitude of payoff Magnitude of probability	Increasing risk aversion with increasing payoff/probability for gains Decreasing risk aversion with increasing absolute payoff/probability for losses
The Advantage model	Reference point Lottery size (probability and payoff) Difference probability – payoff	Risk aversion for gains Risk seeking for losses

Reyna and Brainerd (1991: 249) characterise thinking 'as fluid and ranging, that is, as operating on gist rather than on verbatim details, as parallel rather than linear as in logic, and as fuzzy or qualitative rather than precise in computation'. Framing effects are the result of processing on a qualitative level, only extracting the gist of the information presented.

Take again the Asian disease problem as an example: *200 people will be saved* would, according to Fuzzy-trace theory reduce to *some people will be saved.* The risky option *1/3 probability that 600 people will be saved and 2/3 probability that no people will be saved* would reduce to *some people probably will be saved and some people probably will not be saved.*

Since *some people will be saved is* definitely better than *some people probably will be saved and some people probably will not be saved*, this leads to a preference for the risk averse option. For the negative framing, the picture reverses: *some people will die* is definitely worse than *some people probably will die and some people probably will not die.* Hence the preference for the risk seeking option.

Elaboration theory

Maule (1989, 1995) holds that in most situations subjects will use more elaborated frames than just the simple ones given to them. He argues that such elaboration is more likely to occur in important situations where more cognitive activity is invested. Elaboration theory offers no account for framing effects *per se*, but questions untested assumptions that the imposed frames are working as intended. Elaboration theory holds that every form of elaboration will reduce framing effects.

Probabilistic mental model theory

Kühberger (1995) applied Probabilistic mental model theory (Gigerenzer *et al.*, 1991) to framing. Probabilistic mental model theory also holds that people work with richer and more variable models than warranted by the bare formal structure. The focal idea is that, in order to make frequency based inferences, people construct a reference class for the problem at hand. Different problems may induce different reference classes. Probabilistic mental model theory thus can predict a framing effect or not, depending on the respective problem content. For the Asian disease problem, the theory assumes that, in order to make decisions, people construct a reference class like 'programs for fighting disasters', for instance. In this problem context an essential element of the relevant domain is time. Experience tells us that fighting disasters takes time. As time goes by things may change. After an initial number of people have been saved (killed), in the following days some additional people may be saved (killed). The crucial difference between the two programmes lies in the possibility that such an additional gain (loss) can happen. This difference discriminates the two programmes from one another: *200 people will be saved (and later maybe more)* would then be the better choice in the domain of gains and *400 people will die (and later maybe more)* would be the worse choice in the domain of losses.

Positive–negative asymmetry

According to Peeters and Czapiński (1990), positive and negative stimuli are evaluated asymmetrically. A positivity bias reflects something like subjectively anchored optimism. A negativity effect, on the other hand, holds that more weight is accorded to potential losses than to potential gains, and that negative stimuli are weighted more than positive stimuli in the forming of an overall evaluation (affective negativity-effect). Furthermore, an informational negativity-effect is posited, which holds that individuals strive to gain control over potentially harmful stimuli, resulting in extra attention to, and cognitive work with, those negative stimuli. This view has two implications: first, losses should be weighted more heavily than formally equivalent gains because of their greater information value. Second, neutral presentations of a problem should be more easily framed as gains than as losses, because it should be cognitively easier to frame situations as gains than as losses.

Table 8.2 summarises these cognitive models, with their main concepts and predictions.

Table 8.2 Prominent concepts and predictions for cognitive models

Theory	*Prominent concepts*	*Predictions*
Fuzzy-trace theory	Gist extraction Fuzzy processing	Risk aversion for gains Risk seeking for losses
Elaboration theory	Elaboration	Increasing inconsistency in risk attitude with increasing elaboration
Probabilistic mental model theory	Reference class	Risk attitude depends on reference class
Positive–negative asymmetry	Positivity bias Negativity effect	Not related to risk attitude (mainly in message compliance studies)

Motivational modelling: hopes and fears

Security-potential/aspiration theory

Some researchers have applied Lopes' (1987) Security-potential/aspiration theory to framing effects (Schneider, 1992; Maule, 1995). Security-potential/aspiration theory holds that two factors determine risky choice. The first factor is security-potential, which reflects the relative attention that an individual pays to security and/or potential. In terms of framing, security seeking would lead one to avoid the worst outcomes and potential seeking would lead one to approach the best outcomes. The second factor is the aspiration level. This reflects the individual's hopes and needs and is more influenced by the situation. In the domain of gains both factors generally favour risk avoidance, whereas with losses the two factors act in opposite ways. Security favours the choice of the certain alternative, but this alternative is often below the aspiration level and is thus not acceptable.

Security-potential/aspiration theory is not purely motivational. It also has a formal component which is meant to parallel cognitive processes. The motivational component is meant to explain why these processes occur.

Self-discrepancy theory

The core concept of Self-discrepancy theory (Higgins, 1987; Tykocinski *et al.*, 1994) is self-belief. Individuals hold their self-concept, or actual self, their representations of goals, ideals, wishes, hopes and aspirations (ideal self-guide) as well as their representations of beliefs about duties, obligations and responsibilities (ought self-guide). Self-regulation in terms of the ideal self-guide orients people towards positive outcomes. They thus tend to maximise the presence of positive outcomes and minimise their absence. Self-regulation in terms of the ought self-guide orients individuals towards negative outcomes; they tend to maximise the absence of negative outcomes or minimise their presence. Note that different types of framing are indicated here: positive or negative valence is not only dependent on the type of outcome but also on the presence or absence of the outcome.

Table 8.3 summarises these motivational models and their main concepts and predictions.

Metaphorical models

Framing is usually described in terms of concepts that are closely related to decision theory. There are some models, however, that describe it by using a conceptual language which stems from more or less different

Table 8.3 Prominent concepts and predictions for motivational models

Theory	*Prominent concepts*	*Predictions*
SP/A theory	Security-potential Aspiration	Risk aversion for gains Inconsistent risk attitude for losses
Self-discrepancy theory	Actual, ideal, ought self-guide	Individual difference in sensitivity to domains: risk aversion for gains (actual–ideal) risk-seeking for losses (actual–ought)

scientific backgrounds. Such metaphorical models may not be within the realm of cognitive psychology or even within the realm of psychology at all. These models include behavioural models (Rachlin *et al.*, 1986; March, 1996), which exploit the correspondence between the concept of probability and the concept of delay. Other metaphorical models are neural network models (Grossberg and Gutowski, 1987), which use connectionist terminology to explain framing and many other phenomena of risky decision making, and Catastrophe theory, which makes predictions for framing in the case of multiple decisions (Svyantek *et al.*, 1991).

EVALUATING THE MODELS

It is surprising to see that so many different theories are cited to account for framing. But how should those theories be evaluated? In this section some of the specific merits and difficulties associated with each of them are discussed.

Amount of empirical attention

In terms of the amount of empirical attention, the case is settled: Prospect theory is, by far, the winner. Out of approximately 130 empirical papers on framing in risky situations, more than 100 use Prospect theory as the theoretical background. The other theories have been tested either in one single or, at most, in two to three experiments. Because of this, empirical support may not be an adequate standard for evaluating models, for two reasons. First, the empirical base to date is too sparse. However, experiments testing formal models are often very similar to each other. This should, in principle, enable the test of formal models against each other, although this has not yet been done. Second, a new theory for framing will probably only be published if the data support it. That is, in published research, predictions generally tend to be confirmed. As a consequence, most results for the only sparsely tested models are supportive.

Empirical support

For cognitive models, predictions may depend on how important a problem is, on the degree of expertise, or on problem content. Importance and involvement are relevant to Fuzzy-trace theory, since they may influence the degree of fuzziness in processing. Higher importance or involvement can be operationalised by using real as opposed to hypothetical stakes, or by specifying that the decision maker, as opposed to another person, is influenced. It is predicted that this will lead to more effort in information processing and thus to less fuzzy processing: no fuzzy processing, no framing effect. However, the findings either: (1) do not indicate an effect of measured, rated, or assumed degree of involvement or importance (e.g., Levin *et al.*, 1988; Roszowski and Snelbecker, 1991; van der Pligt and van Schie, 1990); or, to the contrary, (2) show low framing effects with low involvement (Meyerowitz and Chaiken, 1987; Rothman *et al.*, 1993), and higher effects for high importance (Wilson *et al.*, 1987). Such findings are inconsistent with Fuzzy-trace theory.

Expertise and involvement are of relevance to Elaboration theory. Both are assumed to reduce the framing effect. Importance and involvement do not reduce framing, as shown above. The same is true for knowledge and expertise. Generally, experiments that compare students with experts in their fields and with different grades of expertise, do not find differences (Kühberger, 1996). Expertise or familiarity with the problem domain does not make the framing effect disappear. Elaboration theory is thus not supported by the data.

Problem content is relevant to Probabilistic mental model theory. There should be evidence that the framing effect appears or disappears with different problem content. As reviewed by Goldstein and Weber (1995), content dependency has been demonstrated in many different areas of psychology. Direct evidence on this is sparse, but recent experiments demonstrate the relevance of content to decision making in general (Huber and Kühberger, 1996) and framing in particular (Schneider, 1992; Wagenaar *et al.*, 1988). Goldstein and Weber (1995) offer strong arguments that future research will show that content is central to understanding judgement and decision making.

The cognitive models are very closely related with respect to the notions of elaboration and of domain-specificity. For elaboration, Fuzzy-trace theory holds that people act on more simplified structures than those presented, whereas Elaboration theory and Probabilistic mental model theory hold that they act on richer structures than those presented. However, positive–negative asymmetry implies that richer structures are elaborated only for negative frames. Thus, framing can be seen as a consequence of elaboration by simplification or elaboration by complication. The reasons for elaboration differ between the models. We simplify because our processing system is built to prefer to act on simple structures, says Fuzzy-trace theory. We elaborate because our processing system more or less automatically uses information from our knowledge base which has been relevant in our learning history, say both Fuzzy-trace theory and Probabilistic mental model theory (this latter account resembles in a remote way the ideas in behavioural models, in which the learning history is focal). Finally, positive–negative asymmetry argues that we elaborate the negative because evolution has shaped our cognitive system in a way that makes it more susceptible to the negative, be it affective or be it informational. This is because, usually, the negative is more relevant for survival.

Domain-specificity is the second notion which is relevant. All cognitive models rely on prior knowledge to guide encoding, organisation and manipulation of information, and thus predict that framing should be content specific. However, they differ in how the semantic content of stimuli can affect psychological processing. Content specificity can result from (i) domain-specific encoding and representation of information (Fuzzy-trace theory, Elaboration theory), (ii) domain-specific rules for manipulating encoded information (Probabilistic mental model theory), and (iii) domain-specific attentional mechanisms (positive–negative asymmetry).

The predictions of motivational models depend on individual differences. This may prove promising, given Decision theory's traditional tendency to overlook individual differences. The core concepts of the motivational models are hopes, fears and wishes, which lead individuals to be more receptive either to gains (potential in SP/A theory and ideal self-guide in Self-discrepancy theory) or to losses (security in SP/A theory and ought self-guide in Self-discrepancy theory). Positive–negative asymmetry also acknowledges the driving force of hopes, fears and wishes. The positivity bias is something like a subjectively anchored optimism. Positive–negative asymmetry thus has a motivational component which is similar to SP/A and Self-discrepancy theory. If adequately measured, these motivational processes can contribute significantly to the understanding of the framing effect (Maule, 1995; Schneider, 1992; Tykocinski *et al.*, 1994). There are numerous unsuccessful findings too, however. Many different global personality characteristics have been tested with framing: beliefs about the self (Meyerowitz and Chaiken, 1987; Robberson and Rogers, 1988; Rowe and Puto, 1987; Tykocinski *et al.*, 1994; Wilson *et al.*, 1990), appraisals of threat and coping (Bier and Connell, 1994; Maheswaran and Meyers-Levy, 1990; Meyerowitz and Chaiken, 1987; Steffen *et al.*, 1994; Tykocinski *et al.*, 1994), field-dependency (Fagley and Miller, 1990), susceptibility to others (Lalor and Hailey, 1990), life-orientation (Bier and

Connell, 1994; Lauver and Rubin, 1990), locus of control (Bier and Connell, 1994), need for cognition (Bier and Connell, 1994), decision making style (Duchon *et al.*, 1989), and risk taking propensity (Elliott and Archibald, 1989; Fagley and Miller, 1990; Rowe and Puto, 1987). Significant influences on framing, however, have hardly ever been reported. The problem with these personality characteristics seems to be that they are often measured too globally to be applied to motivational models directly.

A preliminary synthesis of these models shows that, while many different models for framing exist, they share common concepts to a great extent. Pure formal models offer a means to describe most findings of framing, but they are at the level of merely describing behavioural products rather than psychological processes. The cognitive and motivational models add the flesh to the formal bone. Cognitive models do so by stressing the concept of elaboration and by specifying task and content effects which serve to enhance or reduce elaboration. Motivational models do so by highlighting the hedonic motivational dynamics of hopes, fears and wishes which are said to determine the weight that individuals allocate to the positive or the negative. While cognitive and motivational models offer interesting predictions, their empirical support is generally weak. It will be necessary for cognitive and motivational models to measure the concepts which underlie their predictions better so that decisive data can be obtained.

Generalisability of models

Good theories are not insular molecular ones; rather, they should apply to more domains and topics than just one. In framing, however, very insular theories are brought forward, which are hardly ever related to each other or to other similar phenomena by their inventors. Take the context of persuasion, for example. In a sense, the first framing experiment was carried out in this context (McCroskey and Wright, 1971). Similarly, the framing of survey questions is an important research topic (Fine, 1992). Framing is also discussed in more applied domains such as risk taking and driving (Cvetkovich and Earle, 1988), consumer decision making (e.g., Hempel and Daniel, 1993), and other applied topics (Spears *et al.*, 1992). This research uses the term 'framing' in many different and divergent senses for manipulations in tasks, contexts and contents. Or take the studies on the framing of acts or contingencies (the many studies of mental accounting), or problem solving, where a large body of literature on problem isomorphs exists (e.g., Simon and Hayes, 1976). Where is the framing theory that could provide and would attempt to provide an overall account for this research? As Hogarth (1986: 442) puts it:

> The theoretical challenge is not simply to explain the current 'anomalies'; rather it is to make predictions that take us beyond these

phenomena. However, this can only be done if investigators construct their models by considering implications of a wider range of environmental circumstances than has been the case to date.

CONCLUDING REMARKS

In this chapter, a review of the literature on framing has revealed a diversity of paradigms and models put forward to describe or explain the effects. The overall framing effect is considerable in size, but depends on the methodology used to elicit it. Prospect theory is by far the most influential account of framing, and empirical research with respect to other models is sparse. The numerous different models of framing can be grouped on the basis of their emphasised aspects into formal, cognitive, motivational and metaphorical models. These groups have fuzzy boundaries, however. Cognitive and motivational models are often thought to provide a more psychological description of the *how* and *why* of formal models. Formal theories may adequately describe the robust findings in the paradigm of Tversky and Kahneman's Asian disease problem. However, in order to test cognitive or motivational models and to clarify the pragmatic significance of the framing effect, researchers have been increasingly motivated to enrich problems in content and structure. While being formally irrelevant, such task and content effects tend to reveal some of the shortcomings of pure formal models and to demonstrate the progress resulting from cognitive and motivational viewpoints. The synthesis presented in this chapter shows that most models within groups share their prominent concepts. Most cognitive models centre around the concept of elaboration, but differ on the reason and the direction of the influence of elaboration on framing. A further similarity between cognitive models is that they all predict framing to be content-specific. Most motivational models emphasise the influence of hedonic factors like hopes, fears and wishes, but run into difficulties when they try to relate those motivational concepts to framing findings. The framing phenomenon cannot be understood adequately within purely formal theories, especially with respect to the striving of decision research to come to grips with more natural decision processes. Research within cognitive and motivational models, though as yet empirically weak, offers promise for an understanding of the phenomenon at the level of psychological processes rather than at the level of overt behaviour.

REFERENCES

Barton, S.L., Duchon, D. and Dunegan, K.G. (1989) 'An empirical test of Staw and Ross's prescription for the management of escalation of commitment behaviour in organizations', *Decision Sciences*, 20: 532–44.

Bateman, T.S. and Zeithaml, C.P. (1989) 'The psychological context of strategic decisions: a model and convergent experimental findings', *Strategic Management Journal*, 10: 59–74.

Bier, V.M. and Connell, B.C. (1994) 'Ambiguity seeking in multiattribute decisions: effects of optimism and message framing', *Journal of Behavioral Decision Making*, 7: 169–81.

Christensen, C. *et al.* (1991) 'Framing bias among expert and novice physicians', *Academic Medicine*, 66(9, Suppl.): 76–8.

Coombs, C.H. (1975) 'Portfolio theory and the measurement of risk', in M.F. Kaplan and S. Schwarz (eds) *Human Judgment and Decision Processes*, New York: Academic Press.

Cvetkovich, G. and Earle, T.C. (1988) 'Decision making and risk taking of young drivers: conceptual distinctions and issues', *Alcohol, Drugs and Driving*, 4: 9–19.

De Dreu, C.K.W., Emans, B.J.M. and van de Vliert, E. (1992) 'Frames of reference and cooperative social decision making', *European Journal of Social Psychology*, 22: 297–302.

Duchon, D., Dunegan, K.J. and Barton, S.L. (1989) 'Framing the problem and making decisions, the facts are not enough', *IEEE Transactions on Engineering Management*, 36: 25–7.

Elliott, C.S. and Archibald, R.B. (1989) 'Subjective framing and attitudes towards risk', *Journal of Economic Psychology*, 10: 321–8.

Fagley, N.S. and Miller, P.M. (1990) 'The effect of framing on choice: interactions with risk-taking propensity, cognitive style, and sex', *Personality and Social Psychology Bulletin*, 16: 496–510.

Fine, T.S. (1992) 'The impact of issue framing on public opinion: toward affirmative action programs', *Social Science Journal*, 29: 323–34.

Gigerenzer, G., Hoffrage, U. and Kleinbölting, H. (1991) 'Probabilistic mental models: a Brunswikian theory of confidence', *Psychological Review,* 98: 506–28.

Goldstein, W.M. and Weber, E.U. (1995) 'Content and discontent: indications and implications of domain specificity in preferential decision making', *The Psychology of Learning and Motivation*, 32: 83–136.

Grossberg, S. and Gutowski, W.E. (1987) 'Neural dynamics of decision making under risk: affective balance and cognitive–emotional interactions', *Psychological Review*, 94: 300–18.

Hempel, D.J. and Daniel, H.Z. (1993) 'Framing dynamics: measurement issues and perspectives', *Advances in Consumer Research*, 20: 273–9.

Higgins, E.T. (1987) 'Self-discrepancy: a theory relating self and affect', *Psychological Review*, 94: 319–40.

Hogarth, R.M. (1986) 'Generalization in decision research: the role of formal models', *IEEE Transactions on Systems, Man, and Cybernetics*, 16: 439–49.

Hogarth, R.M. and Einhorn, H.J. (1990) 'Venture theory: a model of decision weights', *Management Science*, 36: 780–803.

Huber, O. and Kühberger, A. (1996) 'Decision processes and decision trees in gambles and more natural decision tasks', *Journal of Psychology*, 130: 329–39.

Kahneman, D. and Tversky, A. (1979) 'Prospect theory: an analysis of decision under risk', *Econometrica*, 47: 263–91.

Komorita, S.S. and Carnevale, P.J. (1992) 'Motivational arousal vs. decision framing in social dilemmas', in W. Liebrand, D. Messick, and H. Wilke (eds) *Social Dilemmas*, New York: Pergamon.

Kühberger, A. (1995) 'The framing of decisions: a new look at old problems', *Organizational Behavior and Human Decision Processes*, 62: 230–40.

Kühberger, A. (1996) 'The influence of frames on risky decisions: a meta-analysis', Paper submitted for publication.

Lalor, K.M. and Hailey, B.J. (1990) 'The effects of message framing and feelings of susceptibility to breast cancer on reported frequency of breast self-examination', *International Quarterly of Community Health Education*, 10: 183–92.

Lauver, D. and Rubin, M. (1990) 'Message framing, dispositional optimism, and follow-up for abnormal Papanicolaou tests', *Research in Nursing and Health*, 13: 199–207.

Lerman, C. *et al.* (1992) 'The impact of mailing psychoeducational materials to women with abnormal mammograms', *American Journal of Public Health*, 82: 729–30.

Levin, I.P., Schnittjer, S.K. and Thee, S.L. (1988) 'Information framing effects in social and personal decisions', *Journal of Experimental Social Psychology*, 24: 520–9.

Lopes, L.L. (1987) 'Between hope and fear: the psychology of risk', in L. Berkowitz (ed.) *Advances in Experimental Social Psychology Vol. 20*, New York: Academic Press.

McCroskey, J.C. and Wright, D.W. (1971) 'A comparison of the effect of punishment-oriented and reward-oriented messages in persuasive communication', *Journal of Communication*, 21: 83–93.

Maheswaran, D. and Meyers-Levy, J. (1990) 'The influence of message framing and issue involvement', *Journal of Marketing Research*, 27: 361–7.

March, J.G. (1996) 'Learning to be risk averse', *Psychological Review*, 103: 309–19.

Markowitz, H. (1952) 'The utility of wealth', *Journal of Political Economy*, 60: 151–8.

Maule, A.J. (1989) 'Positive and negative decision frames: a verbal protocol analysis of the Asian disease problem of Tversky and Kahneman', in H. Montgomery and O. Svenson (eds) *Process and Structure in Human Decision Making*, Chichester: Wiley.

Maule, A.J. (1995) 'Framing elaborations and their effects on choice behaviour: a comparison across problem isomorphs and subjects with different levels of expertise', in J.P. Caverni, M. Bar-Hillel, H.F. Barron and H. Jungermann (eds) *Contributions to Decision Making I*, Amsterdam: North-Holland.

Meyerowitz, B.E. and Chaiken, S. (1987) 'The effect of message framing on breast self-examination: attitudes, intentions, and behavior', *Journal of Personality and Social Psychology*, 52: 500–10.

Peeters, G. and Czapiński, J. (1990) 'Positive–negative asymmetry in evaluations: the distinction between affective and informational negativity effects', *European Review of Social Psychology*, 1: 33–60.

Rachlin, H., Logue, A.W., Gibbon, J. and Frankel, M. (1986) 'Cognition and behavior in studies of choice', *Psychological Review*, 93: 33–45.

Reyna, V.F and Brainerd, C.J. (1991) 'Fuzzy-trace theory and framing effects in choice: gist extraction, truncation, and conversion', *Journal of Behavioral Decision Making*, 4: 249–62.

Robberson, M.R. and Rogers, R.W. (1988) 'Beyond fear appeals: negative and positive persuasive appeals to health and self-esteem', *Journal of Applied Social Psychology*, 18: 277–87.

Roszkowski, M.J. and Snelbecker, G.E. (1991) 'Effects of "framing" on measures of risk tolerance: financial planners are not immune', *Journal of Behavioral Economics*, 19: 237–46.

Rothman, A.J., Salovey, P., Antone, C., Keough, K. and Martin, C.D. (1993) 'The influence of message framing on intentions to perform health behaviors', *Journal of Experimental Social Psychology*, 29: 408–33.

Rowe, D. and Puto, C.P. (1987). 'Do consumers' reference points affect their buying decisions?', *Advances in Consumer Research*, 14: 182–7.

Schneider, S.L. (1992) 'Framing and conflict: aspiration level contingency, the status quo, and current theories of risky choice', *Journal of Experimental Psychology: Learning, Memory, and Cognition*, 18: 1040–57.

Shafir, E., Osherson, D.N. and Smith, E.E. (1993) 'The advantage model: a comparative theory of evaluation and choice under risk', *Organizational Behavior and Human Decision Processes*, 55: 325–78.

Simon, H.A. and Hayes, J.R. (1976) 'The understanding process: problem isomorphs', *Cognitive Psychology*, 8: 165–90.

Spears, R., Abraham, S.C.S., Abrams, D. and Sheeran, P. (1992) 'Framing in terms of "high-risk groups" versus "risky practices" and prognoses of HIV infection', *European Journal of Social Psychology*, 22: 195–201.

Steffen, V.J., Sternberg, L., Teegarden, L.A. and Shepherd, K. (1994) 'Practice and persuasive frame: effects on beliefs, intention, and performance of a cancer self-examination', *Journal of Applied Social Psychology*, 24: 897–925.

Svyantek, D.J., DeShon, R.P. and Siler, M.T. (1991) 'The illusion of certainty: a catastrophe model of decision framing', *Current Psychology Research and Reviews*, 10: 199–209.

Tversky, A. and Kahneman, D. (1981) 'The framing of decisions and the psychology of choice', *Science*, 211: 453–8.

Tversky, A. and Kahneman, D. (1992) 'Advances in prospect theory: cumulative representation of uncertainty', *Journal of Risk and Uncertainty*, 5: 297–323.

Tykocinski, O., Higgins, E.T. and Chaiken, S. (1994) 'Message framing, self-discrepancies, and yielding to persuasive messages: the motivational significance of psychological situations', *Personality and Social Psychology Bulletin*, 20: 107–15.

Urbany, J.E. and Dickson, P.R. (1990) 'Prospect theory and pricing decisions', *Journal of Behavioral Economics*, 19: 69–80.

van der Pligt, J. and van Schie, E. (1990) 'Frames of reference, judgement and preference', in W. Stroebe and M. Hewstone (eds) *European Review of Social Psychology, Vol. I*, New York: Wiley.

Wagenaar, W.A., Keren, G. and Lichtenstein, S. (1988) 'Islanders and hostages: deep and surface structures of decision problems', *Acta Psychologica*, 67: 175–89.

Wilson, D.K., Kaplan, R.M. and Schneiderman, L.J. (1987) 'Framing of decisions and selections of alternatives in health care', *Social Behaviour*, 2: 51–9.

Wilson, D.K., Wallston, K.A. and King, J.E. (1990) 'Effect of contract framing, motivation to quit, and self-efficacy on smoking reduction', *Journal of Applied Social Psychology*, 20: 531–47.

Chapter 9

Beyond gambles and lotteries

Naturalistic risky decisions

Oswald Huber

The main argument of the present chapter is that the lottery model does not fit naturalistic decision making *in general*. Instead, the decision process resembles a problem solving process, in which the decision maker engages in risk management by trying to eliminate or to reduce the risk of a negative event or its consequences by applying one or several *defusing* operators. The chapter first summarises two experiments and their results, which show that behaviour in naturalistic tasks differs distinctly from that expected according to traditional decision theory. An outline of *risk management* as a central subprocess in the decision process is then presented, with an outline of the role of uncertainty and the representation of naturalistic decision tasks. Finally, some aspects of research on naturalistic risky tasks are discussed.

Decision making under risk and uncertainty has been one of the central topics of research in decision theory since its beginnings. Most of the experiments on risky decision behaviour have used and are using simple lotteries (gambles or bets). However, despite the undisputed advantages of lotteries in an experiment (experimenter's control over outcomes, probabilities, etc.), there is an increasing concern about the relevance of these results for natural decisions and the applicability of the SEU model and others anchored in the lottery paradigm (such as Prospect theory, Kahneman and Tversky, 1979) in natural decision situations. There is a nagging suspicion that the essence of what naïve decision makers do is missed by such models. Discussions of different aspects of the problem can be found, for example, in Dörner and Wearing (1995), in some of the contributions in Klein *et al.* (1993), in Huber *et al.* (1997), Kühberger (1994), Larrick (1993), Smithson (1989) or Wagenaar (1988). Beach (1990) argues that in general high-powered and very precise models are not adequate to capture the manner in which natural decisions are made. Despite interesting new approaches like Image theory, the theory of Explanation-Based Decisions (Pennington and Hastie, 1993), or theories about the decision behaviour of expert decision makers (Klein *et al.*, 1993), at present no 'general' theory of risky decision making in naturalistic tasks is available.

In contrast to mainstream decision theory, risk research has always been interested mainly in natural situations. Risk research has shown clearly that many more aspects are relevant in the perception and evaluation of subjective risk than the utility of the negative outcome and subjective probability. Examples are: voluntariness of exposure, controllability of consequences, or discounting of time (see, for example, Yates, 1992). Even if risk research generally is not so interested in modelling individual decision behaviour, its results are highly relevant for our topic and cannot be ignored in the long run. Yates (1992) reports observations that decision makers try to form new options that reduce risks without sacrificing advantages.

Management research also contributes to the doubts about the relevance of the lottery paradigm (Bromiley and Curley, 1992). Shapira (1994) found that managers place more importance on monetary amounts and less on probabilities. Business executives make clear distinctions between risk taking and gambling, where gambling is something to avoid in business (March and Shapira, 1987).

In the 1950s, decision theory was interested also in gambles involving skill (for example, Cohen and Hansel, 1959). Skill is related to the concept of control. There are many everyday decisions which involve some combination of skill and chance. This topic was investigated in depth in research on achievement motivation, but in decision theory, interest in the chance vs. skill theme somehow died out.

Surprisingly, there seem to exist hardly any experiments comparing directly behaviour in choices among gambles and in naturalistic choice tasks. Huber and Kühberger (1996) found gambling tasks to differ systematically from naturalistic decision tasks, and suggested topics where the differences should be investigated in more detail, such as the cognitive representation of the decision situation, the components of the decision process, and the role of subjective probabilities. Huber (1995) varied the decision maker's perceived control in an alternative with ambiguous probabilities, and found ambiguity avoidance without control and ambiguity seeking with control.

Altogether, results from different sources suggest that research on risky decision behaviour should turn to naturalistic tasks, in order to avoid decision research becoming an area encapsulated in artificial tasks bearing no relevance to most daily life.

In this chapter, I concentrate on individual decisions of non-expert decision makers. First, I discuss some differences between the gambling or betting tasks used in standard experiments and naturalistic risky tasks. Then I introduce a new method of information presentation we use in our experiments, and the reason for adopting this method. Then, the designs of our two first experiments are presented, and the tasks used in these experiments are described. After a summary of the main results

I will discuss the following: an outline of risk management as a central subprocess in the decision process, the role of uncertainty, and the representation of the task.

I concentrate my discussion of the differences between the lottery tasks and naturalistic risky tasks on three aspects, which I consider as especially important in my context: the structuring of the task, the decision maker's background knowledge, and the topic of control.

(1) In a standard experiment, the experimenter structures the task for the decision maker: which alternatives are available, which events are relevant, which outcomes may occur. As research on the framing effect shows, the structure the experimenter imposes may influence the choice. In contrast, in a natural decision situation the decision maker usually has to develop her or his own structure, which is often a demanding task.

(2) In a standard gambling experiment, the decision maker's background knowledge is not relevant. Such experiments are usually designed so as to prevent the decision maker from gathering experience. For example, the chosen gambles are not played until the decision maker has made all decisions. In contrast, background knowledge plays an important role in naturalistic tasks, for example in finding out which alternatives exist, what consequences they have, or how the decision maker can avoid a negative outcome. The view of background knowledge as an undesirable extraneous variable ignores the fact that background knowledge is an important source of information generally in our thinking, reasoning, problem solving, and so on.

(3) In an experiment within the lottery paradigm, after the choice has been made, decision makers have no control whatsoever over the outcome. In many naturalistic situations, however, they have at least partial control, or believe they have control. For example, if I decide to travel into a region where an epidemic disease rages, then I can possibly interrupt the causal chain between the infection and the outbreak of that disease by a vaccination. In some situations, the decision maker can take precautions against negative consequences, for example by saving important computer files on a backup disk. The decision maker may also exert control by preparing a worst-case plan for what to do when the negative outcome occurs. I personally think that the neglect of the topic of control is the most serious deficiency of traditional risky decision theory.

The differences between gambles and bets and naturalistic tasks can be summarised by stating that naturalistic decision tasks are ill-structured problems in knowledge-rich domains, where causal relations and attributions and the decision maker's control beliefs are relevant.

The differences between lotteries and natural decision tasks lead to consequences on the theoretical level. In lotteries and theories based on the lottery paradigm two types of variables are central: subjective values (utilities) of outcomes and their subjective probabilities. In these respects, natural decision tasks may differ from gambles in three ways:

1 Variables relevant in gambling tasks may be less important in the subjective representation constructed for a naturalistic task. This is presumably the case for numerical probabilities of outcomes. Shapira (1994) found that managers place more importance on monetary amounts than on probabilities.
2 Variables not extant or relevant in gambling tasks may be important in the subjective representation of a naturalistic task, for example the topic of control beliefs, or the search for additional alternatives.
3 Variables may be relevant in lotteries as well as in naturalistic tasks, but may serve different purposes in the decision process. Here too, subjective probability is a possible candidate.

METHOD OF ACTIVE INFORMATION SEARCH

Experiments within the lottery paradigm differ from natural situations not only in the type of decision task, but also in how information is presented to the decision maker. In such experiments, complete presentation of information is the standard. Usually, all outcomes and probabilities are displayed simultaneously to the decision maker. An exception is the work of Payne *et al.* (1993) on accuracy and effort in decision processes.

The complete presentation of information (CPI) does not allow a generalisation to natural situations, because here we have to search actively for information we – not an experimenter – consider as relevant. If a subject uses a certain piece of information in an experiment with CPI, there is no guarantee that he or she would use that information also in a natural situation. A subject may utilise a specific item of information, for example because he or she believes it to be important as the experimenter (who is obviously an expert) takes the effort to present it, or simply because that piece of information is there. Amount and quality of information may shape the process, therefore the manner of information presentation may be crucial.

Consequently, research on naturalistic decision behaviour needs a procedure which does not force the use of a specific item of information on decision makers, but leaves it to them which information is inspected and which is not. In multidimensional decision theory, the problem has been solved in a satisfactory manner with the help of the alternative by dimensions matrix. There are several operationalisations of such a matrix (see Chapter 2 and Payne *et al.*, 1993) which enable an analysis of what information a subject has inspected (and what not) in which sequence. There is no comparable standardised method available for risky decision making. Engländer and Tyszka (1980) used a question-asking method in multiattribute choice, where the experimenter acted as an expert, whom the subject could ask for information. We adapted this method to our method of Active Information Search.

In the method of Active Information Search (AIS), the subject is first presented with a minimal description of the decision situation. Then he or she can ask the experimenter questions, in order to obtain more information. The subject can ask any question, and also repeat questions any time. The question is recorded, and the answer is presented printed or written on a small card. This style of answering the questions was adopted in order to eliminate effects of verbalising the answer by the experimenter, and to avoid non-verbal influences. Note that the *subject* asks the questions, not the experimenter.

The application of the AIS method necessitates the use of pilot studies for each decision task, for two reasons: (a) the minimal description has to be optimised, and (b) to find out as many as possible of the questions subjects ask. The latter is desirable for having an answer prepared, and also for having the answer cards ready. Answers to new questions have to be improvised by the experimenter during the experiment, therefore the probability of new questions should be small.

EXPERIMENTAL INVESTIGATION OF NATURALISTIC RISKY DECISIONS

In order to investigate decision behaviour in naturalistic risky tasks, our research group in Fribourg have run – up to now – two experiments. In the following I report only the most important aspects of these experiments and their main results. For details, refer to the cited papers.

The main research question in both experiments was to investigate decision behaviour in naturalistic risky tasks. A second was the investigation of the AIS method. In Experiment 1 we compared the AIS method with the 'standard' method of CPI. In Experiment 2 we developed *structured* versions of the AIS method, where the subject is presented with a list of questions and can select and present to the experimenter in sequence as many of them as wanted. We compared these structured AIS versions with the basic version as described above. I do not go into details here concerning the investigation of the AIS method and its variations.

Experiment 1

Subjects were thirty-two non-students of different age groups, professions and levels of education.

Subjects were run individually. After a warm-up decision task, the two tasks described below were presented in a random order. For one half of the subjects, information was presented according to the AIS method as described above. For the others in the condition with CPI a task description was presented which contained all the information of the prepared answer cards.

Post Office task

The subject acts as the new provisional manager of the post office in the village H. Next year, this manager's performance is to be evaluated, and based on that evaluation the superiors will decide whether the provisional manager becomes the permanent manager or not.

The post office has very cramped conditions, and has faced the following problem for several years: in November and December, it has to deal with many parcels. Conditions may become unbearable if the number of parcels to be handled becomes too large.

The village administration offers the manager now (in spring/summer) the opportunity to rent the local meeting hall for sFr 12,000 (about $10,000). The decision has to be made today, because there are other applicants. This hall would be ideal for the post office, because it is very close and there are no other possibilities to rent enough space nearby.

Whether it pays off to rent the hall depends on the number of parcels to be handled before Christmas. If the amount of parcels to be handled is high, then renting the hall is necessary, because otherwise the delivery of the parcels would be delayed, and complaints from customers would have to be expected. Furthermore, working conditions for the employees would become very bad. If, however, the number of parcels to be handled is low, then it would not be necessary to rent the hall. The sFr 12.000 would have been wasted. The probability that the number of parcels is high is 60 per cent.

The subject has to decide whether to rent the hall or not.

This decision task is a realistic one, which was used by the German Post Department in training its middle management. It was also applied in Huber and Kühberger (1996).

Machine task

The subject has to assume the role of the owner of a small factory which produces a kind of weatherproof credit card for ski lifts. The order books are so well filled that it is necessary to buy an additional high-capacity machine for production to meet the great demand.

After an initial screening of the relatively few offers, two machines remain on the shortlist. Both are approximately equal in price and overheads. There are differences in how prone the machines are to interruptions caused by breakdowns. Of course, such interruptions are very undesirable, because they disturb the production process and may cause a failure to meet deadlines.

Machine A is a well-established type based on traditional technology. Statistics of the Swiss Federal Institute of Technology (ETH Zürich) show that the probability of interruptions caused by machine breakdown is low (15 per cent).

Machine B is a new type. The probability of a breakdown is higher than that of Machine A (22 per cent). The probability of a machine breakdown is influenced by careful operation and regular maintenance.

This task has been used in Huber (1995).

We selected the two tasks, because they seem to be conceptually different. The Post Office task can be structured very well according to a lottery. There are two critical states of nature (the number of parcels is high or is low) which are exhaustive and mutually exclusive, and determine the outcomes. The Machine task can also be mapped into a lottery, but this is not as straightforward as in the Post Office task. On the other hand, it can easily be structured as a multiattribute choice task, with the likelihood of a breakdown as one attribute, and the probabilities as aspects of this attribute, with each machine having one aspect.

Experiment 2

Sixty non-students of different ages, professions and levels of education were run individually. They started with the Post Office task as a warm-up task. Then the two main tasks described below were presented in a random order. Subjects were assigned randomly to the basic version or one of the structured AIS versions. The whole experiment lasted approximately 60 minutes.

Ticks task

The subject acts as the director of a centre for allergic children. The children are accommodated in a building which is owned by a Swiss tycoon. Recently, this man has died, and the heirs are in disagreement about how to divide the estate. If they do not reach an agreement, then the building has to be sold in order to enable a division. In this case, the centre has to move out, and the director has to find another location for the centre for allergic children which meets the requirements for treating allergies.

Now, the foundation *Children for the Future* offers to donate a home to the centre. It is a large house in the forest. All the necessary adaptations for children and the provision of special facilities would be financed by the foundation. The problem is that the forester's house stands in a wood which is contaminated with a specific kind of tick. These ticks can cause meningitis, with grave consequences for health.

The subject is informed that he or she can accept the donation with its associated risk or can choose to decline the donation and stay in the present building with the risk of having to search a new place for the centre in the near future.

Precision mechanics task

In this task, the subject plays the role of the owner of a small factory specialising in precision mechanics. Apart from the administrative staff, the firm employs eleven precision mechanics. In the last two years orders have been shrinking. Up to now all the precision mechanics could be retained. The situation, however, is now so bad that the owner has to let some of them go.

Now the firm has been offered a new order, which could change the whole situation. An electronic firm wants to order parts for micromachines. This order would keep the firm working at capacity for one and a half years. The problem is that the firm would have to buy a new machine for the production of these micromachine parts. This would mean that the firm would have to use all its financial reserves and, in addition, would have to take out a substantial loan. The question is whether, after the 1½ years of guaranteed work, there will be enough additional orders to pay back the loan. If not, the firm would have to dismiss even more of the precision mechanics than it is currently envisaging.

The subject has to decide whether he or she will accept the order of the electronic firm in spite of the uncertainty of getting enough orders afterwards, or whether he or she will decline the order and dismiss some of the precision mechanics now.

Both tasks can be structured according to a lottery. In the Ticks tasks both alternatives have uncertain consequences, in the Precision mechanics task one of the alternatives has a sure consequence (fire some of the precision mechanics now).

Summary of main results

The questions asked by the subjects provide the data for further analyses. Each question was assigned to one of the following codes:

1 *Situation*: All questions demanding (background) information about the decision situation, for example, 'What can I find out about the employees of the firm?'
2 *Consequences*: Questions about the consequences of choosing a specific alternative, for example, 'What are the disadvantages of the forester's house?' Questions about certain and uncertain consequences, respectively, were distinguished.

3 *New alternatives*: Questions aiming at options not presented by the experimenter, for example, 'Are there other alternatives?', 'Could I rent some big containers?'
4 *Probability*: Questions interested in the probability of an event or the prognoses of an event, for example, 'Which machine has a higher breakdown probability?', 'How large is the risk of getting bitten by a tick?'
5 *Control*: Questions dealing with the decision maker's control over the external event or over negative consequences, for example, 'Can I protect the children from getting the disease?'
6 *Worst-case plans*: Questions demanding information about what can be done in case a negative event occurs, for example, 'If it comes to the worst, I could always sublet the hall to clubs or firms who want to make a Christmas celebration or dinner or a New Year's party, couldn't I?'

In this chapter, I concentrate on the question types Probability, New Alternatives, Control and Worst-case plans. The dependent variable is the mean percentage of subjects who asked at least one question in the respective category. The mean percentages obtained with the basic AIS version are summarised in Table 9.1.

An average of less than half of the subjects asked at least one question about probability, the maximum being 40 per cent in the Ticks task, the minimum 6 per cent in the Post task. This is quite different from what we would have expected according to traditional decision theory. Probability-questions were especially rare in the Post and the Precision mechanics tasks.

Questions concerning New alternatives, Control and Worst-case plans are indicators of cognitive processes involving risk management. The search for new alternatives, testing for control and the development of Worst-case plans are cognitive operators which enable the decision maker to defuse the risk of a negative event or its consequences.

Table 9.1 Mean percentage of subjects with at least one question in the respective category[1]

	Tasks			
Question type	*Post*	*Machine*	*Ticks*	*Precision mechanics*
n =	16	16	20	20
Probability	6	38	40	10
New alternative	44	6	55	50
Control	6	25	60	0
Worst-case plan	0	0	10	0

Note: 1 Data from Experiment 1 and 2 combined, basic AIS version only

Nearly all subjects attempted risk management and applied one or more defusing operators. On average, about half of the subjects tried to find a new alternative. Control was the defusing operator used most often in the Ticks task, whereas in the Precision mechanics task the operator New alternative was more relevant. Also Worst-case plans were asked, but played a minor role compared with New alternative and Control. Worst-case plans were much more frequent in the structured versions of AIS.

Most people asked Probability-questions in combination with at least one of the defusing operators (Control, Worst-case plans and New alternative). We interpret this to mean that many subjects use the probability information to evaluate whether it is necessary or not to apply a defusing operator. However, a high proportion of subjects used the defusing operators without additional information about probability. Altogether, these results also show that defusing operators are more relevant than probabilities in the decision process.

In Experiment 2, we analysed also the differences between the chosen and the not chosen alternative. These results fit well into the general picture. More information in total is processed for the chosen alternative, which is congruent with well-established results in multiattribute decision theory (for example, Payne *et al.*, 1993). However, the increase in the processed information is not distributed uniformly among question types. Many more Control and Worst-case plan operators were applied with the chosen alternative than with the not chosen one. This indicates that these operators served to defuse the negative consequences of the alternative with the desirable outcomes. Negative aspects of the not chosen alternative were, however, well noted. There is no difference in Consequences uncertain and Probability-questions between the two alternatives.

AN OUTLINE OF THE SUBPROCESS *RISK MANAGEMENT*

We assume that in the decision process the decision maker constructs a mental representation of the situation and the alternatives (see next section). The subprocess *risk management* is activated if there is uncertainty about which outcome will result from the choice of a promising alternative. The decision maker attempts to solve the problem by employing risk management. That is, he or she attempts to defuse the danger of the situation by applying one or more *defusing operators*. This subprocess can be incorporated into general models of decision making. For reasons of space, I do not go into details here.

The first step in the subprocess is uncertainty *detection*. A quite coarse evaluation of uncertainty is adequate (see next section). It is sufficient to know whether the occurrence of a negative outcome is in fact possible.

If this is the case, then *risk management* is activated. As outlined above, the defusing operators used in active risk management observed in our experiments are: Control (a test of whether the danger of a negative outcome can be reduced by exerting control over relevant variables), New alternative (searching for a new alternative, which keeps the positive aspects but avoids the negative outcomes), and Worst-case plans (searching for an action or sequence of actions which would be able to neutralise negative outcomes when they are about to occur). Another defusing operator is Precautions: taking precautions against negative consequences, for example by buying insurance. This operator occurred only rarely in our experiments, but is well known in everyday risky decision making. Figure 9.1 depicts these general ideas.

While the other defusing operators attempt risk management within the framework of a promising alternative, New alternative is risk management by broadening the problem space on the level of the formation of alternatives.

Our assumptions about the function of the defusing operators in the decision process are confirmed by the results concerning chosen and not chosen alternatives. Whereas the negative aspects of chosen and not chosen alternatives are noted equally well, defusing operators were applied much more often with the chosen alternative.

The subprocess *risk management* is triggered off by uncertainty about the outcomes, but the role of the subjective probability of the negative outcome is very different from its role in the lottery paradigm. Theories rooted in the SEU tradition usually postulate some function concatenating utilities and subjective probabilities into a kind of overall value for the alternative, which then determines the choice. Nothing of the kind is assumed in our model. The goal of *risk management* is to eliminate risk or at least to reduce it below some threshold of relevance.

Another type of uncertainty may be relevant in connection with defusing operators, namely uncertainty as to whether the application of a specific defusing operator produces the intended result (see below).

The application of a specific type of defusing operator is probably at least in part governed by background knowledge. Background knowledge about a specific topic may suggest a test of control. For example, in the domain of infectious diseases probably many lay persons come up with the idea that there may exist a vaccine. On the other hand, if the relevant condition in a decision situation is the weather in my country in April, my background knowledge would screen out in advance the possibility of control.

Furthermore, some kind of cost–benefit considerations are probably relevant in accepting or not a specific defusion operator. If the costs of preventing a negative event are too high, the decision maker may search for other defusing possibilities.

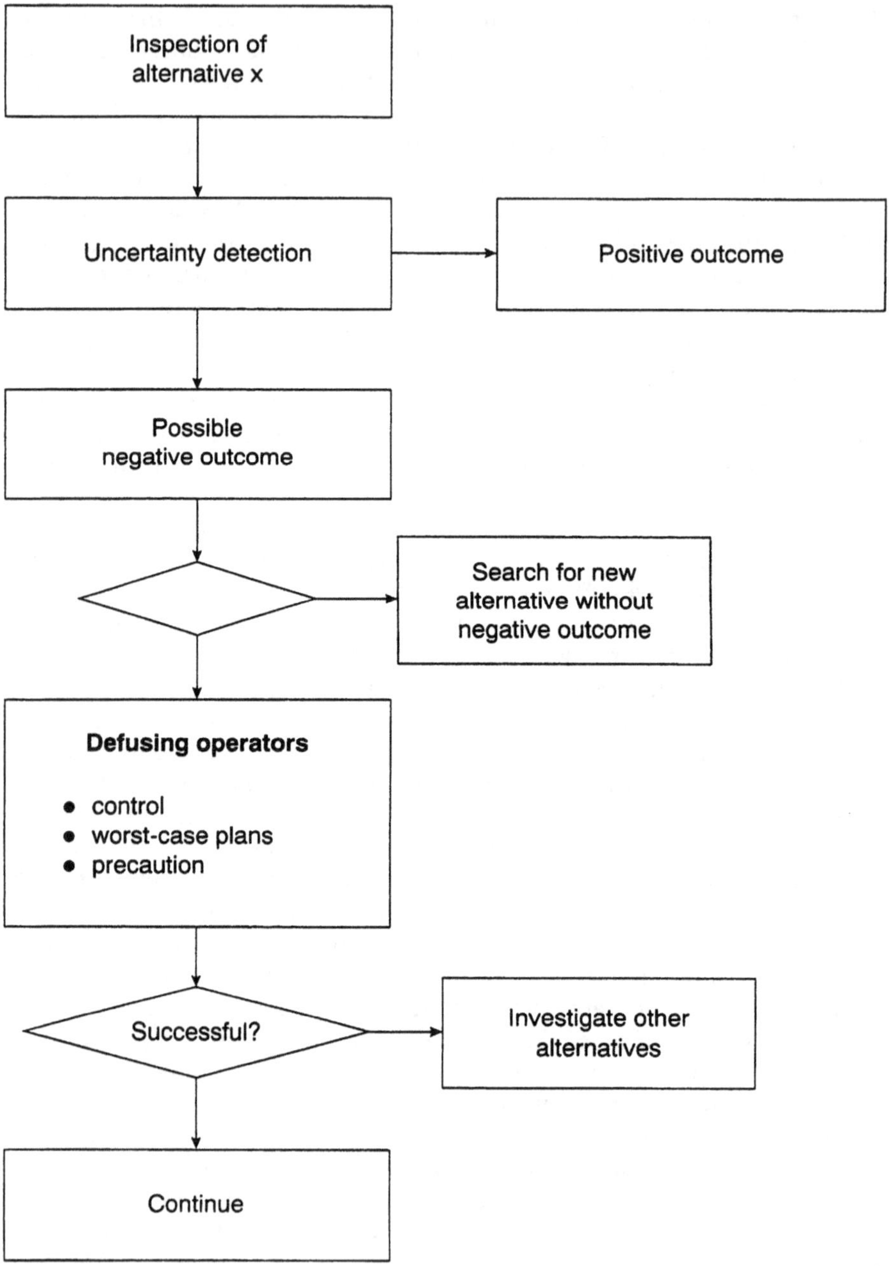

Figure 9.1 Flow chart of risk management

THE ROLE OF PERCEIVED UNCERTAINTY

Perceived uncertainty may be relevant in a risky decision process in several ways. Here I concentrate on two aspects only: uncertainty about events and outcomes, and about the effect of a defusing operator.

Uncertainty about events and outcomes

This is the manner in which uncertainty is usually incorporated in risky decision theory. I think that such a concept of perceived uncertainty is necessary in order for the decision maker to realise that, for example, some negative outcome could happen. Precise subjective probability representations are presumably relevant only in specific decision tasks, like lotteries or situations with natural frequencies (e.g., sporting events). In most natural situations vague or even ordinal probability information is the best we can get. I presume that in most such situations it is sufficient for the decision maker to know that an event *may* happen. This means that three coarse levels of uncertainty could be enough: practically certain, possible, practically impossible. In our experiments, only two of our seventy-six subjects with the AIS method were interested actively in precise (numerical) probability. Moreover, one should bear in mind that most of the subjects using information about probability also employed defusing operators.

In Experiment 1 (Huber *et al.*, 1997) we also tested the possibility that decision makers get information about probabilities independent of asking questions, for example by inferring it from available information and background knowledge. If this were the case, those decision makers *not* asking for probabilities should have more probability items in the verbal protocol; in other words, there should be a negative correlation. The correlation, however, turned out to be significantly positive. There-fore, this explanation can be ruled out as a general one.

Uncertainty about the effect of a defusing operator

The effect of a certain control measure may be uncertain; for example, whether the decision maker really can prevent the negative event, or whether the attempted Worst-case plan really works. For example, a vaccination may be ineffective in 20 per cent of the cases. In such situations, the decision maker has to decide whether the confidence that the defusing operator will work effectively is sufficiently high. The threshold for sufficiency is probably affected by several aspects. One is the desirability of outcomes. If an outcome is very desirable, the decision maker may be tempted to lower the threshold, thus being satisfied with a lower confidence. Furthermore, characteristics of the decision situation may be relevant, for example time pressure, the importance of the decision, or the duration of the decision process so far.

THE REPRESENTATION OF THE DECISION TASK

In a naturalistic decision situation, how the decision maker cognitively represents the task becomes a fundamental question. Our results lead us to conclude that the lottery paradigm is not even an approximately adequate representation for risky decision situations in general.

The best assumption at the moment seems to be that the subject represents the situation by a (complex) system, in which causal relations may exist between external events or actors and specific states or consequences. Especially important in this representation are causal relations involving acts of the decision maker her- or himself, thus allowing (some) control over the system. In our experiments, we found people attempted to exert control in three ways: (1) by controlling the occurrence of the negative event, for example, by killing all the ticks with a chemical; (2) by interrupting the causal chain between the event and the negative consequence (e.g., vaccination); (3) by designing a Worst-case plan, which is initiated when the negative event is about to happen. Uncertainty about a causal link may be part of the representation.

Figure 9.2 depicts the representation of an alternative a_i according to these ideas. Only one alternative branch of a basic decision tree is expanded. Note that this expansion contains only the most simple *general* structure for representing a naturalistic alternative. For a specific alternative and a specific event, not all the control and worst-case actions may be realised. For example, if event e_{jl} is a particular economic situation in Australia five years from now, the decision maker's action space may not contain a control action for this event. A standard gamble in this general framework is a special case with no available control or worst-case actions, where the causal structure between event e_{jl} and outcome o_{jl} is deterministic. The representation of Figure 9.2 depicts the situation only at the level of the alternative. The search for a New alternative requires an expansion of this conception.

It might be useful for a theoretical analysis to represent the decision process at least in some phases as a problem solving process, with a state having positive but not negative outcomes as the goal. The decision maker would then search whether this goal state can be reached (with the help of defusing operators) from an alternative. This search would presumably start with the presented alternative(s), but if a connection to the goal state cannot be found easily, new alternatives would be searched for or invented. In the context of subjective representation, it might be useful to combine decision theoretical ideas with those of theories of complex problem solving (e.g., Frensch and Funke, 1995) and of decision scenarios (Biel and Montgomery, 1989).

The construction of a representation is an integral part of the decision process. This construction process is not just something like an

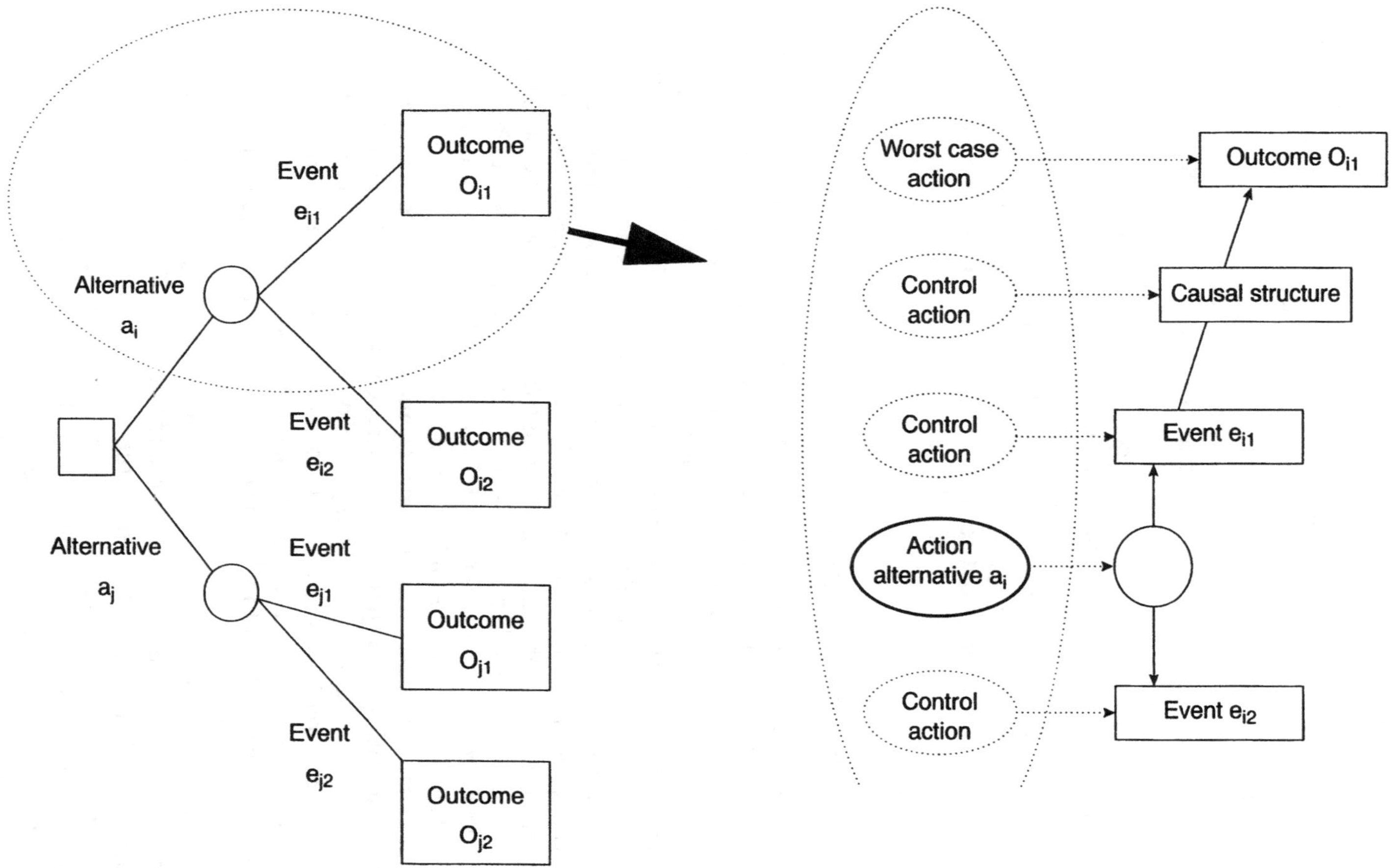

Figure 9.2 Representation of a naturalistic alternative

editing-phase (see, for example, Prospect theory, Kahnemann and Tversky, 1979), where a given basic representation of the task is revised by the decision maker, and then – in a second phase – the components are evaluated.

In a naturalistic task, usually the decision maker her- or himself has to create the basic representation of the situation in which the decision has to take place, and of the alternatives and their consequences. The construction process cannot be considered as a clear-cut phase. It rather goes hand in hand with evaluation processes, tests of defusing operators, etc. For example, if an alternative has very desirable consequences, it is worth while to try to defuse negative aspects, but the construction of the representation of an alternative will probably be terminated when it turns out to have real bad outcomes. Therefore, the subjective representation cannot be expected to remain stable during the decision process.

CONCLUDING REMARKS

Despite the observed differences among the four tasks in our experiments, the general picture emerging about the decision process is similar. The lottery model cannot be considered as a general model for naturalistic decisions as well. It ignores completely the topic of risk management and overemphasises the role of relatively fine-grained subjective probabilities. Its basic assumption, that decision makers somehow concatenate utilities and subjective probabilities into an overall value which determines the choice, seems not to be adequate. Consequently, biases in probability judgement are probably not very relevant for most naturalistic decisions, in particular if one takes into account that extremely few subjects are interested in *precise* probability information. The decision process in naturalistic tasks rather resembles a problem solving process, in which the decision maker engages in risk management by trying to eliminate or reduce the risk of a negative event or its consequences by applying one or several defusing operators. Risky decision theory should therefore focus attention also on biases in causal judgements and control estimations. It is a task for further research to find out which findings from gambles and bets can be generalised to what types of naturalistic decisions, and under what circumstances.

The observed differences between the four tasks also constitute a strong argument for investigating a broad range of different tasks in future experiments. This should help us in the identification of possible types of risky tasks and in the development of a formal language to describe such tasks. I do not exclude the possibility that there are naturalistic tasks which are adequately represented by a lottery (for example, stock exchange decisions, some types of medical decisions).

Our results provide also some hints for the construction of decision aids for naturalistic risky tasks. Such a decision aid should in the first place help the decision maker to construct a representation of the situation, which includes the causal structure. Therefore a standard decision tree is not sufficient. Probably one of the computer programs enabling a graphical representation of a system and defining the relations among the components would be most adequate. Providing a structure is not sufficient, however. Huber and Kühberger (1996) found in their experiment that subjects who drew a decision tree introduced less of their background knowledge and were more prone to biasing than those subjects who did not. Therefore, aiding the construction of a representation has to be accompanied, for example, by tools to avoid biasing evaluations as well as the result of the application of a defusing operator. I want to emphasise that the application of defusion operators must be considered as rational behaviour. It would be rather irrational *not* to test possibilities of controlling negative events, for example, if there exists a chance to be able to do so. However, in some circumstances decision makers may be prone to biasing the result of the application of a defusing operator. For example, they might overestimate their own control.

I want to close this chapter by making a plea for decision theory to take on the challenge presented by decision tasks outside the lottery paradigm. Clearly, there exist decision situations where decision makers engage actively in risk management (for example, by searching for control) instead of just evaluating values and probabilities. In my opinion, such tasks are more frequent in daily life than lottery tasks. However, I do nevertheless assume that there also exist tasks which are essentially lotteries, for example a patient's choice between two types of treatment. I furthermore believe that there are natural tasks where decision makers base their choice on probabilities. Thus, one task for decision theory seems to be to work out a classification of decision tasks. Another is to investigate and to compare decision behaviour in different types of tasks. Opening up decision theory to non-lottery tasks would force us to broaden our theoretical orientation, and offers a rich variety of new research questions.

ACKNOWLEDGEMENTS

The experiments reported in this chapter were financed by a grant from the *Schweizerischer Nationalfonds zur Förderung der Wissenschaft, Project* No. 11–37315.93. Project collaborators were: Claudia Beutter, Odilo W. Huber, Jorge Montoya and Roman Wider.

I want to thank Ray Crozier, Rob Ranyard, Alex Wearing and an anonymous reviewer for their helpful comments.

REFERENCES

Beach, L.R. (1990) *Image Theory: Decision Making in Personal and Organizational Contexts*, Chichester: Wiley.

Biel, A. and Montgomery, H. (1989) 'Scenario analysis and energy politics: the discourse of causal structures in decision making', in H. Montgomery and O. Svenson (eds) (1989) *Process and Structure in Human Decision Making*, Chichester: Wiley, 243–60.

Bromiley, P. and Curley, S.P. (1992) 'Individual differences in risk taking', in F. Yates (ed.) *Risk-Taking Behaviour*, New York: Wiley, 87–132.

Cohen, J. and Hansel, C.E.M. (1959) 'Preference for different combinations of chance and skill in gambling', *Nature*, 183: 841–42.

Dörner, D. and Wearing, A.J. (1995) 'Complex problem solving: towards a (computer simulated) theory', in P.A. Frensch and J. Funke (eds) *Complex Problem Solving: The European Perspective*, Hillsdale, N.J.: Erlbaum, 65–99.

Engländer, T. and Tyszka, T. (1980) 'Information seeking strategies in an open decision situation', *Acta Psychologica*, 56: 113–23.

Frensch, P.A. and Funke, J. (eds) (1995) *Complex Problem Solving: The European Perspective*, Hillsdale, NJ: Erlbaum.

Huber, O. (1995) 'Ambiguity and perceived control', *Swiss Journal of Psychology*, 54: 200–10.

Huber, O., Beutter, C., Montoya, J. and Huber, O.W. (1996) 'Risk management or probability based decisions in naturalistic tasks?', Paper submitted for publication.

Huber, O. and Kühberger, A. (1996) 'Decision processes and decision trees in gambles and more natural decision tasks', *Journal of Psychology*, 130: 229–36.

Huber, O., Wider, R. and Huber, O.W. (1997) 'Active information search and complete information presentation in naturalistic risky decision tasks', *Acta Psychologica,* 95: 15–29.

Kahneman, D. and Tversky, A. (1979) 'Prospect theory: an analysis of decision under risk', *Econometrica*, 47: 263–91.

Klein, G.A., Orasanu, J., Calderwood, R. and Zsambok, C.E. (eds) (1993) *Decision Making in Action: Models and Methods*, Norwood, NJ: Ablex.

Kühberger, A. (1994) 'Risiko und Unsicherheit: zum Nutzen des Subjective Expected Utility-Modells' [Risk and uncertainty: about the utility of the Subjective Expected Utility model], *Psychologische Rundschau*, 45: 3–23.

Larrick, R.P. (1993) 'Motivational factors in decision theories: the role of self-protection', *Psychological Bulletin*, 113: 440–50.

March, J.G. and Shapira, Z. (1987) 'Managerial perspectives on risk and risk taking', *Management Science*, 33: 1404–18.

Payne, J.W., Bettman, J.R. and Johnson, E.J. (1993) *The Adaptive Decision Maker*, Cambridge: Cambridge University Press.

Pennington, N. and Hastie, R. (1993) 'Reasoning in explanation-based decision making', *Cognition*, 49: 123–63.

Shapira, Z. (1994) *Managerial Risk Taking*, New York: Russell Sage.

Smithson, M. (1989) *Ignorance and Uncertainty: Emerging Paradigms*, Berlin: Springer.

Tversky, A. and Kahneman, D. (1992) 'Advances in prospect theory: cumulative representation of uncertainty', *Journal of Risk and Uncertainty*, 5: 297–323.

Wagenaar, W.A. (1988) *Paradoxes of Gambling Behavior*, Hillsdale, NJ: Erlbaum.

Yates, J.F. (ed.) (1992) *Risk-Taking Behavior*, New York: Wiley.

Part IV

The time dimension

Introduction to Part IV

Time is an ever present and prominent dimension in all human decision making. Decisions are oriented towards future time, they take time to make, their consequences develop over time, and they are sometimes thought about for a long time afterwards. This section includes chapters about human decision making, all of which emphasise the time dimension.

Chapter 10 by Gärling, Karlsson, Romanus and Selart presents research in which the past time perspective is highlighted. They summarise research on the impact of information about earlier decisions and their outcomes on subsequent decisions. In their review, the authors cover research including multistage decision making and decisions in a sequence of escalation of a failing course of action (also called entrapment). Effects of prior decisions and outcomes on later decisions include sunk cost effects and the status quo phenomenon. Empirical results, such as the finding that prior outcomes tend to affect evaluations of losses rather than gains in a subsequent decision, known as the loss sensitivity principle, are related to different theoretical explanations in the second part of the chapter.

In many professional and personal situations time is a scarce resource. This explains why so many decisions are made under time pressure. Maule and Edland focus in Chapter 11 on the time it takes to make a decision and how lack of time may affect the decision process. The effects of time pressure on decision making as compared with decisions made under no time pressure imply that, in most cases, but not in all, the quality of the decisions deteriorates under time pressure. This chapter also looks at changes in cognitive strategy under time pressure, focusing on adaptive changes in micro-strategy (acceleration of process, filtration and omission) and macro-strategy (changes in the balance of the goals for the decision process, changes from compensatory to non-compensatory rules, changes in cost–benefit evaluations of effort and accuracy, etc.). Finally, the Variable State Activation Theory broadens the perspective and integrates the field.

Kerstholt and Raaijmakers (Chapter 12) analyse a series of sequential decisions in a dynamic environment developing over time. This approach moves the research focus closer to many real-life decision making situations in which a sequence of decisions is needed to navigate in interaction with a continuously changing environment. Dynamic tasks change over time, require several interdependent decisions and provide feedback from these decisions. The authors present the main research findings in this area including timing of decisions, strategy selection, perception of feedback, and information selection over time. The results indicate, for example, that people typically rely on the present state and are less skilled in taking rate of change into account in dynamic decision making, that strategies seem to be more judgement-oriented when a more action-oriented approach would be more effective, and that delayed feedback is particularly harmful to optimal decision making. The chapter points out that dynamic situations are difficult to investigate because of the lack of control resulting from the great number of different trajectories that subjects may activate through the decision space. The recommendation is to design simpler task environments than those utilised in research today.

Chapter 13 by Svenson and Hill provides an overview of previous empirical research related to Differentiation and Consolidation Theory. This theory was briefly presented in Chapter 3. In an attempt to extract information about decisions in interaction with a dynamic environment, Svenson and Hill measured the attractiveness of decision alternatives in a real-life situation at different points in time. The authors followed a career decision over five months, and measured the attractiveness on different attributes (characterising the different career alternatives and selected by the subjects themselves), both before the decision was made and after it had been made but not yet implemented. The results illustrate how a value conflict, in which the chosen alternative is worse than its closest competitor on an important attribute, is solved by means of a value reversal changing a prior disadvantage into an advantage after the decision has been made.

In Chapter 14, Zakay focuses on confidence, that is, the feeling that what one is doing or has done is or was correct. Feelings of confidence are important for current decisions and behaviour and for how past decisions and behaviour are evaluated. The author points out that inappropriate feelings of confidence may lead to suboptimal behaviour, as, for example, in the case of the decision maker who is too confident in his or her preliminary choice and ignores information which would have changed that decision. The author covers different areas in which inappropriate confidence has been demonstrated, including eyewitness testimony, post-decision confidence, forecasting and overconfidence in different knowledge domains. Different theoretical explanations for the empirical findings are offered in the chapter. Finally, Zakay presents an account of an empirical study of expert judgements, the results of which imply, for example, that the faster an answer is retrieved, the more confident is the judge.

Chapter 10

Influences of the past on choices of the future

Tommy Gärling, Niklas Karlsson, Joakim Romanus and Marcus Selart

A ubiquitous characteristic of decision making is its future orientation: choices are made of courses of action with consequences in the future. This future orientation may explain the relative neglect in previous research of influences of the past.

There are several types of influences of the past (Elster and Loewenstein, 1992). One is learning from the past. For instance, decision strategies are learnt, and so, to varying degrees, are the basic information-processing skills entailed by decision strategies (Payne *et al.* 1993). It may be true that the quality of decisions is not always improved by learning (Camerer and Johnson, 1991). Nevertheless, there is little reason to question its important role.

Learning is, however, not the focus of this chapter. Its concern is both more general and more specific. We ask what the influences of the memory of outcomes of past decisions are on decisions made in the present. If such memories are mentally related to the conditions under which the decisions were made (e.g., the use of decision strategy), then they constitute a potential source of learning (Hogarth, 1981). However, for experienced decision makers there may be no or little transfer to subsequent decision making. Yet, as we shall see, they are influenced by the outcomes of past decisions.

We consider memory of prior outcomes to be a prerequisite for the kind of influences of the past which we will discuss in the following. As illustrated in Figure 10.1, if an outcome (O_1) of a prior decision (D_1) is remembered, it may change the evaluation of the set of outcomes ($\{O_2\}$) of a decision (D_2) to be made at the present time (t_0). Somewhat loosely, we call such a change *integration*. More specific definitions will be given below.

Although we primarily confine ourselves to integration across time, the concept of integration applies more generally (Thaler, 1980, 1985; Thaler and Johnson, 1990). For instance, in the Jacket and Calculator problem (Ranyard and Abdel-Nabi, 1993; Tversky and Kahneman, 1981), where subjects choose between buying a jacket and a calculator in a nearby store

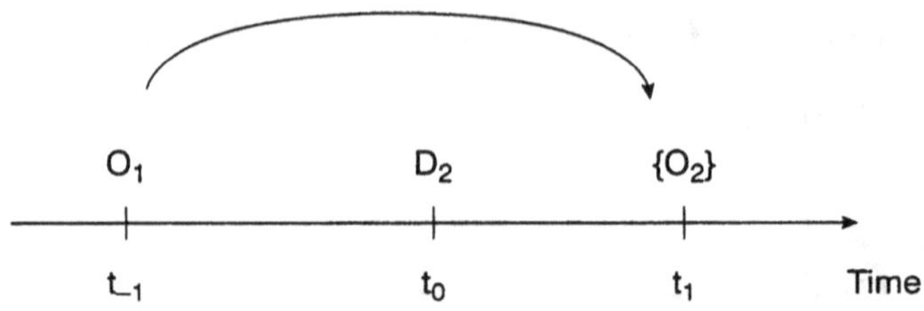

Figure 10.1 Possible influences of a prior outcome on a current decision

or at a discount rate in a more distant store, the issue is whether the outcomes of two simultaneous choices (of buying the jacket and the calculator) are integrated or segregated.

According to our analysis, remembering prior outcomes is a necessary but not sufficient condition for integration. A primary aim of this chapter is therefore to delimit what we believe are sufficient conditions. In the next section we review several known phenomena in which influences of the past seem to play an important role. We label them phenomena of integration of outcomes across time. Then, in the following section, we examine the explanations which have been offered for the different integration phenomena. In a concluding part we attempt to integrate the different explanations in a process model.

PHENOMENA OF INTEGRATION OF OUTCOMES ACROSS TIME

There are several phenomena with different names which seem to have in common that integration of outcomes takes place across time. The aim of this section is briefly to review these phenomena which include multistage betting, impacts of prior outcomes, sunk cost effects, and escalation.

Review of previous research

Multistage betting

Everyday examples of multistage betting include playing a game of poker, betting at the race track, or managing a stock portfolio. A new bet is usually made after outcomes of previous bets are known. Research examples include performance in the multistage betting game where subjects choose the amount to stake in a series of bets (Funk *et al.*, 1979; Huber, 1990, 1994). The outcome of each trial is added to or deducted from the subjects' capital. The unit of analysis is the betting strategy rather than single bets. An optimal strategy is to invest a constant proportion of the current capital (Rapoport and Jones, 1970). However, betting is affected empirically by previous wins and losses, by the size of the capital, and by the probability of winning (Huber, 1990). Perceived control is still another factor which Huber *et al.* (1990) demonstrated to be of importance.

Effects of prior outcomes

Although interesting results have emerged from studies of multistage betting (see also Brehmer (1992), for a review of the related research on dynamic decision making), it has proved difficult to investigate integration of outcomes across time. We therefore turn to studies in which subjects have encountered (or, rather, have been asked to imagine that they have encountered) only a single prior outcome when they are facing a new choice. In such a paradigm there needs to be little concern that subjects do not remember the prior outcome. Cognitive limitations may still play a role since integration also requires transformations of the information. An illustration is provided by the following empirical examples from Kahneman and Tversky (1979: 273):

> (Example 1) In addition to whatever you own, you have been given 1,000. You are now asked to choose between (A) a 50 per cent chance of winning 1,000 or nothing, and (B) winning 500 for sure;
>
> (Example 2) In addition to whatever you own, you have been given 2,000. You are now asked to choose between (A) a 50 per cent chance of losing 1,000 or nothing, and (B) losing 500 for sure.

A majority of subjects made different choices (B and A, respectively), despite the fact that the options in both cases are a 50 per cent chance of winning 2,000 or 1,000 versus winning 1,500 for sure when the amounts which were given in advance (the prior outcomes) are added to the outcomes of the current choice. It is unlikely, then, that subjects added the prior outcomes to the current outcomes. This form of integration of the prior outcomes was thus not demonstrated.

Laughhunn and Payne (1984) note that a decision frequently involves two or more sequential risky choices at different points in time. This applies to decision making in business organisations as well as to personal decision making. At each stage of the decision making process following the first, the decision maker (DM) may have observed outcomes of prior choices. In an experiment, managers were asked to make fictitious decisions concerning risky investments with very high stakes. There were three different conditions: for identical choice problems subjects were told that they had experienced a gain, a loss, or no prior outcome. In some choice problems the options were to continue or discontinue investments, in others to decide how to dispose of an asset. Subjects were also presented with similar problems referring to personal financial decisions with lower stakes. Indicating an effect of prior outcome, substantial percentages of choices were changed when subjects were told that they had experienced a prior gain or loss as compared to when there was no prior outcome. This tendency was stronger for personal than for corporate choices. In the latter cases, the tendency was even stronger for prior losses than for prior gains. The impact of prior losses was stronger for continuing/discontinuing than for disposal decisions. With the aim of illuminating how prior outcomes are integrated, whether subjects changed from risk seeking to risk aversion or the reverse was assessed. Unfortunately, in this respect no definite conclusion was reached. Still, in contrast to the results reported in Kahneman and Tversky (1979) (see the examples given above), an impact of a prior outcome was quite lucidly demonstrated. An important reason why different results were observed may be that the choice problems were embedded in real-life scenarios, making the historical contexts salient.

A series of similar experiments was performed more recently by Thaler and Johnson (1990) using as subjects master's degree students in business administration and psychology undergraduate students. The choice problems were very similar in content and structure to those described above, taken from Kahneman and Tversky (1979). As in the Laughhunn and Payne (1984) study, effects of prior outcomes were demonstrated, in this case irrespective of whether subjects gambled for real or hypothetical money. In the scenarios presented to subjects, a prior outcome was described as 'You have just won X' instead of 'In addition to whatever you own, you have been given X' in Kahneman and Tversky (1979). By referring to a betting sequence, the former wording may emphasise that subjects need to keep track of gains and losses. This change may account for the differences in results.

Although none of several possible accounts of how prior outcomes are integrated received ample support, the results obtained by Thaler and Johnson (1990) unequivocally showed that prior gains led to risk seeking whereas prior losses led to risk aversion. The former effect was referred to in gambler jargon as 'playing with the house money'. Thaler and Johnson also observed a 'break-even' effect: if subjects could win an amount which exactly covered a prior loss, they were more likely to gamble than they were otherwise after such a loss or no loss.

Another phenomenon which appears to involve an effect of a prior outcome is the status-quo bias (Samuelson and Zeckhausen, 1988). When the options are to choose or replace a previously chosen option (status quo), subjects tend to choose the status quo. A bias is demonstrated if the chosen option is preferred to another option when it is the status quo but not otherwise.

Whether a previously chosen option being compared to one or several new options is equivalent to a choice between a prior gain and expected future gains or losses was recently investigated by Karlsson *et al.* (1996).[1] Consistent with the status-quo bias, subjects would prefer a prior gain to gambles with the same expected values. However, the results did not show that, not even when several manipulations were undertaken to increase the salience and value of the prior gain. In keeping with the results of Thaler and Johnson (1990) and those of several other experiments (Gärling and Romanus, 1996; Gärling *et al.*, 1994; Romanus *et al.*, 1996a, 1996b), a prior gain instead led to increased risk seeking or likelihood to gamble. In a similar vein, the validity of the status quo bias has more recently been questioned (Ritov and Baron, 1992; Schweitzer, 1994). Although evidence suggests that status quo increases in value (Kahneman *et al.*, 1990), the status-quo bias may reflect a preference for inaction or inertia. The bias may thus be consistent with the impact of a prior outcome when the latter entails a choice to continue or discontinue a course of action.

Sunk cost effects

Situations exist when a DM chooses between continuing or discontinuing an endeavour in which investments of money, effort, or time (sunk costs) have been made. It is irrational to base a choice on anything else but the consequences of the current choice (Baron, 1994; Dawes, 1988). A sunk cost affects all these outcomes in the same way and should therefore be ignored.

Arkes and Blumer (1985) demonstrated sunk cost effects in a series of studies. For instance, in one of several questionnaire experiments subjects imagined that they had purchased two weekend ski trips but were unable to make both. Subjects then chose to cancel the less expensive although they were told that they would like it better. A field experiment was also conducted in which half of the subjects were offered a discount on a subscription to a series of theatre plays whereas the other half paid the full price. Demonstrating external validity of the findings of the questionnaire experiments, those subjects who paid the full price attended more theatre plays than those who received the discount.

Escalation

Escalation refers to a persistent commitment to a failing course of action. Examples include continuing to wait for a bus although walking would be faster, not breaking up a souring romantic relationship or, at an organisational or national level, refusing to discontinue a commitment although finding oneself 'knee-deep in the big muddy', which many international conflicts or unsuccessful business ventures testify to. Such situations have in common that they entail sunk costs incurred by an originally chosen course of action (Staw and Ross, 1987). Furthermore, distinguishing escalation from sunk cost effects which are one-shot matters, it involves ongoing sequences of choices of persisting or withdrawing. Simple withdrawal is, however, not an obvious solution since it results in losses. Persistence at least holds the promise of an eventual gain. Thus, in escalation situations, losses are suffered in a course of action where the consequences of continuing or discontinuing are uncertain.

Empirical research on escalation is reviewed by Brockner (1992). Most of the research uses experimental simulations of actual escalation situations occurring in business organisations. In a typical study (Staw, 1976), students role-played that they were the financial vice-president of a company. Their task was to decide what resources to allocate to continued investments. Prior to making decisions half of the subjects were told that a previous allocation decision had been successful, the other half that it had been unsuccessful. Half of the subjects in each of the groups were furthermore told that they were responsible for the previous decision, the other half that they were not responsible. The group of responsible subjects who were led to believe that the previous decision was unsuccessful allocated more resources to the previous course of action than did the other groups. More recent research includes a study by Davies and Bobko (1986) demonstrating that responsible subjects were more persistent when the outcome of a previous decision was framed as a loss than when it was framed as a gain.

In another review of research findings concerning antecedent factors of escalation or entrapment, Staw and Ross (1987) distinguished project factors (expected benefits and costs) from psychological factors such as responsibility and information feedback, social factors relating to the need for self-justification, and structural factors at an organisational level, exemplified by corporate pride and administrative inertia. A generalisation appears to be that these types of factors come into play sequentially. Project benefits may dominate initially, a desire to recover sunk costs at a later stage when such costs become known, and at still later stages, when failure seems certain, self-justification and responsibility diffusion triggering a host of structural factors.

Summary

A factor distinguishing between the different phenomena is whether one or several choices are made. Another factor is whether or not the DM has incurred losses. In addition to those two factors (see Table 10.1), a third may be what relationship exists between the prior and current choices. However, although some relationship probably must exist for

Table 10.1 Phenomena of integration of outcomes over time

	Single choices	*Sequential choices*
Prior loss(es)	Sunk cost effects	Escalation
Prior loss(es) or gain(s)	Effects of prior outcome	Multistage betting

integration to occur, it is unclear that the different phenomena differ in this respect.

The impact of a single outcome of a prior choice on a subsequent choice is a limiting case of sequential decision making such as multistage betting. A special case of this limiting case is when the prior outcome is a sunk cost, that is, when the prior outcome is a loss. Escalation constitutes a special case of multistage betting where each preceding outcome is a sunk cost.

The logical relations between the different phenomena do not necessarily imply that identical or similar explanations would apply to all. It may still be argued that a theoretical analysis should focus on the impact of one or several prior outcomes on a single choice. It is a limiting case of sequential decision making (multistage betting, escalation) which is still tractable using single decisions as the unit of analysis. It subsumes a special case such as the sunk cost effect. In the following section different explanations which have been offered are examined with respect to how they explain the impact of a prior outcome on a single choice.

EXPLANATIONS

The editing phase of prospect theory

A complete explanation of integration of outcomes across time must specify when, how and why integration takes place, preferably based on principles embraced by a general theory. Several explanations are discussed by Laughhunn and Payne (1984). Since prospect theory (Kahneman and Tversky, 1979; Tversky and Fox, 1995; Tversky and Kahneman, 1991, 1992) figures in several, we begin with explanations related to this major theory of decision making under risk and uncertainty.

Prospect theory is similar to expected utility theory (von Neumann and Morgenstern, 1947; Savage, 1954) in assuming that a DM first assigns a utility or value $v(x)$ to each outcome x, then chooses the option with the highest sum of values across all outcomes. An important difference is, however, the assumption that a DM edits options prior to assigning values to outcomes. Editing operations include framing of outcomes as gains or losses relative to a reference point. Framing also entails segregating or integrating prior outcomes (Kahneman and Tversky, 1984; Tversky and Kahneman, 1981). A decision frame based on a 'minimal account' implies that outcomes of a particular choice are evaluated independently of prior outcomes (i.e., segregated). Such a decision frame may frequently be employed because it '(i) simplifies evaluations and reduces cognitive strain, (ii) reflects the intuition that consequences should be causally linked to acts, and (iii) matches the properties of hedonic experience which is more sensitive to desirable and undesirable changes than to steady states' (Tversky and Kahneman, 1981: 457).

A comprehensive account is an alternative to a minimal account which encompasses prior outcomes (Ranyard, 1995; Tversky and Kahneman, 1981). Why is such a frame not adopted in the editing process? Of the three reasons noted by Tversky and Kahneman (1981), the last one appears to be the most compelling because it may relate to biological adaptiveness (Barkow *et al.*, 1992). Strong biologically relevant incentives are perhaps therefore needed to force attention to steady states instead of changes. Basically, the ability to remember recent events is a prerequisite for adaptation. At least under some circumstances, biological importance also seems to govern what is remembered (Lachman and Lachman, 1979). Similarly, as a DM judges probabilities on the basis of ease of memory retrieval of past events using the availability heuristic (Tversky and Kahneman, 1973), prior outcomes may be assumed to be integrated if they are easy to retrieve from memory. Thus, factors which improve memory of a prior outcome should enhance its integration with current outcomes. Recency is perhaps the most important single such factor. It should be noted that, despite integration of one or more prior outcomes, a DM still responds to changes from a reference point. Take as an example a sequence of prior outcomes $x_1 \ldots x_n$ which a DM is known to have encountered. Assume that the subset of recent prior outcomes denoted $\{x_{ij}\ i < n\}$ retrieved from memory is integrated with the current outcomes. If integration means that the prior outcomes are added, the value of a current outcome y is evaluated as $v(y + \Sigma x_i)$. In other words, the reference point is neither zero nor the total assets but the sum of the subset of prior outcomes. A special case is that this subset contains only a single prior outcome.

A host of other factors are also likely to enhance memory of prior outcomes and thus to increase the likelihood that they are integrated with current outcomes. The magnitude of a prior outcome is one possible such factor. Although negative events are in general processed more comprehensively (Taylor, 1991; Weber, 1994), a positive prior outcome may still be easier to remember than a negative one (Isen, 1987). Any perceptual or cognitive feature making a prior outcome stand out should furthermore enhance its recall. Some of these other factors may override recency.

Sometimes an old prior outcome is therefore integrated with current outcomes whereas a new one is not.

Yet, although memory retrieval is a necessary factor, it cannot be sufficient since, as already mentioned, a prior outcome is sometimes segregated when no memory retrieval is involved (Kahneman and Tversky, 1979). A primary aim of the editing phase proposed in prospect theory is cognitive simplification, thereby alleviating cognitive strain for the DM. In research on both problem solving and decision making, it has been argued that subjects are sometimes unwilling to change the external representation of a problem. In a similar vein, Slovic (1972) proposed a 'concreteness principle' stating that a DM tends to use explicitly available information in its current format. Thus, a DM may frequently not allocate the cognitive resources required either for searching for more information or for changing the format of the information. Gilbert (1991) has more broadly argued that the encoding of information in the given format is pervasive and perhaps unavoidable. According to the concreteness principle, no integration of prior outcomes would be expected unless the format of the decision problem is changed. Empirical evidence in support of this proposition has recently been obtained (Romanus *et al.*, 1996b). Different groups of undergraduates serving as subjects were presented with different descriptions of gambling choices. In one set of descriptions a prior gain or loss was added to the status quo (not gambling), in another set it was added to the potential gain, and in still another set it was added to the possible loss. A finding which will be discussed further below was that ratings of satisfaction with the different outcomes of not gambling, gambling and winning, and gambling and losing, showed that the prior outcomes were integrated with the current loss across all sets of descriptions. However, in support of the concreteness principle, in the remaining cases subjects only integrated the prior outcome when it was explicitly added to the current outcome.

Sometimes less cognitive effort is required to perform a task if its mental representation is changed. Jones and Schkade (1995) actually found that subjects translated a problem from the initial representation in which it was presented to a more familiar or convenient one. A prior outcome retrieved from memory may still be ignored if the DM believes it will have identical effects on all current outcomes. Such cancellation (Kahneman and Tversky, 1979) is a means of transforming a choice problem to render it cognitively simpler. It may account for segregation of prior outcomes.

At a specified point in time, the outcomes of a prior decision are perhaps not yet known. As shown by Tversky and Shafir (1992) and Shafir and Tversky (1992), a prior outcome may then have no impact on a subsequent choice. The conditions appear to be similar to when a prior outcome has no impact because it cannot be retrieved from memory. However,

Tversky and Shafir's finding that subjects segregated an unknown prior outcome was replicated in Gärling and Romanus (1996, Experiment 2) when the probability of a prior gain was stated to be equal to the probability of a prior loss (0.50). A prior gain was also found to be segregated in another condition where it was stated to be 0.75 as well as in a third condition where it was stated to be 0.25. In each case there are still several outcomes. Thus, a reason for the difficulty may be that subjects are unable to think through all of them.

If difficulties in imagining uncertain or risky prior outcomes lead to their being ignored, logically this should extend to the outcomes of a current choice. Since it does not (Gärling and Romanus, 1996), there may be a difference between prior and current outcomes. In the case of a prior outcome, a choice has already been made, whereas current outcomes are directly related to the choice faced by the DM. As a consequence, the editing process may start with the current outcomes, which are those which will be evaluated first. To the extent that prior outcomes are known and easy to retrieve from memory, they will be added to the current outcomes. However, if there are many current outcomes which are risky or uncertain, a preferred cognitive simplification may still be to segregate the prior outcomes.

Whether or not a prior outcome is seen as being connected to the evaluation of current outcomes is a factor promoting integration which needs to be added. In an illustrative empirical study it was found that a majority of subjects chose not to replace a lost theatre ticket although they chose to buy one after having lost an equivalent sum of money (Tversky and Kahneman, 1981). The question is why losing money was not seen as connected to the choice to buy a theatre ticket whereas losing it was. Thaler (1980, 1985) claims that people use mental or psychological accounts to keep track of gains and losses incurred by sequential choices. A negative balance on an account is assumed to have a different effect on a related choice than has a positive balance. However, outcomes one keeps track of in another account have no effect. In the example, although losing a theatre ticket means losing as much money as losing a bill, the latter is registered on a different account.

In drawing parallels between mental accounting and categorisation, Henderson and Peterson (1992) show that principles known to govern categorisation apply to mental-accounting phenomena. In this vein, we identify mental accounting with categorisation of events on some other basis than temporal contiguity. Like temporal integration it serves some biological or psychological purpose. We want in particular to emphasise the role of goals and aspirations in determining the 'mental accounts' a DM uses (Ranyard, 1995). For instance, if a primary goal is to earn a fortune, any monetary loss or gain is likely to be registered and integrated. In contrast, many people prefer to keep track only of large losses, making sure they avoid misfortune. Also, in many cases monetary outcomes are means rather than goals. As implied by the reasons for their choices stated by subjects presented with the lost theatre ticket scenario (Henderson and Peterson, 1992), unless one really wanted to see the play, paying twice the amount for the ticket did not seem to be a good way of spending money on entertainment since it would reduce other opportunities. However, other bases for categorising events should not be ruled out. Whether or not a prior outcome is compatible (e.g., expressed in the same unit) with the current outcomes is one such basis. The important role of compatibility has been demonstrated in many other circumstances (see Selart, Chapter 4, for a review).

Categorisation is, however, more encompassing than adding values or utilities. It also serves the purpose of identifying and inferring other valuable information. Examples include inferring an expected average outcome (Kahneman and Miller, 1986) or identifying increasing or decreasing trends or recurrent patterns in outcome sequences (Varey and Kahneman, 1992). A temporal and content basis for integrating prior outcomes is frequently available simultaneously. As shown in a recent study by Klaar (1995), the content basis may dominate. However, such a dominance should also be affected by changes in the memory representation of a prior outcome as a function of time.

Thaler and Johnson (1990) asked subjects how much a monetary loss would hurt after they had incurred another loss. As the results showed, the same monetary loss was more unpleasant when it was preceded by either a smaller or larger loss. A small to modest loss thus appears to sensitise, a large loss to numb subjects to subsequent losses. The latter may also be labelled a contrast effect. Independent evidence presented in Thaler and Johnson indicated that the pairs of losses were segregated. In Tversky and Griffin (1991) subjects rated how happy they thought a person would be on a day when he or she experienced a neutral event knowing that a positive or negative, connected or unconnected event had occurred the week before. The impact of the prior event on the ratings was larger when it was unconnected than when it was connected. Inconsistent with Thaler and Johnson (1990), it was concluded that integration does not depend on connectedness but that contrast effects do.

In a recent study[2] we were interested in whether Tversky and Griffin's (1991) conclusion would generalise to the integration of prior outcomes in risky choices. We chose a fictitious horse-race betting task to study the impact of prior gains and losses. Participants were thirty-two undergraduates who received a modest monetary compensation. The bets were presented in a booklet in which subjects indicated how likely they were to gamble in the current race. Half of the subjects imagined on different trials that in the prior race they had won a specified amount (prior gain), lost a specified amount (prior loss), or withheld from gambling (no prior outcome). A prior gain was never large enough to cover a possible loss incurred by the current choice to gamble. Likewise, a prior loss was not large enough to jeopardise the potential gain of the current choice. Thus, we attempted to avoid the break-even effect and to reduce the playing-with-the-house-money effect (Thaler and Johnson, 1990). Yet, consistent with what Thaler and Johnson found, subjects rated that they were more likely to gamble when the prior outcome was a gain and less likely when it was a loss (see Table 10.2). The remaining half of the subjects were not told that the prior gain was a win in the preceding race but the same amount of money which they previously had lent to a friend who unexpectedly paid it back. The prior loss was incurred by lending the same amount of money to a friend despite the fact that he or she was very unlikely to repay it. If contrast effects depend on connectedness, we expected less integration of the prior outcome. However, as Table 10.2 shows, integration was in fact stronger. This finding is consistent with the notion that money transactions between friends are kept track of in a mental account other than gambling money.

Extending the editing phase of prospect theory

Thaler and Johnson (1990; see also Thaler, 1980, 1985) suggested that prospect theory should incorporate a hedonic editing rule which integrates or segregates prior outcomes. Whereas other editing rules are employed for the sake of cognitive simplification, the goal of such a rule is to maximise value. Thus, the distinction is blurred between an editing phase and an evaluation phase.

No effect of integrating a prior outcome should be expected if options are evaluated according to a linear function mapping an outcome x on value v, that is, if $v(x) = a + bx$. Apparently, in this case the difference in value between $v(x_1)$ corresponding to one option and $v(x_2)$ corresponding to another option is exactly the same as the difference between $v(x_1 + z)$ and $v(x_2 + z)$ where a prior outcome z has been added. However, since the value function proposed in prospect theory is concave for gains and

Table 10.2 Mean ratings of likelihood to gamble (on a scale from −50 to 50) for no prior outcome, a prior loss, or a prior gain which were connected or unconnected to the current outcomes

	Connected		*Unconnected*	
	M	*SD*	*M*	*SD*
No prior outcome	7.4	63	3.8	58
Prior loss	−14.4	20	−5.3	38
Prior gain	9.9	67	8.4	59

convex and steeper for losses (Kahneman and Tversky, 1979), the difference in value will be different when the prior outcome is added. It is generally true that either $v(x + z) > v(x) + v(z)$ or the reverse. Integrating rather than segregating a prior outcome will therefore lead to a higher or lower value. If the goal of hedonic editing is to maximise value, editing operations should ensure that the prior outcome is added to (integrated with) some outcomes and not added to (segregated from) other outcomes before being evaluated according to the value function. Value is maximised if a loss is added to a loss but not if a gain is added to a gain. Value is also maximised if a small loss is added to a large gain (a mixed gain). Whether or not value is maximised if a small gain is added to a large loss (a mixed loss) depends on the relative sizes of the gain and the loss.

The empirical results obtained by Thaler and Johnson (1990) only partially supported the hedonic editing rule. An alternative account labelled the renewable resources model was therefore offered by Linville and Fischer (1991).[3] The point of departure is still that a DM maximises value. Since a gain is believed to buffer a loss, outcomes entailing a large gain and a small loss, or the reverse, are integrated. However, awareness of his or her limited but renewable resources to cope with large losses, results in multiple losses being aversive to the DM, who will therefore segregate them. Gain-saving resources are also perceived to be limited but renewable. Consequently, multiple gains are segregated.

By asking subjects whether they would prefer two events to occur on the same day (integration) or on different days (segregation), Linville and Fischer (1991) obtained empirical support for the predictions from the renewable resources model. The events were either financial (monetary losses or gains), academic (successes or failures in exams), or social (positive or negative encounters with people). Almost identical results were obtained within each domain. Some evidence was also found for integration across domains (e.g., if one event was financial and the other social).

As noted by Larrick (1993), in risky choices a DM is perhaps often more concerned about avoiding negative outcomes than attaining positive ones. Therefore, it may be questioned whether the renewable resources model accurately predicts integration when subjects make risky choices. If the goal is to avoid the negative impact of losses, subjects evaluating risky outcomes presumably attend to and process more thoroughly expected losses (Taylor, 1991; Weber, 1994). If they do, a compatible loss-sensitivity principle of integration may be to add prior outcomes to expected losses rather than to add prior gains to expected losses and prior losses to expected gains (Table 10.3). In contrast, the prior outcomes may be segregated from expected gains. The effect of a prior loss is therefore to increase the dissatisfaction with a possible loss and the effect of a prior gain to decrease it. Direct empirical support for these predictions has been obtained in several previous studies (Gärling and Romanus, 1996; Gärling *et al.*, 1994; Romanus *et al.*, 1996a, 1996b). Similar results are presented in Figure 10.2, showing the mean ratings of satisfaction with not gambling, gambling and winning, and gambling and losing, respectively, obtained from one of the groups of participants in our study described above. In accordance with the loss-sensitivity principle, these ratings indicate that only dissatisfaction with the expected loss was affected by the prior outcomes.

Table 10.3 Two sets of predictions of integration of prior outcomes with current outcomes in risky choices

	Renewable resources model[1]		*Loss-sensitivity principle*[2]	
	Expected gain	*Expected loss*	*Expected gain*	*Expected loss*
Prior gain	no	yes	no	yes
Prior loss	yes	no	no	yes

Sources: 1 Linville and Fischer, 1991
2 Gärling and Romanus, 1996

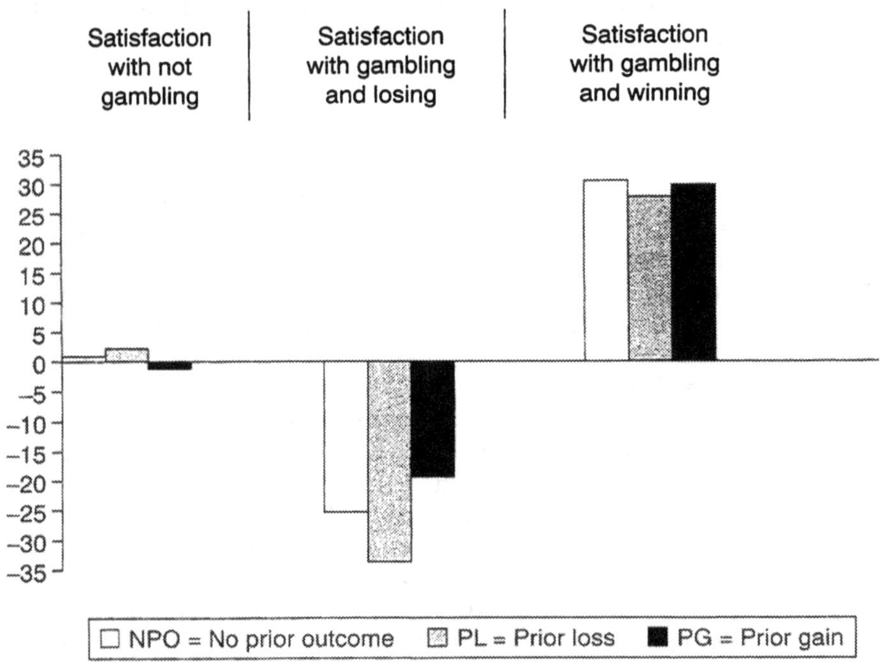

Figure 10.2 Mean ratings of satisfaction in gambling outcomes

Explanations unrelated to prospect theory

Explanations based on prospect theory rely on mechanisms of information processing leading to various forms of biases. Although Whyte (1986) has suggested that such mechanisms may also account for escalation (see Schaubroek and Davies, 1994, for empirical support), an alternative explanation in terms of self-justification or desire to appear rational was originally proposed by Rubin and Brockner (1975) and Staw (1976). Brockner (1992) concludes that this explanation is supported by many empirical studies of escalation in which the need for self-justification has been manipulated. Yet Brockner admits that it is unlikely that self-justification is a sufficient explanation of escalation. Is self-justification a viable general explanation of effects of prior outcomes? The need for self-justification appears to be confined to situations where losses are due to prior decisions for which one is responsible. However, if presenting oneself as being consistent is another important ingredient of the need for self-justification, it may perhaps be evoked as an explanation in the somewhat broader class of situations where a DM has a choice of continuing or discontinuing a course of action after having faced a prior outcome. In addition to being confined to a limited number of situations, the concept of self-justification does not seem to offer more than an alternative description of the observed phenomenon.

In a similar vein, Arkes and Blumer (1985) suggested that sunk cost effects in many cases reflect a DM's wish to avoid appearing wasteful. However, despite being consistent with some of the reported data, neither does this explanation seem to be a candidate for a more general account of effects of prior outcomes. It may also be noted that Garland and Newport (1991) argued, on the basis of experimental evidence, that sunk cost effects primarily reflect biased information processing.

It is conceivable that a prior outcome alters a DM's mood state. If so, the prior outcome may have an influence on the process of making a current choice although there is no integration of the prior outcome with the expected outcomes (but note that Romanus *et al.* (1996a), found that a positive mood may increase integration). A distinction is frequently made between an enduring temperament to react emotionally in certain ways, transitory moods or affect, and emotional reactions to situational factors (Russell and Snodgrass, 1987). A prior outcome may trigger an emotional reaction resulting in a transitory mood, perhaps more easily in people who are disposed to react in a certain way or already are in a certain mood.

A positive mood has been found to lead to optimism in judging probabilities (Isen and Geva, 1987; Johnson and Tversky, 1983). Presumably because subjects do not want to jeopardise their positive mood, the dissatisfaction with an expected loss has also been shown to increase (Arkes *et al.*, 1988). In Isen and Geva (1987), the net effect was increased risk aversion. Arkes *et al.* (1988) and Isen and Patrick (1983) found that positive affect increased risk aversion when subjects were offered an insurance policy in which the loss was salient. However, increased risk seeking was observed when subjects in a positive mood were offered lottery tickets for which the loss was less salient. Presumably, in this case risk seeking was caused by optimism.

If subjects react to a prior gain with positive affect, a reduced likelihood to gamble should be expected, consistent with the results obtained by, for instance, Isen and Geva (1987). The reverse was, however, observed in experiments conducted by Gärling and Romanus (1996), Gärling *et al.* (1994), and Romanus *et al.* (1996a, 1996b). On the other hand, Laughhunn and Payne (1984) concluded that their results concerning risk taking were consistent with a mood effect. In none of the cited studies did subjects experience real prior outcomes. It is therefore doubtful that mood was induced. A more plausible possibility is that a prior gain (or loss) did not alter mood but nevertheless induced optimism (or pessimism). Consistent with this interpretation, optimism and pessimism have been assumed to change the decision weights a DM assigns to risky or uncertain outcomes (Hogarth and Einhorn, 1990).

Some of the explanations of effects of prior outcomes based on prospect theory which were examined in the previous subsection (hedonic editing, the renewable resources model, and the loss-sensitivity principle) make allowance for the effects of different motives on information processing. In contrast, the explanations examined in this subsection do not go far in specifying the consequences of differences in motives for how information is processed. A potential contribution is instead to suggest motives (self-justification or desire to appear rational, maintaining a positive mood) which should be added to maximising value or avoiding negative outcomes.

An integration of explanations

A summary of the different explanations is given in Table 10.4. In this table only explanations which seem to have some generality are included. Some refer to cognitive limitations on why integration does not occur. Failure to retrieve a prior outcome, a description of the decision problem which does not include the prior outcome, cancellation, and uncertainty about the prior outcome all belong to this category. Connectedness, hedonic editing, the renewable resources model, the loss-sensitivity principle, and mood are explanations which focus on motivational or affective reasons why integration of a prior outcome sometimes occurs and sometimes does not occur. Optimism is categorised as a cognitive explanation because it may reflect a cognitive bias (Gilovich *et al.*, 1985). However, it

Table 10.4 Summary of major explanations of integration of prior outcomes in risky choices

Type	*Specific effect*	*Non-specific effect*
Cognitive	Concreteness (Slovic, 1972)	Optimism (Hogarth and Einhorn, 1990)
	Cancellation (Kahneman and Tversky, 1979)	
	Uncertainty (Tversky and Shafir, 1992)	
	Availability (Tversky and Kahneman, 1973)	
Motivational	Connectedness (Thaler, 1980, 1985; Tversky and Kahneman, 1981)	Mood (Isen, 1987)
	Hedonic editing (Thaler & Johnson, 1990)	
	Renewable resources model (Linville & Fischer, 1991)	
	Loss-sensitivity principle (Gärling & Romanus, 1996)	

also qualifies as a motivational explanation if optimism is induced by a positive mood (Isen and Geva, 1987).

Some of the explanations make the assumption that there are specific effects of a prior outcome on assessments of likelihoods, decision weights, or values. In effect the DM chooses among different sets of options than he or she would do otherwise. Non-specific effects imply that the prior outcome changes the DM's state which in turn affects his or her processing of the current options. Anything other than a prior outcome will have the same effect. Again, the optimism explanation is difficult to classify. Its effect is specific if a prior outcome leads to optimism which changes the subjective probabilities or decision weights assigned to outcomes. However, it may be more appropriate to classify the effect as non-specific if it is assumed that optimism induced in some other way has the same effect. As an example, consider the possibility that a lucky outcome in one domain (winning a game of poker at a friend's house) generalises to another (taking risks when driving home). It may be noted that if motivational explanations presuppose specific effects (hedonic editing, the renewable resources model, and the loss-sensitivity principle), they make the assumption that cognitive limitations can to some extent be overcome by increased effort. No such assumption is entailed by motivational explanations (mood) presupposing non-specific effects.

The proposed explanations appear to be complementary rather than conflicting. An exception is hedonic editing and the renewable resources model, which attempt to explain the same observations in different ways.

According to the loss-sensitivity principle, a DM attempts to avoid negative outcomes rather than to maximise value as the hedonic editing rule and the renewable resources model presuppose. Thus, the loss-sensitivity principle is complementary since a DM may sometimes maximise value and sometimes attempt to avoid negative outcomes. Highlighting the complementary nature of the explanations, Figure 10.3 outlines a process model. Goals and aspirations constitute one factor which determines how options are evaluated, including whether or not current options should be edited so that prior outcomes are integrated with the expected outcomes of those options. Of course, the prior outcomes must be retrieved from memory. Memory retrieval of prior outcomes may also directly influence editing of the options. Likewise, editing may be directly influenced by how the choice problem is described. Mood and optimism may both be affected by prior outcomes and influence evaluations of the options.

CONCLUDING REMARKS

The review of previous research in this chapter shows that the past in the form of outcomes of prior decisions influences choices. Such influences have been labelled effects of or integration of prior outcomes (Thaler and Johnson, 1990), sunk cost effects (Arkes and Blumer, 1985; Laughhunn and Payne, 1984), multistage betting (Funk *et al.*, 1979), and escalation (Brockner, 1992). As noted, these phenomena are closely related. Yet they may have different explanations.

In the review it was possible to identify ten general explanations which have been or may be proposed concerning the integration of prior outcomes in risky choices. These explanations encompass both specific cognitive limitations and motivational or affective factors with specific as well as non-specific effects. It is suggested that most of them are complementary, and that it is possible to integrate them in a process model.

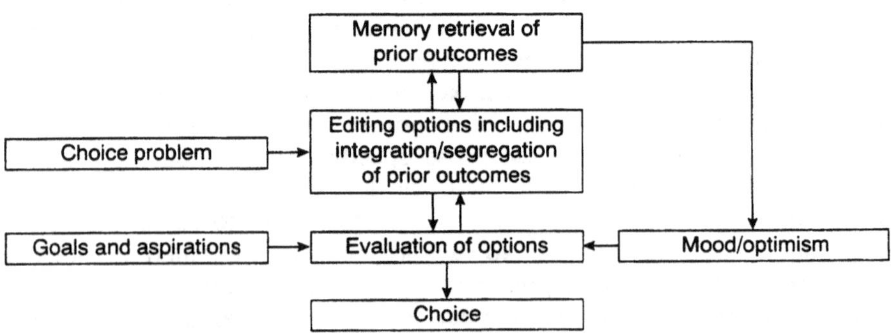

Figure 10.3 Process model encompassing compatible explanations

Although our previous research (Gärling and Romanus, 1996) has shown that the loss-sensitivity principle is a viable motivational explanation based on the assumption that a DM attempts to avoid negative outcomes rather than to maximise value, the present review suggests that a thorough understanding of effects of prior outcomes on risky choices requires a broader approach. It is hoped that valuable directions for such an approach are suggested by the diverse sets of possible explanatory factors.

NOTES

1 Although perhaps not natural, it is not logically excluded that status quo constitutes a loss which is compared to other losses, some of which are as bad or less bad.

2 This study has not been reported elsewhere. For further details, see Gärling and Romanus (1996) who used an almost identical procedure.

3 Thaler and Johnson (1990) also proposed a quasi-hedonic editing rule which accounted for their empirical findings. However, this rule will not be discussed since it does not seem to have the same solid theoretical rationale and makes the same predictions as the renewable resources model.

ACKNOWLEDGEMENTS

Preparation of this chapter as well as the research reported therein was financially supported by grants to the first author from the Swedish Council for Research in the Humanities and Social Sciences (no. 244/92, no. 6/93, and no. 12/94). The authors thank the editors and an anonymous reviewer for valuable suggestions, and Ole C. Boe for assistance with the literature review.

REFERENCES

Arkes, H.R. and Blumer, C. (1985) 'The psychology of sunk cost', *Organizational Behavior and Human Decision Processes*, 35: 124–40.

Arkes, H.R., Herren, L.T. and Isen, A.M. (1988) 'The role of potential loss in the influence of affect on risk-taking behavior', *Organizational Behavior and Human Decision Processes*, 42: 181–93.

Barkow, J.H., Cosmides, L. and Tooby, J. (eds) (1992) *The Adapted Mind*, New York: Oxford University Press.

Baron, J. (1994) 'Nonconsequentialist decisions', *Behavioral and Brain Sciences*, 17: 1–10.

Brehmer, B. (1992) 'Dynamic decision making: human control of complex systems', *Acta Psychologica*, 81: 211–41.

Brockner, J. (1992) 'The escalation of commitment to a failing course of action: toward theoretical progress', *Academy of Management Review*, 12: 39–61.

Camerer, C.F. and Johnson, E.J. (1991) 'The process–performance paradox in expert judgment', in K.A. Ericsson and J. Smith (eds) *Toward a General Theory of Expertise*, Cambridge: Cambridge University Press.

Davies, M. and Bobko, P. (1986) 'Contextual effects on escalation processes in public sector decision making', *Organizational Behavior and Human Decision Processes*, 37: 121–38.

Dawes, R.M. (1988) *Rational Choice in an Uncertain World*, San Diego, CA: Harcourt Brace Jovanovich.

Elster, J. and Loewenstein, G. (1992) 'Utility from memory and anticipation', in J. Elster and G. Loewenstein (eds) *Choice over Time*, New York: Russell Sage Foundation.

Funk, S.G., Rapoport, A. and Jones, L.V. (1979) 'Investing capital on safe and risky alternatives: an experimental study', *Journal of Experimental Psychology: General*, 108: 415–40.

Garland, H. and Newport, S. (1991) 'Effects of absolute and relative sunk costs on the decision to persist with a course of action', *Organizational Behavior and Human Decision Processes*, 48: 55–69.

Gärling, T. and Romanus, J. (1996) 'Integration and segregation of prior outcomes in risky decisions', *Göteborg Psychological Research*, 26, no. 1.

Gärling, T., Romanus, J. and Selart, M. (1994) 'Betting at the race track: does risk seeking increase when losses accumulate?', *Perceptual and Motor Skills*, 78: 1248–50.

Gilbert, D.T. (1991) 'How mental systems believe', *American Psychologist*, 46: 107–19.

Gilovich, T., Vallone, R. and Tversky, A. (1985) 'The hot hand in basketball: on the misperception of random sequences', *Cognitive Psychology*, 17: 295–314.

Heath, C. (1995) 'Escalation and deescalation of commitment in response to sunk costs: the role of mental accounting', *Organizational Behavior and Human Decision Processes*, 62: 38–54.

Henderson, P. and Peterson, P. (1992) 'Mental accounting and categorization', *Organizational Behavior and Human Decision Processes*, 51: 92–117.

Hogarth, R.M. (1981) 'Beyond discrete biases: functional and dysfunctional aspects of judgmental heuristics', *Psychological Bulletin*, 90: 197–217.

Hogarth, R.M. and Einhorn, H.J. (1990) 'Venture theory: a model of decision weights', *Management Science*, 36: 780–803.

Huber, O. (1990) 'Cognitive processes in a multistage investment task', in K.J. Gilhooly, M. Keane, R.H. Logie and G. Erdos (eds) *Lines of Thinking: Reflections on the Psychology of Thought*, vol. 1, Chichester: Wiley.

Huber, O. (1994) 'Decision behavior in a multistage investment task', *Acta Psychologica*, 85: 139–54.

Huber, O., Debeutz, A., Pratscher, J. and Quehenberger, I. (1990) 'Perceived control in a multistage decision task', *Journal of Behavioral Decision Making*, 3: 123–36.

Isen, A.M. (1987) 'Positive affect, cognitive processes, and social behavior', *Advances in Experimental Social Psychology*, 20: 203–53.

Isen, A.M. and Geva, N. (1987) 'The influence of positive affect on acceptable level of risk: the person with a large canoe has a large worry', *Organizational Behavior and Human Decision Processes*, 39: 145–54.

Isen, A.M. and Patrick, R. (1983) 'The effect of positive feelings and risk taking: when the chips are down', *Organizational Behavior and Human Performance*, 31: 194–202.

Johnson, E.J. and Tversky, A. (1983) 'Affect, generalisation, and the perception of risk', *Journal of Personality and Social Psychology*, 45: 20–31.

Jones, D.R. and Schkade, D.A. (1995) 'Choosing and translating between problem representations', *Organizational Behavior and Human Decision Processes*, 61: 214–23.

Kahneman, D., Knetsch, J.L. and Thaler, R. (1990) 'Experimental tests of the endowment effect and the Coase theorem', *Journal of Political Economy*, 98: 1325–48.

Kahneman, D. and Miller, D.T. (1986) 'Norm theory: comparing reality to its alternatives', *Psychological Review*, 93: 136–53.

Kahneman, D. and Tversky, A. (1979) 'Prospect theory: an analysis of decision under risk', *Econometrica*, 47: 263–91.

Kahneman, D. and Tversky, A. (1984) 'Choices, values, and frames', *American Psychologist*, 39: 341–50.

Karlsson, N., Romanus, J. and Gärling, T. (1996) 'The status-quo bias and integration of prior outcomes in risky decisions', *Göteborg Psychological Research*, 26, no. 4.

Klaar, Y. (1995) 'Segregate gains, integrate losses: an information perspective', Paper presented at the 15th Research Conference on Subjective Probability, Utility and Decision Making (SPUDM15), Jerusalem, Israel, August.

Lachman, J.L. and Lachman, R. (1979) 'Theories of memory organization and human evolution', in C.R. Puff (ed.) *Memory Organization and Structure*, New York: Academic Press.

Larrick, R.P. (1993) 'Motivational factors in decision theories: the role of self-protection', *Psychological Bulletin*, 113: 440–50.

Laughhunn, D. and Payne, J.W. (1984), 'The impact of sunk cost on risky choice behaviour', *INFOR (Canadian Journal of Operations Research and Information Processing)*, 22: 151–81.

Linville, P.W. and Fischer, G.W. (1991) 'Preferences for separating or combining events', *Journal of Personality and Social Psychology*, 60: 5–23.

Payne, J.W., Bettman, J.R. and Johnson, E.J. (1993) *The Adaptive Decision Maker*, New York: Cambridge University Press.

Ranyard, R. (1995) 'Mental accounts in financial decision making: a cognitive-psychological approach', Paper presented at the 15th Research Conference on Subjective Probability, Utility and Decision Making (SPUDM15), Jerusalem, Israel, August.

Ranyard, R. and Abdel-Nabi, D. (1993) 'Mental accounting and the process of multiattribute choice', *Acta Psychologica*, 84: 161–77.

Rapoport, A. and Jones, L.V. (1970) 'Gambling behavior in two-outcome multi-stage betting games', *Journal of Mathematical Psychology*, 7: 163–87.

Ritov, I. and Baron, J. (1992) 'Status-quo and omission biases', *Journal of Risk and Uncertainty*, 5: 49–61.

Romanus, J., Hassing, L. and Gärling, T. (1996a) 'A loss-sensitivity explanation of integration of prior outcomes in risky decisions', *Acta Psychologica*, 93: 173–83.

Romanus, J., Karlsson, N. and Gärling, T. (1996b) 'Loss-sensitivity and concreteness as principles of integration of prior outcomes in risky decisions', *Göteborg Psychological Research*, 26: no. 2.

Rubin, J.Z. and Brockner, J. (1975) 'Factors affecting entrapment in waiting situations: the Rosencrantz and Guildenstern effect', *Journal of Personality and Social Psychology*, 58: 1040–7.

Russell, J.A. and Snodgrass, J. (1987) 'Emotion and the environment', in D. Stokols and I. Altman (eds) *Handbook of Environmental Psychology*, vol. 1, New York: Wiley.

Samuelson, W. and Zeckhausen, R. (1988) 'Status quo bias in decision making', *Journal of Risk and Uncertainty*, 1: 7–59.

Savage, L.J. (1954) *The Foundations of Statistics*, New York: Wiley.

Schaubroek, J. and Davies, E. (1994) 'Prospect theory predictions when escalating is not the only chance to recover sunk costs', *Organizational Behavior and Human Decision Processes*, 57: 59–82.

Schweitzer, M. (1994) 'Disentangling status quo and omission effects: an experimental analysis', *Organizational Behavior and Human Decision Processes*, 58: 457–76.

Shafir, E. and Tversky, A. (1992) 'Thinking through uncertainty: nonsequential reasoning and choice', *Cognitive Psychology*, 24: 449–74.

Slovic, P. (1972) 'From Shakespeare to Simon: speculations and some evidence about man's ability to process information', *Research Monograph* 12, No. 2, Oregon Research Institute, Eugene, OR.

Staw, B.M. (1976) 'Knee-deep in the Big Muddy: a study of escalating commitment to a chosen course of action', *Organizational Behavior and Human Performance*, 16: 27–44.

Staw, B.M. and Ross, J. (1987) 'Behavior in escalation situations: antecedents, prototypes, and solutions', *Research in Organizational Behavior*, 9: 39–78.

Taylor, S.E. (1991) 'Asymmetrical effects of positive and negative events: the mobilization-minimization hypothesis', *Psychological Bulletin*, 110: 67–85.

Thaler, R.H. (1980) 'Toward a positive theory of consumer choice', *Journal of Economic Behavior and Organization*, 1: 39–60.

Thaler, R.H. (1985) 'Mental accounting and consumer choice', *Marketing Science*, 4: 199–214.

Thaler, R.H. and Johnson, E.J. (1990) 'Gambling with the house money and trying to break even: the effects of prior outcomes on risky choice', *Management Science*, 36: 643–60.

Tversky, A. and Fox, C.R. (1995) 'Weighing risk and uncertainty', *Psychological Review*, 102: 269–83.

Tversky, A. and Griffin, D. (1991) 'Endowment and contrast in judgments of well-being', in F. Strack, M. Argyle and N. Schwarz (eds) *Subjective Well-Being*, Oxford: Pergamon.

Tversky, A. and Kahneman, D. (1973) 'Availability: a heuristic for judging frequency and probability', *Cognitive Psychology*, 5: 207–32.

Tversky, A. and Kahneman, D. (1981) 'The framing of decisions and the psychology of choice', *Science*, 211: 453–8.

Tversky, A. and Kahneman, D. (1991) 'Loss aversion in riskless choice: a reference-dependent model', *The Quarterly Journal of Economics*, 106: 1039–61.

Tversky, A. and Kahneman, D. (1992) 'Advances in prospect theory: cumulative representation of uncertainty', *Journal of Risk and Uncertainty*, 5: 297–323.

Tversky, A. and Shafir, E. (1992) 'The disjunction effect in choice under uncertainty', *Psychological Science*, 3: 305–9.

Varey, C. and Kahneman, D. (1992) 'Experiences extended over time: evaluation of moments and episodes', *Journal of Behavioral Decision Making*, 5: 169–85.

Von Neumann, J. and Morgenstern, O. (1947) *Theory of Games and Economic Behavior*, New York: Wiley.

Weber, E.U. (1994) 'From subjective probabilities to decision weights: the effect of asymmetric loss function on the evaluation of uncertain outcomes and events', *Psychological Bulletin*, 115: 228–42.

Whyte, G. (1986) 'Escalating commitment to a course of action: a reinterpretation', *Academy of Management Review*, 11: 311–21.

Chapter 11

The effects of time pressure on human judgement and decision making

A. John Maule and Anne C. Edland

Time is a critical resource in human judgement and decision making. Without sufficient time many activities assumed to underpin good judgement and choice cannot be executed. The present chapter considers how people adapt when time is in short supply, or what we shall refer to as time pressured situations. Recent research indicates that time pressure is a very common feature of professional and personal decision situations (Maule *et al.*, in preparation) and that complaints of insufficient time are the most frequently reported of the everyday minor stressors or hassles by all except the elderly (Chamberlain and Zika, 1990). The primary aim of the present chapter is to review research on the effects of time pressure on the judgement and decision making of individuals in static decision situations (i.e., situations involving a single decision where relevant information is available at the point of choice). Kerstholt and Raaijmakers (Chapter 12) have reviewed decision making in dynamic task environments (i.e., situations involving several decisions taken in the context of a continuously changing environment), so this area will be excluded from the present chapter. Modes of adapting to time constraints are also known to vary systematically across different individuals (e.g., Kaplan *et al.*, 1993; Stiensmeier-Pelster and Schurmann, 1993), and affect decision making in groups (e.g., Janis, 1982), negotiations (Carnevale *et al.*, 1993) and organisations (Bronner, 1972), but these also lie outside the scope of the present chapter.

The present chapter extends an earlier review by Edland and Svenson (1993) of this small but expanding area. This chapter draws on a wider range of studies on time pressure and, in the later sections, presents an integrative perspective for interpreting previous findings and for guiding future research.

THE EFFECTS OF TIME PRESSURE ON CHOICES AND JUDGEMENTS

Time pressure and the quality of judgement and decision making

There appears to be a general assumption that time pressure reduces the quality of decision making. For instance, Isenberg (1984) showed that managers and other professionals judge time pressure to be a major constraint on the quality of their decision making. There has, however, been comparatively little evidence directly evaluating these beliefs. Payne *et al.* (1993, 1995) reviewed a series of their own studies on the effects of time pressure on gambling decisions. Quality was operationalised in terms of the proportion of occasions that respondents chose the alternative with the highest expected value (maximising expected value is commonly assumed to be the basis for rational decision making). They showed that time pressure reduced the quality of decision making and that this reduction varied as a function of the strategy used. Zakay and Wooler (1984) defined quality in a similar way and showed that respondents initially taught to use the optimal expected value decision rule did not actually use this rule when they were subsequently required to make decisions under time pressure. Rouse (1979), in the context of a fault finding task, also showed that time pressure disrupted a previously learned optimal strategy. In his study, time pressured subjects resorted to a 'brute-force' strategy leading to an increase in diagnostic errors. These two studies suggest that knowledge of the optimal rule for non-pressured situations is not sufficient to overcome the disruptive effects of time pressure on the quality of performance.

Rothstein (1986) investigated the effects of time pressure on accuracy in multiple cue probability learning. Judgements made by respondents were compared with the actual or true states, and through feedback they learned to develop a strategy for combining sources of information in order to make accurate judgements. Results indicated a general lowering in the quality of judgement under time pressure, and this was due to a disruption in the implementation of the derived strategy ('cognitive control') rather than a disruption in the learning of the appropriate strategy ('cognitive matching').

Three further studies indicate that the relation between time pressure and accuracy is, however, not as straightforward as suggested by the studies reviewed above. Svenson and Benson (1993a) found that the framing bias was weaker under time pressure. Given that such biases are taken to reflect a lowering of decision accuracy, this finding suggests that time pressured decisions were more accurate. Galotti *et al.* (1986) showed that the imposition of time constraints had a more detrimental effect on the problem solving performance of good as opposed to poor problem solvers. Finally Maule (in preparation) investigated the effects of time pressure on evaluative judgements of job applicants. Each of twenty-one applicants was described in terms of four attributes (e.g., management skill) and each was presented twice. A measure of judgement accuracy was determined in terms of the consistency across these pairs of judgements. For one group, the second set of judgements was made under time pressure. This time pressured group showed the same level of consistency as a control group without any time restriction. There was, however, a significant relationship between the degree of consistency and the mode of adapting to time pressure. In particular, there was less consistency when the primary mode of adapting was based on processing less task relevant information as compared with processing the same amount of information but at a quicker speed. This suggests that the effects of time pressure on accuracy may depend crucially upon mode of adapting.

Finally, Smith *et al.* (1982) and Bockenholt and Kroeger (1993) showed that confidence in the quality of the decision taken declines under time pressure. Smith *et al.* (1982) presented evidence suggesting that this reduction in confidence occurs for two reasons: first, because of the increased use of simpler decision strategies (decision makers would, from experience, know that simpler strategies are associated with lower accuracy); and second, because there is an increased likelihood that there would be insufficient time to implement completely the adopted cognitive strategy (process feedback of this kind is likely to be interpreted as indicating an insufficient decision process).

Overall, the studies reviewed in this section do suggest that time pressure may reduce both the actual quality of judgement and decision making and an individual's confidence in the quality of this activity. This occurs even when individuals have been previously taught the optimal strategy. However, some studies show no effect or even a reverse effect. The evidence strongly suggests that the effects of time pressure on quality depend crucially on the strategy adopted, suggesting the possibility that, in the future, we may be able to assist decision makers by advising them which strategy to use to minimise the detrimental effects of time pressure.

Time pressure and risk preferences

Initially, studies suggested that time pressure induced people to become less risky. Ben-Zur and Breznitz (1981) used a simple two-alternative gambling task to show that time pressured respondents were less likely to choose an option with a low probability of winning a large amount, instead preferring an option with a high probability of winning a small amount. Busemeyer (1993), however, showed that the relationship between time pressure and risk taking is more complex than this. He showed no effect of time pressure on risk taking in a gambling situation when the spread of probabilities was low (i.e., all outcomes had approximately similar likelihoods of occurrence), but changes in risk-taking when the spread was high (i.e., some outcomes were much more likely to occur than others). The nature of these changes varied according to whether the overall expected value (EV) of the gambles was positive or negative. When the EV was positive there was increased risk-taking under time pressure, but when it was negative there was a decrease in risk taking. This may be related to Prospect theory (Kahneman and Tversky, 1979), which states that people put greater weight on losses than on gains. Thus, people subjectively experience losses as more negative than the same amount of gains are experienced as positive. In summary, the findings in this section suggest that although time pressure may influence risk taking, the precise nature of this influence may vary across different decision situations.

Time pressure and polarisation of judgements

Kaplan *et al.* (1993) reported an experiment showing that, under time pressure, judgements of the likeableness of people described in terms of positive or negative traits were less extreme. To explain this finding they argued that time pressure induces a shift in the focus of processing from external to internal sources of information. They draw on research showing that, under time pressure, internal sources of information such as racial and gender stereotypes become more important, and external information in the form of presented person descriptions become less important. Further, Kaplan *et al.* argue that since internal sources are more neutral, time pressured judgements are less extreme. A priority for future research should be to evaluate the extent to which these effects extend to other judgmental situations.

Time pressure and attribute weights

Several studies have investigated the effects of time pressure on attribute importance ratings (see Edland 1993, 1994). The pattern of findings has, however, been rather contradictory. For instance, Svenson *et al.* (1985) asked respondents to judge the attractiveness of apartments described in terms of three attributes. There were two primary effects of time pressure. First, it increased the importance of the negative aspects of the most important attribute (i.e., long travelling time to the university). Thus alternatives with poor aspects on this attribute became much less attractive under time pressure. Second, it led to a general decrease in the attractiveness of all alternatives. However, subsequent work has revealed somewhat different findings. Edland (1993, 1994) used a task requiring participants to choose candidates for a university programme and found that time pressure enhanced the importance of positive information. Edland (1992) suggests that these contradictory findings may be explained by focusing on the goal of the decision. The earlier studies asked participants to choose something for their own purposes (apartments), whereas the later studies for someone else's purposes (university programme). In the former, there is less need to be able to justify the choice to someone else, so the avoidance of negative aspects is more important. In the latter, the perceived need to explain why a candidate was chosen will increase the importance of the positive information. Thus, time pressure may enhance the importance of the most important attribute, which may vary from task to task.

Changes in cognitive strategy under time pressure

A second area of research has focused on the effects of time pressure on the processes underlying judgement and decision making. Research has identified three broad modes of adapting to time pressure. Maule and Hockey (1993) have classified the first two in terms of changes in micro-strategy, since they assume relatively minor modifications in cognitive processing, and the third in terms of changes in macro-strategy, since it involves major changes to the underlying strategy.

Micro-strategy changes

The first type of micro-strategy change, acceleration, involves an increase in the tempo or speed of activity associated with either a faster rate of information processing and/or elimination of pauses, rests and other interruptions in task-related activity. There is evidence showing that acceleration is commonly used to adapt to time pressure (e.g., Benson and Beach, 1996; Ben-Zur and Breznitz, 1981; Maule and Mackie, 1990; Payne *et al.*, 1993). The second micro change, selectivity, involves a reduction in the total amount of information processed and is discussed in two ways. The first of these, filtration, is characterised by a reduction in the proportion of total attribute information that is processed. Filtration occurs selectively, with early research suggesting a high priority given to and thereby relatively less reduction in the processing of negative information (e.g., Wright, 1974). However, more recent research suggests that priority is accorded to important information regardless of whether it is positive or negative (see Edland, 1993). Maule and Mackie (1989), however, found no evidence for filtration. The second way of discussing selectivity, omission, involves neglecting whole categories of information, e.g. completely ignoring one or more attributes across all alternatives. Maule and Mackie (1990) show evidence for omission behaviour in decision making situations.

The evidence strongly indicates that acceleration, filtration and omission are important modes of adapting to time pressure. However, Maule and Hockey (1993) identify three criticisms of the work to date in this area. First, there is a lack of theory to explain when and why particular modes of adapting are adopted. Second, there is no explanation why people implement these modes in different ways (e.g., filtering may occur in favour of negative information or positive information). Third, there has been little attempt to link this work to related areas of cognitive psychology concerned with stress and strategy change.

A rather different description of micro-strategy changes has been developed in the context of Criteria Dependent Choice (CDC) models (Bockenholt and Kroeger, 1993). These models have been developed to explain how people choose in situations involving just two relatively simple choice alternatives. The two alternatives are defined in terms of a number of key attributes, and the choice process based on a series of pairwise comparisons of the alternatives along each attribute, in the order from most to least important. Each comparison results in an attractiveness difference; these differences, in turn, are summed over successive comparisons until the accumulated attractiveness in favour of one alternative exceeds a predetermined criterion. At this point the process stops and the favoured alternative is chosen. The value of the criterion is set by the decision maker at the outset of the process. Bockenholt and Kroeger (1993) argued that people adapt to time pressure by lowering the criterion. This mode of adapting, which can be thought of as a change in micro-strategy, would lead to a reduction in the time needed to make a decision, and reduce the attributes informing choice to those that were relatively important. Further, they argued that, since many of the classic decision rules are readily mimicked by CDC models, the resulting pattern of information acquisition under time pressure is often erroneously interpreted as indicating that people adapt by changing the decision rule (cf. Payne and co-workers reviewed below) rather than the decision criterion. They present experimental data in broad support of their model, but do concede that its applicability is limited to binary choice situations. The extent to which the CDC approach provides a serious challenge to competing theories assuming that people adapt to time pressure by changing decision rules depends upon being able to develop the approach in the context of complex multi-alternative choice situations.

Macro-strategy changes

In their review of the decision strategy literature Ford *et al.* (1989) suggested that time pressure induces a change in strategy involving a switch from compensatory to non-compensatory decision rules and an increased use of attribute-based rather than alternative-based processing.

These changes in strategy have been explained in the context of contingency theories of strategy selection (e.g., Beach and Mitchell, 1978). Decision makers are assumed to have a repertoire of decision rules and, in a particular situation, adopt one or more of these on the basis of a cost–benefit analysis. Costs are associated with the resources necessary to implement the strategy, involving both internal resources (e.g., energetic resources to meet workload demands) and external resources (e.g., finance). Benefits are associated with the value accruing to the decision maker if the strategy is adopted. It is assumed that for every decision situation there will be a strategy which optimises the cost–benefit calculations. For example, a decision that is important with relatively high potential benefits for the decision maker will justify the use of a relatively complex strategy involving a high resource budget.

The imposition of a time constraint is assumed to change the cost–benefit analysis, leading to a change in strategy. For instance, the value of a strategy may change because there is now insufficient time to implement it fully. Payne *et al.* (1995) showed that under time pressure it is optimal to use simpler strategies involving a basic search and evaluation of some of the relevant information about each alternative, focusing, in the first instance, on more important attribute information. This ensures that, at the point of choice, there is some information about each alternative to base the decision on, and this information is relatively important. Alternatively, time pressure may increase costs. For example, time pressured decision makers may accelerate information processing in order to implement a preferred strategy within the deadline. This increased speed of processing would be expected to increase costs in terms of workload demands.

In both examples described above, time pressure induces a decrease in the relative value of high-information load, time-consuming compensatory strategies and an increase in the relative value of simpler, less time-consuming non-compensatory strategies (Christensen-Szalanski, 1980). An important feature of this approach is that time is treated as a task characteristic similar in kind to other characteristics such as the number of alternatives or attributes. Though the term 'time pressure' is used, this approach ignores the possibility that time pressure may be associated with a change in affective state which may, in itself, change the nature of the decision process and its quality.

Combination of micro and macro approaches

Payne and his co-workers have further developed the cost–benefit approach in a series of studies which consider changes in cognitive strategy at both the micro and macro levels (for a review see Payne *et al.*, 1993, 1995). They identified a set of elementary information processes (EIPs) necessary to execute decision strategies (e.g., reading a particular item of information, or comparing two items of information). Then they identified the type and order of EIPs necessary to implement particular compensatory and non-compensatory strategies in a simple gambling task. They also identified the costs and benefits of utilising each strategy in the task. Costs were defined in terms of the workload associated with resourcing the EIPs necessary to implement the strategy (assessed in a number of different ways, the simplest of which was a count of the number of EIPs needed to implement the strategy). The benefits were assessed in terms of the accuracy of the strategy, where accuracy was calculated by deriving the proportion of occasions that the adoption of the strategy led to a choice of the alternative with the highest expected value (EV).

In a series of studies, based on both experiments and computer simulations, Payne and his associates showed that time pressure induced a general decrease in decision accuracy (i.e., benefits). This occurred regardless of the decision strategy adopted. The simulation work showed that compensatory strategies consistently led to a greater reduction in accuracy than non-compensatory strategies. Indeed, across different variants of the gambling task, the greatest accuracy under time pressure was always achieved by one of the simpler non-compensatory strategies. As indicated above, the relatively high accuracy of non-compensatory strategies is due to the fact that these strategies ensure that some information about every alternative (usually important information) is available at the point of choice. The experimental findings revealed that people first tried to adapt to time pressure by means of acceleration, without any change in decision strategy. If this was insufficient to meet the demands of the time constraint, then more radical changes were adopted involving an increased use of non-compensatory strategies. People showed a strong propensity to switch to the particular non-compensatory strategy that the simulation indicated was of greatest accuracy in that situation. This suggests that their strategy change was essentially adaptive.

In a recent study Payne *et al.* (1996) provided further evidence for their effort/accuracy approach, in a situation where time stress was due to the opportunity cost of delaying decisions, and where task goals emphasised either accuracy or saving effort. They showed that experimental participants were generally adaptive to opportunity-cost time pressure, processing less information, being more selective and processing more by attribute. In addition, when the task goals emphasised choice accuracy, time pressured participants received a lower expected payoff than when the goals emphasised savings in effort. It was suggested that this rather paradoxical finding was due to the fact that the greater emphasis on task goals would increase the value assumed to accrue from the use of more complex compensatory strategies. Since these are not appropriate in time pressured situations, the emphasis on task goals would lead to non-adaptive changes in underlying decision strategy.

Work undertaken by Payne and his associates over the last ten years has considerably enhanced our understanding of the effects of time pressure on decision making. There are, however, three important limitations to this work. First, similar to the contingency theory of Beach and Mitchell considered earlier, the approach is essentially 'cold'. Time pressure is conceptualised as a task characteristic which, when varied, leads to changes in cognitive strategy mediated by effort/accuracy calculations. However, time pressure may also be conceptualised as a stressor which induces changes in emotional and bodily states. These changes in state are known to affect the nature of cognition and, therefore, are likely to be an important factor determining how people adapt to time pressure. In a recent discussion, Payne *et al.* (1995) have highlighted the importance of including affect in the model, but provide no suggestions about how this should be achieved. There is a need to develop a theoretical approach which incorporates both conceptualisations of time pressure. Second, effort has been evaluated in terms of the number of operations needed to complete a task, neglecting important person-related factors such as the individual's current energetic state (e.g., a state of tiredness as compared with an energised state). These different states will crucially affect the effort needed to implement a strategy, and thereby change the effort/accuracy calculations assumed to underlie strategy determination. This is likely to be a particularly important factor in time pressure situations, since stressors are known to change energetic states (Hockey, 1986). Finally, the model assumes a single evaluation of costs and benefits early on in a decision process, leading to the adoption and implementation of particular decision strategy. Contemporary stress theory strongly suggests that the cost and benefits of particular actions are continuously monitored throughout a task and actions modified when this is appraised as necessary (e.g., Hockey, 1986). Theories of time pressure on decision making need to incorporate these more dynamic aspects of appraisal and strategy determination. In the next section we review a recent approach which takes account of these criticisms, and evaluate it in the context of some recent empirical findings.

Variable State Activation Theory: an integrative approach

Maule and Hockey (1993) suggest that a focus simply on micro and macro changes under time pressure may be too narrow an approach. They present a different theoretical scheme which identifies a much broader set of issues for research in this area. The new scheme, Variable State Activation Theory, has its roots in stress theory. At the heart of this scheme is the view that stressors like time pressure should not be seen as external forces which act upon a passive organism. Rather, in the face of stressors, people are much more active, appraising the situation that they confront and the extent to which they have resources to meet the demands of the situation (Lazarus and Folkman, 1984). A situation which is potentially damaging to an individual will not be stressful if the individual appraises that he/she has resources to cope with the threat. Of central importance to this approach is an appraisal mechanism reflecting the individual's interpretation of the demands of the situation and the extent to which he/she has resources to cope with these demands. If the appraisal indicates that the individual has the resources to cope, then these coping responses are initiated. If the appraisal suggests that the individual is unable to cope, then he/she is likely to show the symptoms of stress manifested at one or more of the physiological, psychological and behavioural levels.

Hockey (1986) used this general approach and developed it in the more specific context of the effects of stress on cognition. He argued that the cognitive system is essentially self-regulatory. The system appraises and adapts to demands, where possible, by means of familiar and routine control mechanisms which are both automatic and associated with a low cognitive cost. Thus, relatively minor changes in speed, timing and memory use occur automatically to meet small changes in demands associated with the task in hand. Demands outside the normal range signal the need for a different mode of control involving supervisory control. This form of control is associated with high levels of cognitive effort, planning and conscious evaluation of goals. In applying this approach to time pressure, Maule and Hockey (1993) argue that, in most instances, time pressure is likely to involve demands that lie outside the normal operating range and thereby involve supervisory control. They identify four modes of supervisory control relevant to time pressured situations.

The first mode involves changes in cognitive state associated with increased effort (i.e., trying harder). In the context of time pressure this involves acceleration. There will be an upper limit to this mode set by the system's maximum speed of operation. Also, this strategy is very costly and is only likely to be employed when the task is important and the period over which this mode is to be employed is short (it is not possible to sustain increased effort over long periods). The second mode involves a reappraisal of task goals so as to reduce the demands placed on the system. In an extreme form this might involve an unwillingness to engage in the task situation at all or, more normally, a lowering of task goals justifying simpler cognitive strategies that can be implemented in the time allowed. Filtration and the switch from compensatory to non-compensatory strategies are consistent with this mode of supervisory control. The third mode involves changing or eliminating the stressor at source, which, in the context of time pressure, might involve renegotiating the deadline or seeking agreement that less is to be undertaken in the time allowed. The final mode involves doing nothing, either because of a lack of involvement on the part of the decision maker or because none of the other modes is appraised as effective. In the latter case a situation may occur where the decision is so important that task goals cannot be reduced, the demands far exceed the maximum cognitive effort available and the deadline is both fixed and strict. These circumstances would lead to extreme states such as panic (Janis and Mann, 1977). Each mode is associated with costs and benefits of implementation and, similar to the effort/accuracy models considered above, an evaluation of these costs and benefits provides the basis for choosing between them (Schonpflug and Battman, 1988).

Maule and Hockey (1993) argued that task demands are continuously monitored, with the possibility that modifications to control activity may be necessary at any point in time during a decision process. This is in contrast with the predominant view in decision research, which has tended to assume that the imposition of time pressure induces a change in strategy which is then implemented without modifications.

Two recent studies provide support for one important aspect of the model – the crucial role of appraisal in mediating time pressure effect (Svenson and Benson, 1993b; Maule and Maillet-Hausswirth, 1995). In the Svenson and Benson study two groups were given the same amount of time to make a decision. However, one group was told that the time available was more than enough and the other group was told that the time was inadequate. The behaviour of the first group was similar to what would be expected if they were time pressured, whereas the behaviour of the second group gave no indication of time pressure. These findings suggest that the different instructions led people to appraise task demands differently, leading them to mobilise cognitive effort to different degrees. Maule and Maillet-Hausswirth (1995) gave different groups of participants either half or double the amount of time usually taken to solve a simple everyday risk problem. Each of these groups were further subdivided into those instructed that the time was insufficient and those told it was sufficient (this was assumed to influence the appraisal process). Results indicated that instructions about sufficiency were much more important than actual time in determining how people adapted to time pressure in this situation. Both studies suggest that it is not the actual amount of time but the individual's appraisal of it that is critical in determining underlying cognitive strategy. VSAT is still in an early stage of development and there is a need for further research to test and extend the theory and to link it more closely to the findings and approaches discussed earlier.

METHODOLOGICAL ISSUES

The studies of time pressure reviewed above have adopted rather similar procedures for inducing time pressure. This procedure has involved establishing the average time taken by a group without any time restriction, reducing this by a fixed percentage, and then using this as the deadline for a time pressured group. There are four important problems with this approach. First, the procedure makes no allowance for differences between respondents in terms of the amount of time they normally take to complete the task when no restrictions are in operation. Thus, respondents who normally require a short time to make a decision may be less pressured. Second, we argued earlier that appraisal plays a crucial role in determining how people adapt to time pressure. That is, it is not the actual amount of time that is critical, but how this is appraised and the extent to which an individual has the appropriate resources to meet the time demands. Thus, a particular deadline may be appraised differently, thereby inducing very different states in individuals under the same time pressure conditions.

Third, the approach assumes there are just two states, 'normal' or 'time pressured'. However, this view may be too simplistic. For instance, there may be states of mild time pressure, associated with an increased urgency and a facilitation of action. In this state, decision makers may judge that they can cope with the situation and execute an appropriate action within the time allowed. The pressure may be beneficial in that it provides the extra urgency necessary to initiate an important activity. Freedman and Edwards (1988) suggest that time pressure may even increase the satisfaction associated with a task by making it more challenging and thereby more pleasurable. Mild time pressure may be contrasted with more extreme states which we would label time stress, associated with negative feelings and general disruptions to behaviour. As indicated above, VSAT suggests that these are likely to occur when the task is important and there are no appropriate control activities available to meet the time demands. There is a need for future research to identify and describe the different states that may be induced as time to make a decision is reduced. Finally, all studies to date have introduced the deadline at the beginning of an experimental session. This represents only one of many different ways in which time pressure occurs in the world. For instance, distant deadlines often appear to offer no threat at the outset, and only induce states of time pressure as they become more imminent and the amount of work to be completed is appraised as too much for the time available. On other occasions, the deadline only emerges half-way through the process, or in the context of managing a large number of other activities within a specified time period. Future research needs to identify the different ways in which time pressure is induced and whether these are associated with different modes of adapting.

The issues discussed above highlight the importance of identifying and describing time pressured states from the perspective of the decision maker, rather than assuming that a fixed deadline induces the same time pressured state in all respondents. In addition, they suggest we need to broaden the ways in which we investigate how restrictions in the amount of time affects judgement and decision making.

CONCLUDING REMARKS

The research reviewed in this chapter suggests that time pressure may change the nature of individual judgement and decision making by: (i) reducing the quality of these activities, (ii) changing the underlying risk-taking propensities, (iii) increasing the importance of internal sources of information at the expense of external sources, (iv) inducing changes in underlying cognitive processing based on some combination of acceleration, filtration, omission, changes in underlying decision rule and an increased use of attribute-based processing, (v) increasing the relative importance of different information sources, (vi) changing the relative importance of positive and negative sources of information, (vii) reducing the overall attractiveness of alternatives. However, the evidence indicates that these changes do not always occur, and that they may depend upon how the decision maker appraises the situation, the nature of the state induced (e.g., time pressure, time stress), the task structure and overall task goals.

The present review has highlighted some important issues critical both to an understanding of the extant research and for the development of future research in this area. First, we have demonstrated the importance of an appraisal process in mediating time pressure effects. An implication of this is that time pressure needs to be defined from the decision maker's perspective. Second, we suggested that appraisal occurs continuously over a decision making process rather than just once at the outset of the process, as implied by the effort/accuracy theories. This has implications not only for theories explaining how people adapt in time pressured situations, but also for theories of how strategies are determined in non-pressured situations as well. In particular, our approach assumes that appraisal underlies strategy determination in all decision situations and may, at any time over a decision process, signal the need to modify current strategy. This implies that the initiation and control of strategy should be described, at least in part, in terms of small-scale process sequences initiated in response to local changes in perceived demands.

Third, we have argued that reductions in the amount of time available to make a decision may induce a number of different states, differentiated in terms of both physiological and psychological factors. On the one hand, the imposition of a deadline may be appraised positively if decision makers believe they have the resources necessary to meet the challenge and are able to attain task goals. On the other hand, the deadline may be so stringent or the task so important that decision makers may judge that they do not have the resources to meet the demands of the situation. Under these circumstances negative emotional states may be induced associated with lack of control and failure. A major priority for future research is to identify and describe these different states.

ACKNOWLEDGEMENT

The authors wish to thank the Swedish Work Environment Fund, Professor Ola Svenson and another anonymous reviewer for their helpful comments.

REFERENCES

Beach, L.R. and Mitchell, T.R. (1978) 'A contingency model for the selection of decision strategies', *Academy of Management Journal*, 3: 439–49.

Benson, L. and Beach, L.R. (1996) 'The effects of time constraints on the prechoice screening of decision options', *Organizational Behavior of Human Decision Processes*, 67: 222–8.

Ben-Zur, H. and Breznitz, S.J. (1981) 'The effects of time pressure on risky choice behaviour', *Acta Psychologica*, 47: 89–104.

Bockenholt, U. and Kroeger, K. (1993) 'The effects of time pressure in multiattribute binary choice tasks', in O. Svenson and A.J. Maule (eds) *Time Pressure and Stress in Human Judgment and Decision Making*, New York: Plenum.

Bronner, R. (1972) *Decision Making under Time Pressure*, Lexington, MA: Lexington Books.

Busemeyer, J.R. (1993) 'Violations of the speed–accuracy tradeoff relation: decreases in decision accuracy with increases in decision time', in O. Svenson and A.J. Maule (eds) *Time Pressure and Stress in Human Judgment and Decision Making*. New York: Plenum.

Carnevale, P.J., O'Connor K.M. and McCusker, C. (1993) 'Time pressure in negotiation and mediation', in O. Svenson and A.J. Maule (eds) *Time Pressure and Stress in Human Judgment and Decision Making*, New York: Plenum.

Chamberlain, K. and Zika, S. (1990) 'The minor events approach to stress: support for the use of daily hassles', *British Journal of Psychology*, 81: 469–81.

Christensen-Szalanski, J.J.J. (1980) 'A further examination of the selection of problem-solving strategies: the effects of deadlines and analytic aptitudes', *Organizational Behaviour and Human Performance*, 25: 107–22.

Edland, A.C. (1992) 'Effects of time pressure on human judgement and decision making', Doctoral dissertation, Stockholm: Akademitryck.

Edland, A.C. (1993) 'The effects of time pressure on choices and judgements of candidates to a university programme', in O. Svenson and A.J. Maule (eds) *Time Pressure and Stress in Human Judgment and Decision Making*, New York: Plenum.

Edland, A.C. (1994) 'Time pressure and the application of decision rules', *Scandinavian Journal of Psychology*, 35: 281–91.

Edland, A.C. and Svenson, O. (1993) 'Judgement and decision making under time pressure: studies and findings', in O. Svenson and A. J. Maule (eds) *Time Pressure and Stress in Human Judgment and Decision Making*, New York: Plenum.

Ford, J.K., Schmitt, N., Schechtman, S.L., Hults, B.M. and Doherty, M.L. (1989) 'Process tracing methods: contributions, problems, and neglected research questions', *Organizational Behavior and Human Decision Processes*, 43: 75–117.

Freedman, J.L. and Edwards, D.R. (1988) 'Time pressure, task performance and enjoyment', in J.E. McGrath (ed.) *The Social Psychology of Time*, London: Sage.

Galotti, K.M., Baron, J. and Sabini, J.P. (1986) 'Individual differences in syllogistic reasoning: deduction rules or mental models', *Journal of Experimental Psychology: General*, 115: 16–25.

Hockey, G.R.J. (1986) 'A state control theory of adaptation and individual differences in stress management', in G.R.J. Hockey, A.W.K. Gaillard and M.G.H. Coles (eds) *Energetics and Human Information Processing*, Dordrecht: Martinus Nijhoff.

Isenberg, D.J. (1984) 'How senior managers think', *Harvard Business Review*, November/December, 81–90.

Janis, I.L. (1982) *Stress, Attitudes and Decision*, New York: Praeger.

Janis, I.L. and Mann, L. (1977) *Decision Making: A Psychological Analysis of Conflict, Choice and Commitment*, New York: Free Press.

Kahneman, D. and Tversky, A. (1979) 'Prospect theory: an analysis of decision under risk', *Econometrica*, 47: 263–91.

Kaplan, M.F., Wanshula, L.T. and Zanna, M.P. (1993) 'Time pressure and information integration in social judgment', in O. Svenson and A.J. Maule (eds) *Time Pressure and Stress in Human Judgment and Decision Making*, New York: Plenum.

Lazarus, R. and Folkman, S. (1984) *Stress, Appraisal and Coping*, New York: Springer.

Maule, A.J. (in preparation) 'Modes of adapting to time pressure: the relation between strategy and accuracy'.

Maule, A.J. and Hockey, G.R.J. (1993) 'State, stress and time pressure', in O. Svenson and A.J. Maule (eds) *Time Pressure and Stress in Human Judgment and Decision Making*, New York: Plenum.

Maule, A.J. and Mackie, P.M. (1989) 'The harassed decision maker revisited', Paper presented at the Third Symposium on Thinking, Aberdeen.

Maule, A.J. and Mackie, P.M. (1990) 'A componential investigation of the effects of deadlines on individual decision making', in K. Borcherding, O.I. Larichev and D.M. Messick (eds) *Contemporary Issues in Decision Making*, Amsterdam: North-Holland.

Maule, A.J. and Maillet-Hausswirth, P. (1995) 'The mediating effects of subjective appraisal, cognitive control and changes in affect in determining the effects of time pressure on risk-taking', Paper presented at the 15th Research Conference on Subjective Probability, Utility and Decision Making (SPUDM15), Jerusalem, August.

Maule, A.J., Pearman, A.D. and Durstone, C. (in preparation) *Taxonomies of Individual Decision Making*.

Payne, J.W., Bettman. J.R. and Johnson, E.J. (1993) *The Adaptive Decision Maker*, Cambridge: Cambridge University Press.

Payne, J.W., Bettman, J.R., Johnson, E.J. and Luce, M.F. (1995) 'An information processing perspective on choice', in J. Busemeyer, R. Hastie and D. L. Medin (eds) *Decision Making from a Cognitive Perspective*, New York: Academic Press.

Payne, J.W., Bettman, J.R. and Luce, M.F. (1996) 'When time is money: decision behavior under opportunity–cost time pressure', *Organizational Behavior and Human Decision Processes*, 66: 131–52.

Rothstein, H.G. (1986) 'The effects of time pressure on judgement in multiple cue probability learning', *Organisational Behavior and Human Decision Processes*, 37: 83–92.

Rouse, W. (1979) 'Problem solving performance of maintenance trainees in a fault diagnosis task', *Human Factors*, 21: 195–203.

Schonpflug, W. and Battman, W. (1988) 'The costs and benefits of coping', in S. Fisher and J. Reason (eds) *Handbook of Life Stress, Cognition and Health*, Chichester: Wiley.

Smith, J.F., Mitchell, T.R. and Beach, L.R. (1982) 'A cost benefit mechanism for selecting problem solving strategies: some extensions and empirical tests', *Organizational Behavior and Human Performance*, 29: 370–96.

Stiensmeier-Pelster, J. and Schurmann, M. (1993) 'Information processing in decision making under time pressure: the influence of action versus state orientation', in O. Svenson and A.J. Maule (eds) *Time Pressure and Stress in Human Judgment and Decision Making*, New York: Plenum.

Svenson, O. and Benson, L. (1993a) 'Framing and time pressure in decision making', in O. Svenson and A.J. Maule (eds) *Time Pressure and Stress in Human Judgement and Decision Making*, New York: Plenum.

Svenson, O. and Benson, L. (1993b) 'On experimental instructions and the inducement of time pressure behavior', in O. Svenson and A. J. Maule (eds) *Time Pressure and Stress in Human Judgment and Decision Making*, New York: Plenum.

Svenson, O., Edland, A.C. and Karlsson, G. (1985) 'The effect of numerical and verbal information and time stress on judgments of the attractiveness of decision alternatives', in L.B. Methlie and R. Sprague (eds) *Knowledge Representation for Decision Support Systems*, Amsterdam: North-Holland.

Wright, P.L. (1974) 'The harassed decision maker: time pressures, distractions and the use of evidence', *Journal of Applied Psychology*, 59: 555–61.

Zakay, D. and Wooler, S. (1984) 'Time pressure, training and decision effectiveness', *Ergonomics*, 27: 273–84.

Chapter 12

Decision making in dynamic task environments

José H. Kerstholt and Jeroen G.W. Raaijmakers

Two decades of process tracing studies have provided one robust conclusion: there is no generally used strategy for a particular choice problem, but the selected strategy is highly contingent upon various task and context factors, such as complexity or time pressure (see, for a review, Ford *et al.*, 1989). Recently, Payne *et al.* (1993) added a further dimension to this conclusion by suggesting that strategy selection is not only contingent but also highly adaptive. They based their conclusion on a comparison of the strategies that subjects selected in various task contexts and the outcomes of simulations in which both effort and accuracy were taken into account. Generally, subjects appeared to select a decision strategy that saves considerable effort at the expense of only a small decline in accuracy.

The conclusion that decision making is quite adaptive is based solely on static decision tasks. Many real-world decision tasks, however, are dynamic in nature, which means that the decision context changes over time. When fire-fighters are controlling a fire, when an operator is trying to find a fault in a production process, or when a physician is diagnosing a disease, decisions must be made in an inherently unstable environment. In such situations the system (the fire, the production process or the patient) changes over time, a factor the decision maker has to take into consideration.

How well do people perform in dynamic tasks? In order to provide a tentative answer to this question we will present an overview of the main findings in dynamic decision making research. First, however, we will describe the characteristics of dynamic task environments.

CHARACTERISTICS OF DYNAMIC TASKS

The following characteristics of dynamic tasks, which are most often mentioned in studies on dynamic decision making, were provided by Edwards (1962: 60): 'The environment in which the decision is set may be changing, either as a function of the sequence of decisions, or independently of them, or both.' More recently, Brehmer (1992) included an additional aspect, namely that decisions need to be made in real time.

This factor added an extra dimension to dynamic decision making, as the decision maker has to consider the dimension of time explicitly. It is not enough to know *what* should be done but also *when* it should be done. Taken together, in dynamic tasks individuals typically control a changing system, they receive feedback about the state of the system and they need to make a sequence of decisions.

Change over time

Dynamic decision situations change over time. A fire spreads and a patient's health deteriorates, but these developments may be corrected by the actions of the decision maker. The main effect of the changing nature of dynamic tasks is that the time dimension has to be taken into account explicitly. In continuously evolving situations, decision makers constantly have to decide when to intervene in the system under control, which also implies that time pressure can result when they wait too long before their intervention. In contrast to static tasks, time pressure in dynamic environments is defined by the changing situation itself (for a review of studies on time pressure in static tasks, see Edland and Svenson (1993), and this volume, Chapter 11). A process operator, for example, will experience more time pressure when the performance of the system under control deteriorates rapidly. Thus, decision makers need to relate system changes to the timing of their own actions.

Availability of feedback

Feedback is one of the most crucial features of dynamic decision tasks. In general, the decision maker will have an overall indication of the state of the system, such as an alarm or the complaints of a patient. An overall performance decline provides the decision maker with a cue that something needs to be done. Furthermore, if actions have been applied, the overall system state can also be used to test whether the action was accurate, i.e., had the desired effect on system performance. In contrast with static tasks, decision makers can, therefore, use feedback to adjust system performance incrementally: they may take small steps at a time and select other actions as soon as the development of the system's performance is not in the required direction (Hogarth, 1981). In this regard, Kleinmuntz (1985) made a distinction between action-oriented strategies and judgement-oriented strategies. When action-oriented strategies are used, subjects just apply actions, observe their effect on the system under control and proceed depending on the observed effect. When judgement-oriented strategies are used, on the other hand, decision makers first try to reduce their uncertainty with regard to the cause underlying performance deterioration by requesting information.

Need to make several (interdependent) decisions

Dynamic situations require multiple decisions, and these decisions affect the system under control. In predicting a future system state the decision maker therefore has to take both the autonomous system developments and the effects of his or her own actions into account. As noted by Huber (1990), one central factor in dealing with such a task is the quality of the mental representation of the system under control. The decision maker needs to have an accurate model of the relations between all system parameters and their temporal characteristics. This facilitates a mental simulation of the system's behaviour and consequently increases anticipation of future outcomes. In control theoretical terms, the possibility of predicting a future system state allows for feedforward control. Whereas feedforward control involves choosing actions on the basis of predictions of the future state of the system, feedback control involves choosing actions on the basis of information about the current system state.

Experimental tasks

These abstract characteristics of dynamic tasks have been translated into a wide range of control environments such as simulated economies (Sterman, 1989), tribes or towns (Dörner, 1987), fire fighting (Brehmer, 1990, 1992) and medical diagnosis (Kleinmuntz and Thomas, 1987). Dependent on the specific research question, the dynamic task features mentioned above are more or less implemented in the experimental task. In most experiments, for example, time has been sliced up into discrete units, and the problems have been presented to the subjects in terms of a series of trials (for example, Dörner, 1987; Kleinmuntz and Thomas, 1987; Mackinnon and Wearing, 1985; Sterman, 1989). After subjects have chosen an action, they are presented with the next system state that reflects both the effect of their action and possible autonomous system developments. Brehmer (1990, 1992) and Kerstholt (1994a, 1995), on the other hand, used a real-time simulation. In such a situation the system changes continuously and there is only limited time to think about the most optimal actions. In Brehmer's task, for example, subjects had to extinguish a developing forest fire by sending out fire fighting units to specific locations in the forest. Whenever new events happened, such as when a fire spread in an unexpected direction or when a new fire started, the subjects had to redeploy their forces.

In addition to the specific task characteristics, dynamic laboratory tasks also differ with regard to their complexity. Most researchers have designed dynamic experimental tasks that are relatively complex. Participants have to take many system parameters into account, and the mutual dependencies between these variables and their dynamic developments are opaque. Because of this confounding between system dynamics and complexity it is indeed questionable to what extent the results of these studies increase our knowledge of dynamic decision making processes in general (Hunt, 1991). In the present chapter we will therefore limit ourselves to experimental studies that focused on dynamic decision making behaviour, rather than complexity as such.

MAIN FINDINGS FROM DYNAMIC DECISION MAKING RESEARCH

In the previous section we mentioned three characteristics of dynamic decision tasks: change over time, availability of feedback and the need to make several (independent) decisions. With regard to change over time, it is important to know when to intervene with the system under control (*timing*), which is, in turn, related to the time that is reserved for diagnosis (*strategy selection*). With regard to the availability of feedback most research has focused on how well people deal with delays (*perception of feedback*). If several decisions need to be made it is important to maintain an accurate mental representation of the system under control. The main findings with regard to this aspect of dynamic decision tasks will be presented in the last section, *information selection over time.*

Timing

One of the main requirements in evolving situations is to relate one's own timing of actions to system evolutions (De Keyser, 1990). Kerstholt (1994a, 1995) investigated the moment subjects started to intervene with the system under uncertain, changing system conditions as a function of the rate of system change. From normative models of the experimental task it could be deduced that the moment of intervention should be adjusted to the time left, that is, the higher the rate of change the earlier one should start with intervention. This is not what was observed. As a matter of fact, subjects based the moment of intervention only upon the current system state and did not take the rate of change into account. As a consequence less time remained for corrective actions if the system rapidly deteriorated, resulting in decreased performance. In another experiment it was found that subjects did adapt the moment of intervention to variations in false alarm rate (Kerstholt, 1995). When the probability increased that a system decline was due to a false alarm, subjects postponed intervention until a later time. In this situation, however, subjects should have intervened at the same system level, i.e., independent of the exact false alarm rate subjects should intervene at the latest point in time that still allowed for system recovery. Even though only a little research has been carried out, the results suggest that people are not very good at selecting the right time for intervention.

In order to time actions accurately it is necessary to have an understanding of the dynamics of the system in relation to one's own time use. In many situations people may have learned from experience when to start with a control action for a particular dynamic system. For example, river pilots know from experience when to start altering course, taking the response delay into account (Schraagen, 1994). By learning input–output relations they may anticipate a future system state. However, in many situations a person may not be able to learn these input–output relations simply because of the uniqueness of the situation he or she has to deal with. This is, for example, the case in modern technological environments where multiple systems have to be supervised and where intervention is only required in sporadically occurring, critical situations. Because of system dependencies, the fault may be propagated through the system while one is working on one particular disturbance. Research has indicated that people have a tendency to deal with multiple problems sequentially. This phenomenon was termed 'cognitive lockup' by Moray and Rotenberg (1989). From their experiment it was not clear, however, whether this tendency was also suboptimal; that is, would subjects have performed more accurately with a different problem solving strategy? In order to shed more light on this topic, Kerstholt *et al.* (1996) conducted an experiment in which subjects were required to supervise four dynamic subsystems and to deal with disturbances whenever they occurred. However, the task was designed in such a way that suboptimal performance would be attained if subjects were to deal with the problems sequentially. The results showed that there were rather large differences in performance. Some subjects performed very accurately, whereas others could not solve the problems within the time constraint. One factor that underlay this difference in performance supported the cognitive lockup phenomenon. Many subjects handled the disturbances strictly sequentially and they consistently ignored auditory alarms that signalled additional disturbances. Subjects who performed accurately, on the other hand, were aware of the dynamic developments of the system. They reacted to an auditory alarm by temporarily disrupting their diagnosis process to stabilise the additional disturbed system first, thereby acknowledging their understanding of the development of a disturbance over time. However, with a training curriculum that provided subjects with the opportunity to build up an accurate mental representation of the dependencies between the various systems, overall performance could be significantly improved (Kerstholt and Passenier, 1995).

Taken together, the results indicate that accurate timing behaviour requires extensive knowledge about the causal and temporal relations between system components. In addition to being able to anticipate dependent system reactions, it is important to relate system developments to one's own use of time.

Strategy selection

Studies that specifically investigated how time is divided between diagnosis and action indicated that individuals prefer a judgement-oriented strategy. Before applying an action, they first search for information that reduces their uncertainty concerning the cause underlying a decrease in system performance (Hogarth and Makridakis, 1981; Kerstholt, 1994a, 1995; Kleinmuntz and Thomas, 1987). In the studies by Kerstholt and by Kleinmuntz and Thomas the optimal decision strategy under various task conditions had been defined and subjects' strategies could therefore be compared to these optimal rules. It turned out that subjects also chose a judgement-oriented strategy in situations where an action-oriented strategy would have led to optimal performance, which suggests that subjects perform more poorly in selecting an appropriate strategy in dynamic tasks than in static tasks (e.g., Ford *et al.*, 1989; Payne *et al.*, 1993). They did not select the strategy that would lead to a better outcome *and* would avoid the effortful information processing phase.

How can we explain this tendency to select the suboptimal, judgement-oriented strategy? One necessary condition for adaptive behaviour is that people should have had the opportunity to learn the relations between strategy and outcome. Plausibly, subjects *a priori* believe that a judgement-oriented strategy (first think, then act) is a better strategy than an action-oriented strategy. If they do not have the opportunity to learn the relations between strategy use and outcome, it seems logical that they would select a judgement-oriented strategy. In order to explore this possibility Kerstholt (1994b) analysed strategy selection under two different practice conditions, a minimal and an extensive practice condition. It turned out that practice did not affect strategy selection. In both practice conditions judgement-oriented strategies were used in the same proportion of trials. In a related study, however, Kerstholt (1996) found that subjects could be induced to switch to an action-oriented strategy. When the costs of information were relatively low, subjects predominantly used a judgement-oriented strategy, but when the costs of information were relatively high, they predominantly used an action-oriented strategy. On the one hand, this shows that subjects were not obliviously engaged in information search and were capable of adjusting their strategy to changes in the cost structure. On the other hand, because their strategy was suboptimal in at least some task conditions, they were apparently not responsive to all relevant task variables.

In the context of her experimental task, Kerstholt (1996) mentioned two additional factors that might determine the superior outcome of action-oriented strategies and to which subjects may be less sensitive. The first one is the relation between the diagnostic value of information and its costs. The relative benefits of information decrease as the costs of information increase. Probably subjects were not aware of this relationship, and concentrated only on the explicit costs of the information and not on its diagnostic value. Surely this problem is not unique to dynamic tasks. Indeed, various studies with static tasks also indicate the difficulties people have in selecting information before making a choice (Connolly, 1988). The second factor is unique to dynamic tasks and concerns the time dimension. A judgement-oriented strategy implies that an action is preceded by an information search phase and, as requesting information takes time, one should start earlier with intervention. In systems that may spontaneously recover, however, this means that the proportion of unnecessary interventions also increases and, as a result, performance deteriorates. Subjects may not have realised that this temporal aspect of a judgement-oriented strategy can reduce its net effect. This last explanation was also put forward by Hogarth and Makridakis (1981). In their experiment, various teams were required to control a number of firms in a dynamic, competitive environment. It turned out that, even though the human teams were engaged in elaborate planning sessions, they were often outperformed by simulated teams that were just carrying out random actions. Because the environment was extremely dynamic and affected by numerous components, not under the influence of the subjects, the future could not easily be predicted. In other words, the time spent on the team's own strategic activities was not tuned to the dynamic development of the systems under control.

As far as strategy selection is concerned, the results therefore indicate that people are not sensitive to all task parameters in selecting the optimal strategy. Even though they do take more superficial factors such as the costs of information and actions into account, they may be less sensitive to the diagnostic value of the information and to the time dimension.

Perception of feedback

A major result from dynamic decision making research is that suboptimal performance often results from misperceptions of feedback (Brehmer, 1992; Diehl and Sterman, 1995; Kleinmuntz, 1993; Sterman, 1989). Performance is particularly affected when the decision maker receives delayed rather than immediate feedback. In Brehmer's fire fighting task, for example, it was found that a larger area of forest burned down when subjects had to take delays in reports from fire fighters into account (Brehmer, 1990). Recently, Diehl and Sterman (1995) varied feedback delay more systematically and they also concluded that subjects largely ignored time delays and were insensitive to feedback structure. Sterman (1989) tried to simulate the behaviour of his subjects in a stock management task in order to extract the main differences between subjects' decision behaviour and the structure of the environment. It appeared that subjects' behaviour could be well simulated by a simple 'hill-climbing' heuristic. According to such a rule the actions are based on only the locally available information. Taken together, the results suggest that people ignore delays in feedback, and react as if information informs them about the current state of affairs (Brehmer, 1990; Diehl and Sterman, 1995; Sterman, 1989). When they are faced with delays, subjects do not switch from feedback control to feedforward control, i.e., they do not base their actions on a prediction of a future system state. However, with feedback control, subjects are always too late with their actions as they base their actions upon an earlier system state.

Even though it has been consistently shown that individuals do not take feedback structures sufficiently into account, there is only limited understanding of the nature and the origin of these misperceptions of feedback (Kleinmuntz, 1993). Why is it so difficult to build up mental models that involve feedback delays?

One possibility is that subjects simply forget to take the delays into account, or are not aware of the presence of feedback delays. In Brehmer's fire fighting task, for example, subjects could infer a delay from the time information on their computer screen, but they were not explicitly informed about it (Brehmer, 1990). Another possibility is that people have not had enough opportunities to build up a representation of the temporal relations between system parameters. In order to interpret delayed feedback accurately, decision makers not only need to have a clear representation of the causal relations between system components but they also need a representation of the exact durations of the delays and to keep track of the temporal developments while controlling the system. The representation of time is not just a by-product of dealing with the task. Brown and West (1990), for example, found that increases in the number of relevant temporal stimuli led to a greater disruption of timing behaviour. In other words, processing temporal information is a controlled rather than an automatic process, requiring attentional resources (Michon and Jackson, 1984; Zakay, 1992). This means that subjects should at least be given sufficient training to acquire knowledge on both the causal and temporal relations between system parameters. Another possible explanation for the difficulty to take feedback delays into account is that subjects were aware of the delay but made miscalculations in relating the information to the actual system state. In this case poor performance does not result from incorrect time representations but from relating this knowledge to the evolving system state.

Information selection over time

Of particular importance for dynamic system control is the ability to keep track of changing system states. Huber (1990, 1994) and Huber *et al.* (1990) investigated subjects' performance in a multistage betting task. In such a task the subjects' goal is to increase their capital by investing some part in a series of trials. It was found that subjects adapted their percentage stakes to the probability of winning but, in disagreement with the normative solution, not to the winning amount (Huber, 1994).

In a totally different domain Lusk and Hammond (1991) analysed how weather forecasters predicted microbursts (brief localised windstorms) while viewing radar data that were updated over time. They found that, even though the weather forecasters became more confident over time, most of them did not become more accurate. The same conclusion was drawn by Tolcott *et al.* (1989). In their experiment they found that army intelligence analysts became more confident after they had received updated information on an evolving situation. However, they interpreted this information in the light of the model they had constructed from early information and as a consequence they did not build up an improved model of the situation across time.

Most research on situation assessment has been carried out in the context of human factors research and has been related to the increased automation of systems in combination with manning reductions. In controlling aircraft or complex systems such as flexible manufacturing systems, refineries and nuclear power plant, operators need an up-to-date model of situational parameters to control the system effectively (Endsley, 1995). Especially in critical situations where active intervention is required of the operator it may be very difficult to build up an accurate model of the situation within a short time span. Not only are the systems under control extremely complex, but in the absence of history information at a lower control level it will take time to trace back the antecedents that led to the actual situation. A major challenge to interface design is to support the operators in maintaining an overview of the process evolution (Passenier and Kerstholt, 1996). Especially when a large number of functions are automated, the operator may not receive adequate feedback to keep track of changing system states. As mentioned by Norman (1990), reduced control possibilities may not be due to automation *per se* but more to an inadequate interface design that provides the operator with too little information on system changes.

To conclude, for efficient system control the operator needs an adequate mental model of both the structure of the system under control and the process evolution. This requires that sufficient feedback of control actions is provided. By giving history and preview information the operator can be further supported in maintaining an overview of the complete system.

HOW ACCURATE IS DECISION MAKING IN DYNAMIC TASKS?

Payne *et al.* (1993) suggested that strategy selection in static tasks is highly adaptive: individuals select a strategy that strikes an efficient balance between effort and accuracy. Given that decision makers have two goals

– attaining accurate performance and investing minimal effort – they are able adaptively to incorporate these goals in their decision process, by taking the choice context into account. The fact that this effort–accuracy trade-off is also found in dynamic task environments (Kerstholt 1995, 1996) suggests that the minimisation of effort is an overall goal of the decision maker.

However, despite the fact that subjects seem to take effort into account, many results from dynamic decision making studies have shown that performance is far from optimal. As we have shown in the overview of research findings, people perform rather poorly on a number of dynamic task dimensions. For example, they neglect feedback delays and tend to use strategies that are both suboptimal *and* require a lot of effort. Does this mean that people cannot deal accurately with dynamic task environments?

One could distinguish three global reasons for suboptimal task performance. First, as is often suggested, poor performance may be explained by the limitations of the information processing system itself. Capacity limitations may force people to use heuristics or to deal with multiple disturbances sequentially, and it may be that the 'design' of our cognitive system is not suitable to represent or process time relations of the kind needed in process control. A second reason for poor task performance, however, is that the subjects do not possess the knowledge that is needed to deal with the decision problem. This knowledge may consist of input–output relations – the decision maker may have learned by experience which control action to take when a particular system state is observed – or it may consist of a model of the system under control, specifying the relations between system parameters and their temporal characteristics. Without this knowledge the subjects will simply not be able to relate the effects of their control actions to overall system performance. The third possible mechanism for poor performance is that the presentation of the problem does not match the mental representation of the decision maker. Mental representations and procedures have been developed in specific task contexts, and adaptive behaviour in a laboratory task can only be assessed when there is a correspondence between these mental knowledge structures and the structure of the problem (Anderson, 1990). Thus, the subjects have the knowledge of how to deal with, for example, temporal information, but their specific representation of this knowledge does not match the structure of the problem as it is presented to them (Gigerenzer *et al.*, 1988).

In trying to map the experimental findings on to these explanations one could tentatively conclude that people are not able to deal accurately with dynamic systems, as they ignore feedback delays and do not time their control actions to conform to normative solutions. Or, as Diehl and Sterman (1995: 214) put it: 'people's ability to infer correctly the behaviour of even simple feedback systems is poor [which is] a fundamental bound on human rationality – our cognitive capabilities do not include the ability to solve systems of high-order nonlinear differential equations intuitively'.

However, despite this conclusion from experimental research, it cannot be denied that experts can deal efficiently with highly complex dynamic systems in real life, such as, for example, manoeuvring a ship through restricted waterways. One difference between these real-life situations and experimental tasks is that people will have had numerous occasions in which knowledge could be acquired concerning the relation between input and actions. The expertise of river pilots, for example, seems to consist more of using specific references (e.g., pile moorings, buoys, leading lines) to check the ship's position and orientation in a particular area than in being able to predict accurately a ship's movements (Schraagen, 1994). In other words, even though people do not seem to build up a mental model of the system dynamics itself, they can accurately control the system after learning the relations between input and output signals (see also Dienes and Fahey, 1996).

Given that the efficient control of dynamic systems requires such extended knowledge and experience, it is rather peculiar that most research on dynamic decision making tends to use rather knowledge-intensive decision tasks, without lengthy practice sessions that give subjects the opportunity to build up their knowledge base. If the aim is to focus on performance measures, how well people perform in dynamic tasks, it seems more fruitful to look at experienced decision makers in a real-world context such as is done in the naturalistic decision making tradition (Klein *et al.*, 1993). On the other hand, if one aims at finding general aspects of dynamic decision making, generalisable to a wide range of task domains, then the experimental task should provide maximal control rather than the mere inclusion of all 'real-life' task parameters. At this level, the design of simple task environments is geared to measuring specific research questions, rather than to measuring performance in complex, dynamic tasks as such. Why, for example, are some people able to maintain an overview of the system under control whereas others fixate too much on a single, local, diagnosis problem (Kerstholt *et al.*, 1996)? Why do some decision makers make accurate use of real-time information whereas others use, less efficiently, predictive, planning information (Eisenhardt, 1989)? Instead of an additional study indicating how poorly subjects perform in dynamic tasks, it seems that the time is ripe for more detailed studies increasing our understanding of the way in which dynamic decision tasks are performed.

REFERENCES

Anderson, J.R. (1990) *The Adaptive Character of Thought*, Hillsdale, NJ: Erlbaum.

Brehmer, B. (1990) 'Strategies in real-time, dynamic decision making', in R.M. Hogarth (ed.), *Insights in Decision Making: A Tribute to Hillel J. Einhorn*, Chicago: University of Chicago Press.

Brehmer, B. (1992) 'Dynamic decision making: human control of complex systems', *Acta Psychologica*, 81: 211–41.

Brown, S.W. and West, A.N. (1990) 'Multiple timing and the allocation of attention', *Acta Psychologica*, 75: 103–21.

Connolly, T. (1988) 'Studies of information-purchase processes', in B. Brehmer and C.R.B. Joyce (eds) *Human Judgment: The SJT View*, Amsterdam: North-Holland.

De Keyser, V. (1990) 'Temporal decision making in complex environments', in D.E. Broadbent, J. Reason and A. Baddeley (eds) *Human Factors in Hazardous Situations*, Oxford: Clarendon Press.

Diehl, E. and Sterman, J.D. (1995) 'Effects of feedback complexity on dynamic decision making', *Organizational Behavior and Human Decision Processes*, 62: 198–215.

Dienes, Z. and Fahey, R. (1996) 'Role of specific instances in controlling a dynamic system', *Journal of Experimental Psychology: Learning, Memory and Cognition*, 21: 848–62.

Dörner, D. (1987) 'On the difficulties people have in dealing with complexity', in J. Rasmussen, K. Duncan and J. Leplat (eds) *New Technology and Human Error*, Chichester: Wiley.

Edland, A. and Svenson, O. (1993) 'Judgment and decision making under time pressure: studies and findings', in O. Svenson and A.J. Maule (eds) *Time Pressure and Stress in Human Judgment and Decision Making*, New York: Plenum Press.

Edwards, W. (1962) 'Dynamic decision theory and probabilistic information processing', *Human Factors*, 4: 59–73.

Eisenhardt, K.M. (1989) 'Making fast strategic decisions in high-velocity environments', *Academy of Management Journal*, 32: 543–76.

Endsley, M.R. (1995) 'Towards a theory of situation awareness in dynamic systems', *Human Factors*, 37: 32–64.

Ford, J.K., Schmitt, N., Schechtman, S.L., Hults, B.M. and Doherty, M.L. (1989) 'Process tracing methods: contributions, problems and neglected research questions', *Organizational Behavior and Human Decision Processes*, 43: 75–117.

Gigerenzer, G., Hell, W. and Blank, H. (1988) 'Presentation and content: the use of base rates as a continuous variable', *Journal of Experimental Psychology: Human Perception and Performance*, 14: 513–25.

Hogarth, R.M. (1981) 'Beyond discrete biases: functional and dysfunctional aspects of judgmental heuristics', *Psychological Bulletin*, 90: 197–217.

Hogarth, R.M. and Makridakis, S. (1981) 'The value of decision making in a complex environment: an experimental approach', *Management Science*, 27: 93–107.

Huber, O. (1990) 'Cognitive processes in multistage decision making', in K.J. Golhooly, M.T.G. Keane, R.H. Logie and G. Erdos (eds) *Lines of Thinking: Reflections on the Psychology of Thought*, vol. I, Chichester: Wiley.

Huber, O. (1994) 'Decision making in a multistage investment task', *Acta Psychologica*, 85: 139–54.

Huber, O., Debeutz, A., Pratscher, J. and Quehenberger, I. (1990) 'Perceived control in a multistage decision task', *Journal of Behavioral Decision Making*, 3: 123–36.

Hunt, E. (1991) 'Some comments on the study of complexity', in R.J. Sternberg and P.A. Frensch (eds) *Complex Problem Solving*, Hillsdale, NJ: Erlbaum.

Kerstholt, J.H. (1994a) 'The effect of time pressure on decision making behaviour in a dynamic task environment', *Acta Psychologica*, 86: 89–104.

Kerstholt, J.H. (1994b) 'Learning effects on strategy selection in a dynamic task environment as a function of time pressure', Report TNO-TM 1994 B-12, Soesterberg: Human Factors Research Institute.

Kerstholt, J.H. (1995) 'Decision making in dynamic situations: the effect of false alarms and time pressure', *Journal of Behavioral Decision Making*, 8: 181–200.

Kerstholt, J.H. (1996) 'The effect of information costs on strategy selection in dynamic tasks', *Acta Psychologica*, 94: 273–90.

Kerstholt, J.H. and Passenier, P.O. (1995) 'Can cognitive lockup in ship operation be overcome by an integrated training?', Report TNO-TM 1995 C-50, Soesterberg: Human Factors Research Institute.

Kerstholt, J.H., Passenier, P.O., Houttuin, K. and Schuffel, H. (1996) 'The effect of *a priori* probability and complexity on decision making in a supervisory control task', *Human Factors*, 38: 65–78.

Klein, G.A., Orasanu, J., Calderwood, R. and Zsambok, C.E. (1993) *Decision Making in Action*, Norwood, NJ: Ablex.

Kleinmuntz, D.N. (1985) 'Cognitive heuristics and feedback in a dynamic decision environment', *Management Science*, 31: 680–702.

Kleinmuntz, D.N. (1993) 'Information processing and misperceptions of the implications of feedback in dynamic decision making', *System Dynamics Review*, 9: 223–37.

Kleinmuntz, D.N. and Thomas, J.B. (1987) 'The value of action and inference in dynamic decision making', *Organizational Behavior and Human Decision Processes*, 39: 341–364.

Lusk, C.M. and Hammond, K.R. (1991) 'Judgment in a dynamic task: microburst forecasting', *Journal of Behavioral Decision Making*, 4: 55–73.

Mackinnon, A.J. and Wearing, A.J. (1985) 'Systems analysis and dynamic decision making', *Acta Psychologica*, 58: 159–72.

Michon, J.A. and Jackson, J.L. (1984) 'Attentional effort and cognitive strategies in the processing of temporal information', in J. Gibbon and L. Allan (eds) *Timing and Time Perception*, New York: New York Academy of Sciences.

Moray, N. and Rotenberg, I. (1989) 'Fault management in process control: eye movements and action', *Ergonomics*, 32: 1319–42.

Norman, D.A. (1990) 'The "problem" with automation: inappropriate feedback and interaction, not over-automation', in D.E. Broadbent, J. Reason and A. Baddeley (eds) *Human Factors in Hazardous Situations*, Oxford: Clarendon Press.

Passenier, P.O. and Kerstholt, J.H. (1996) 'Design and evaluation of a decision support system for integrated bridge operation', Report TNO TM-1996 C064. Soesterberg: Human Factors Research Institute.

Payne, J.W., Bettman, J.R. and Johnson, E.J. (1993) *The Adaptive Decision Maker*, New York: Cambridge University Press.

Schraagen, J.M.C. (1994) 'What information do river pilots use?' Report TNO-TM 1994 C-10, Soesterberg: Human Factors Research Institute.

Sterman, J.D. (1989) 'Misperceptions of feedback in a dynamic decision making experiment', *Organizational Behavior and Human Decision Processes*, 43: 301–35.

Tolcott, M.A., Marvin, F.F. and Lehner, P.E. (1989) 'Expert decision making in evolving situations', *IEEE Transactions on Systems, Man, and Cybernetics*, 19: 606–15.

Zakay, D. (1992) 'On prospective time estimation, temporal relevance and temporal uncertainty', in F. Macar, V. Pouthas and W.J. Friedman (eds) *Time, Action and Cognition*, Dordrecht: Kluwer.

Chapter 13

Turning prior disadvantages into advantages

Differentiation and consolidation in real-life decision making

Ola Svenson and Teci Hill

The present chapter starts with an overview of recent decision research related to Differentiation and Consolidation theory and continues with a study of a real-world decision which fills in some of the gaps in knowledge from earlier research. Because detailed presentations of Differentiation and Consolidation (Diff Con) theory are available elsewhere (Svenson, 1992, 1996) and in Chapter 3 of this volume, a very brief account of the theory will be given in the present context.

Differentiation and Consolidation theory treats both pre- and post-decision processes in a process approach to human decision making (Svenson, 1979, 1990, 1992, 1996; Payne *et al.*, 1992). Diff Con theory acknowledges the following stages in a decision process: (1) detection of the decision problem phase; (2) differentiation phase which contains (a) marker identification (a marker is an aspect which triggers or can be used to start the decision or judgement process), (b) selection of preliminary and/or reference alternative and (c) process and structural differentiation; (3) decision; (4) consolidation phase which contains (a) process and rule consolidation, (b) implementation of decision, (c) post-implementation consolidation, (d) outcome of decision and (e) post-outcome consolidation.

Diff Con theory assumes that a pre-decision process involves the differentiation of a preliminary or hypothetically chosen alternative from its competitors in order that a decision can be reached. The differentiation process can involve quick holistic decisions, the application of different decision rules, restructuring of the decision maker's cognitive representation of the different alternatives, and decision problem restructuring.

The goal of a decision process is to achieve a sufficient degree of differentiation to enable a choice. It is not enough to select the best option, but it is necessary to find or create an alternative which is so much better than its closest competitor that it can be expected to remain better even after the decision. Thus, Diff Con theory explicitly models pre-decision processes as a preparation for the post-decision phase. From experience a decision maker knows that the post-decision period may involve both internal (e.g., regret, change of personal values) and external (e.g., bad outcomes) threats against the superiority of a chosen alternative. Therefore, a sufficiently superior alternative has to be found or created and it is not enough just to find the best alternative.

After the decision has been made, consolidation processes follow to support it. Consolidation is performed by processes of the same kinds as those used in differentiation. Sometimes the consolidation of a decision is not successful and this may lead to different reactions including regret, anxiety and/or the changing of a prior decision.

Holistic differentiation is quick and non-analytic. Often it involves processes which the decision maker is not conscious of. Most habits involve decisions with holistic differentiation. An experienced buyer's choice of milk (e.g., by the colour of the container) in a supermarket could exemplify this kind of decision. In holistic differentiation the decision maker does not need to elicit his or her values each time. This does not mean that values do not play a significant role. It only means that the choice of an alternative in a particular decision situation has been directly linked through learning to that situation.

Process differentiation involves the processing of available information using one or more decision rules (Beach, 1990; Svenson, 1979). An example of a decision rule is the conjunctive rule which implies the setting of a criterion level on an attribute (e.g., costs) and the rejection of those available alternatives that fail to pass the criterion level. Editing of a decision problem also belongs to this phase (Kahneman and Tversky, 1979).

Structural differentiation is of three kinds: attractiveness differentiation, facts differentiation and attribute importance differentiation. Attractiveness differentiation means that, in order to achieve a sufficiently superior alternative, the attractiveness of the decision alternatives are changed in support of a preliminarily chosen alternative. For example, the apparent beauty of an expensive painting may gradually increase in an attractiveness restructuring process until the decision to buy the painting becomes possible. Facts restructuring concerns a change in the representations of facts to support a decision alternative. If, when asked about the price of the earlier mentioned painting, a decision maker gives too low a price or rounds it off downwards, this represents facts restructuring supporting the purchase of the painting. The painting is now represented as more beautiful and less expensive than earlier in the decision process. Finally, attribute importance structuring means that an attribute which supports the chosen alternative is given increased importance in relation to the other attributes.

Problem restructuring is another type of differentiation where new decision alternatives are created in processes also involving problem solving. Here, the set of given decision alternatives is not accepted as such but new options are created in the situation. A very simple case of this is the selection of a holiday trip which involves different travel destinations, travel modes, hotels and so on. More complex examples of differentiation through problem restructuring include many societal, social, scientific and corporate decision making situations.

Most studies of decision making using Diff Con as a framework have examined post-decision processes. In the past, post-decision processes have most often been discussed within the framework of Cognitive Dissonance theory. Diff Con theory connects to the classic cognitive dissonance approach (Festinger, 1957, 1964) but differs from it in several ways. Among the differences are that Diff Con represents decision alternatives by aspects on attributes. Classical dissonance theory used holistic evaluations (Festinger, 1964) or information about the pros and cons of a chosen alternative (Frey, 1986). The importance or weight of each attribute is explicitly included in Diff Con theory but this has no correspondence in most cognitive dissonance approaches. The goal of the decision process is to create a sufficiently superior alternative in Diff Con. In the cognitive dissonance approach it is to create cognitive consistency. Diff Con, originating from a decision theoretic approach, treats pre-decision processes to a greater extent than cognitive dissonance research, which originates from social psychology.

In contrast to Festinger's (1964) view that pre-decision processes are largely impartial, Diff Con theory assumes exactly the opposite. Structural differentiation is the theoretical expression of this assumption. Later researchers in the cognitive dissonance tradition have given up Festinger's assumption about impartial pre-decision information processing (Janis and Mann, 1977). Diff Con theory explicitly presents different decision rules as cognitive principles for processing the information in conjunction with the restructuring processes. The restructuring processes are always performed towards greater differentiation or consolidation through one or more decision rules. Most cognitive dissonance approaches have very few assumptions about decision rules (but see Larrick, 1993).

EARLIER STUDIES

As mentioned above, most studies related to the Diff Con framework have treated post-decision processes and therefore the ensuing summary of earlier studies will focus on post-decision processes. In the first of the Diff Con studies, Svenson and Benthorn (1992) used memory of a prior decision to measure post-decision processes. It was assumed that distortions in the memory of a decision are indicators of a consolidation process. The memory paradigm has been very popular in Diff Con-inspired research; unless an alternative method is indicated, this is the way consolidation has been measured. One implication of using memory in this way is that only one decision task at a time can be studied, making the research quite resource-demanding. Furthermore, the decision problem should be neither extremely easy nor difficult in order to avoid ceiling or floor effects.

The subjects in the Svenson and Benthorn study were asked to make decisions between alternatives which were of great interest to the subjects themselves. The selection of this kind of decision refers to the fact that involvement is needed for differentiation and consolidation according to Diff Con theory. The subjects were children aged 11–12 years so the decisions concerned personal headset stereos and computer games for boys and friends and horses for girls. Each subject was given only one decision problem with two alternatives, each of which was characterised on each of four attributes. To exemplify, the personal stereos were characterised by (1) price, (2) design, (3) sound quality and (4) mechanical and electronic quality.

An alternative was presented with marks on horizontal lines representing each of the four attributes. The lines represented attractiveness from 'very poor' to 'very good'. The two alternatives in a decision were presented side by side on an A4 sheet of paper. The importance of each attribute for the decision was judged on separate scales by the subjects.

Either five minutes or one week after having made a choice of one of the pair of alternatives, the subjects were asked to reproduce the representations of the decision alternatives on which the prior decision had been based. The responses were collected by having subjects mark their responses on a paper exactly like the stimulus sheet but without the marks on the attractiveness scales.

The results showed that in order to find any regularities in group data every subject's attribute importance judgement had to be used. The results showed that subjects differed in what attribute they considered most important. Therefore, it was not sufficient to average across an attribute according to its label (e.g., price). Instead, all judgements on the most important attribute had to be aggregated across subjects and decision problems. Then the data on the second most important attribute were treated in the same way, and so on. This principle for analysing data was the first finding in the series of studies relating to Diff Con theory. The second finding was that consolidation took place on only the two most important attributes. A significant increase in attractiveness supporting the chosen alternative was found only in the condition where one week had elapsed since the decision. To specify, the attractiveness of the non-chosen alternative decreased in the post-decision consolidation process, while the attractiveness of the chosen alternative was approximately constant. This resulted in a significant change in advantage of the chosen over the non-chosen alternative which indicated structural consolidation.

The conditions which foster consolidation were illustrated by an experiment in which subjects were asked to justify their decision later (Svenson *et al.*, 1994, study 1). The design was similar to the earlier study with hypothetical alternatives but here adults served as subjects and the decision concerned a difficult medical care choice. To our surprise the instruction to justify inhibited the consolidation process. This was the case also in a second experiment replicating this result (Svenson *et al.*, 1994 study 2). Thus, this third finding did not support Diff Con theory. The need to justify was not found to be a factor driving consolidation of a prior decision. If, however, subjects were only told to remember their decision until a later occasion, consolidation increased as compared with a condition in which there was no such instruction (Svenson *et al.*, 1994). This was the fourth finding in the series of Diff Con studies. A tentative explanation for the last two findings is that the instruction to remember a decision invites consolidation because it may support the memory of which alternative was chosen. Knowing that one has to defend a decision in a later justification may lead to an attempt not to exaggerate and to try to remember the exact arguments as represented by the attractiveness markings. However, these explanations are *post hoc* and need to be tested empirically.

According to Diff Con theory, all decisions with high involvement could be consolidated even when a dominant alternative (better than or equal to its competitor on all attributes) is chosen. Even if the consolidation is weaker, it should be there if other conditions for consolidation are fulfilled. This prediction contrasts with Dominance Structuring theory (Montgomery, 1983), which predicts no further restructuring. Svenson and Benthorn (1992) found attractiveness restructuring also when a dominating alternative was chosen, thus supporting Diff Con theory. This was the fifth finding of Diff Con research.

The use of visual analogue scales and data aggregated according to the importance of the attributes raises some methodological questions. Because the most important attribute plays the greatest role in determining the choice, there is also a greater chance that this attribute has an attractiveness closer to maximum attractiveness than other attributes. This in turn may produce a ceiling effect with little room for further increase on the most important attribute. Instead, there may be more room for increase in the second most important attribute, which may explain why different studies repeatedly find more consolidation on the second attribute than on the first. However, the ratings for the second most important attribute of the non-chosen alternative may be vulnerable to a judgement bias towards the middle of the scale. This bias of regression towards the midpoint could result in effects which could be erroneously interpreted as consolidation. This bias was therefore investigated by Malmsten in an unpublished study (Malmsten, 1996, study 4). He designed decision alternatives in which the effects of judgement regression effects towards the mean of a response scale were eliminated through a careful design of individual decision tasks for each subject. Malmsten's results indicated genuine consolidation effects, thus validating the earlier results and showing that they are not simply response scale artefacts. Benthorn (1994, study 3) used another response scale in an unpublished study of decisions with alternatives described by different rates of change over time (e.g., salary). He used curves in diagrams as alternatives instead of the regular visual analogue scales used in the other experiments. Benthorn found consolidation also in this case.

The above studies all used hypothetical decision alternatives, and it may be argued that the Diff Con results found in hypothetical decisions only reflect one particular case with no real application outside that situation. Furthermore, the earlier experiments had used alternatives in which the attractiveness values on each attribute were defined by the experimenter's markings on a stimulus sheet, which deviates from reality, where attractiveness representations originate from the decision maker him- or herself.

Svenson and Malmsten (1996) therefore used real physical objects in the following study. They also investigated the effects of decision outcome on consolidation. To make the subjects involved, the decision alternatives were personal headset stereos, which were very valuable to the subjects, aged 11–12 years. At the end of the experiment every subject had a chance to win one of the decision alternatives, which added to the realism of the situation. Subjects rated the attractiveness of the headsets themselves, in terms of their attributes, on horizontal scales from poor to good.

To study the effects of outcome on consolidation, a two-step game was used. First, subjects decided which of two lotteries, with one of the headsets to win in each, they preferred. (If a subject had a ticket there was a one in eight chance to win a headset in each lottery.) Second, each subject threw a dice to decide whether he or she had won a ticket in the lottery of his or her choice. Tickets for the more expensive headset were awarded to a subject if the dice showed one or two spots, and for those subjects who had decided to choose the cheaper headset one, two and three gave a ticket in the lottery.

The results showed that outcome affects consolidation. It speeds up attractiveness restructuring consolidation in comparison to hypothetical choices, a finding that supports Diff Con theory. Furthermore, it was shown that a chosen alternative with a positive outcome (lottery ticket) in the dice throw was consolidated to a greater extent than when the outcome was negative (no lottery ticket). The consolidation was so strong that an average disadvantage for the chosen alternative on the two most important attributes was changed into an advantage after a positive outcome. This is further support for Diff Con theory.

Another way of providing outcome feedback was used by Benson and Svenson (1992). Subjects were asked to make a decision with Asian disease type of alternatives (Kahneman and Tversky, 1979; see also Chapter 8). Here, the framing of the alternatives leads to decisions which contradict normative theory. One group of subjects was debriefed and told that their decisions violated principles of rationality. This group of subjects indicated consolidation of their prior choice and not the 'rational' choice explained to them. This was done through problem restructuring a week later. There were no corresponding effects in the control group which was not exposed to the post-decision threat that the prior decision was wrong. This shows that consolidation may strengthen a prior choice despite or because of arguments threatening the decision.

The role of attribute importance structuring has not played a significant role in research until now. Malmsten (1996, study 2) made a preliminary attempt to investigate it but arrived at no definite conclusion. In a very small sample of subjects he observed attractiveness consolidation but not importance consolidation. This may indicate that the latter is weaker and/or less frequent than the former.

Differentiation studies of pre-decision processes are almost non-existent, indicating a great need for such studies connected to the Diff Con framework. In an early study by Montgomery and Svenson (1983), think-aloud protocols were collected in the pre-decision phase. The results indicated that the alternative that was finally chosen could be identified early in the decision process and that the difference in attractiveness increased gradually over time. But this study did not provide reliable results about the details of the process, as is needed in the Diff Con framework. Recently Russo *et al.* (1996) showed how a preliminary choice leads to increased perceived attractiveness of information which favours that choice over information concerning another alternative. In a study by Svenson and Benson (1993), subjects solved Asian-type decision problems (Kahneman and Tversky, 1979) under time pressure. The results indicated that the differentiation process was disturbed in such a way that the decisions were less biased than those of a control group under no time pressure. This illustrates that differentiation processes may lead to decisions which deviate from normative theory.

Because of the lack of Diff Con-related research covering pre-decision processes and their relation to post-decision processes, the following study was conducted. In order to increase the degree of realism, a real-life decision process was investigated. The general question investigated concerned the extent to which differentiation and consolidation processes can be uncovered in a real-life situation. The more specific research questions were the following: (1) Even though the attributes generated by the subjects themselves have completely different labels, is it possible to find regularities when data are grouped according to attribute importance? (2) Will subjects who have a value conflict on one of the two most important attributes indicate stronger or different differentiation and consolidation than subjects with no value conflict? (3) Will the differentiation and consolidation process stop when a dominant situation has been achieved or will it continue beyond that state? (4) Will differentiation and consolidation be reflected in overall measures of attractiveness and/or in an attractiveness profile restructuring on the most important attributes?

EMPIRICAL STUDY

Method

Subjects

Twenty-one students on a course at Stockholm University called 'The Personnel Administration Educational Programme' participated in the study. After two years of study the students had to choose one of five different areas of continued in-depth study as their third year in the programme. The options were (1) personnel administration, (2) organisation, (3) education, (4) psychology and (5) business administration. This decision was extremely important for future job careers as the alternatives differed very much from each other. The students received 'movie passes' (covering entrance fees worth about 15 US dollars) as payment for their participation in the study.

Decision problem

The students were first asked to select their first and second most preferred alternatives from the five options. Thereafter, they were asked to generate four attributes describing the alternatives on the four most important 'characteristics' for making a decision between these two most attractive alternatives. Each subject was then instructed, for each alternative, to mark its attractiveness on a horizontal 82 mm linear scale for each of the attributes (the names of which were written down by the subject in an open space next to each scale). The scales ranged from 'bad' to 'good'. The two alternatives (the names of which were also written down by the subject in an appropriate place) were presented side by side on an A4 sheet with the longer side horizontal. Figure 13.1 shows a response sheet with the answers of a hypothetical subject. The subjects were then asked to assess the overall attractiveness of the two alternatives respectively. Following this, subjects also estimated (on graphical scales) the importance of each attribute and answered some other questions not in focus here.

Procedure

Altogether the subjects received four questionnaires, two prior to the decision and two after the decision had been made. The first questionnaire was completed in April 1994, and the second in May before the

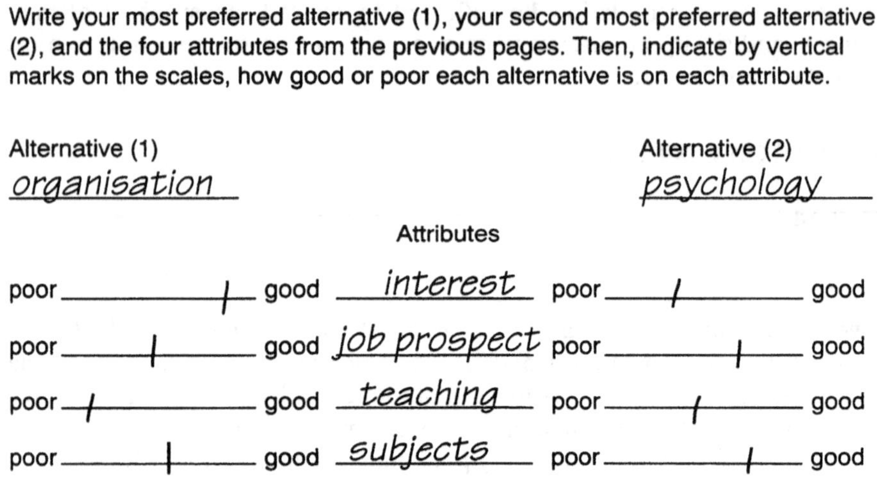

Figure 13.1 Example of attractiveness rating

decision was made. The decision was made through a formal application to the university administration stating what programme alternative the student wanted to follow. The final questionnaire was answered in August of the same year just before the students were starting the studies of their choice.

The first instruction to the students was given in a classroom session. Some subjects filled out the first questionnaire in this session, and the rest took the material home and answered the questions there. The subsequent three questionnaires were sent out by mail, and the subjects were instructed to answer them at home and return the forms immediately by mail.

As mentioned earlier, the students had to select the two best alternatives before the decision was made in order to answer the pre-decision questionnaires (1 and 2). It was emphasised that this was not at all related to the subjects' official decisions and that any alternative could be chosen up to the official university application deadline.

On the second occasion each student received a questionnaire which was identical to the first one, with the exception that the names of the alternatives and attributes, he or she had given the previous time were filled in. For example, if a student had used 'quality of tuition' as an attribute, he or she would get a questionnaire with this attribute name written in for that attractiveness rating scale. The words used were exactly those used by the student on the previous occasion. In addition, there was an option to indicate a fifth attribute if something new had evolved. However, only one subject added another attribute and it was judged least important. Therefore only four attributes will be treated in the following analyses. The second time the subjects also estimated the attractiveness of the alternatives on the attributes and the importance of the attributes. Subjects were asked the same questions in exactly the same way as in the first session. Following the decision, the third and fourth questionnaires were identical to the second questionnaire, the only difference being that some sentences were rephrased to take account of the fact that the students now had made their real official decisions.

Results

Overall evaluations

All of the twenty-one subjects kept the same alternative as the most preferred and finally chosen alternative through all four sessions. The overall evaluations indicated that the chosen alternative was rated to be, on average (arithmetic mean), 13 units more attractive than the second best non-chosen alternative on the 82-unit scale. This difference did not change across the four sessions. Thus, no progressive changes in overall attractiveness could be found in an aggregation of data across attributes and subjects.

Attributes generated

In all there were nineteen different attributes generated by twenty-one subjects. In this count similarly formulated attributes were treated as the same. The attributes were grouped into eight meta-attributes which were the following: (1) programme quality (content), (2) programme quality (process-teachers, etc.), (3) personal interest, (4) own ability, (5) future-oriented attractiveness ('what I want to work with'), (6) instrumentality for future ('usefulness for future work'), (7) social attributes (e.g., same choice as significant other) and (8) prior information about programmes (e.g., official presentation of programmes – this category contained only four cases).

The diversity of the attributes and the possible interpretation each decision maker reads into them illustrates the variability which appears when decision makers are free to choose their own representations of decision problems. Personal interest and usefulness for future work were judged as the most important attributes. The conflicts appeared when one of the following attributes did not support the chosen alternative: (i) quality of programme (two cases), (ii) curriculum quality, (iii) apprenticeship quality, (iv) personal interest (three cases), (v) usefulness for future work (two cases) and (vi) usefulness for the future in general. To illustrate a conflict, attribute (iv), personal interest, was judged to be the most important attribute by two subjects and yet they did not choose the alternative which interested them most. A third subject judged personal interest second most important and chose an alternative which was not supported by this attribute.

For each subject the most important attribute was identified. In the same way the second most important to the fourth most important attributes were also identified. Then the difference in attractiveness ratings between the chosen and non-chosen (the second choice) alternatives were computed for each attribute identified as 1, 2, 3, or 4 in rank order of importance across subjects. To illustrate, a difference in ratings given by a subject who had 'personal interest' as the most important attribute was grouped with another person's difference in ratings of 'usefulness for future work' because this was the most important attribute for that person. The difference favouring a chosen alternative over its closest competitor is called the *attractiveness advantage* of the chosen alternative over the non-chosen alternative on a given attribute.

Attribute importance

Across sessions the most important attribute was rated on average 74.6 in attribute importance and the following attributes 68.7, 60.9 and 51.3, respectively. This suggests that all attributes were considered quite important for the decision made since they were all rated above the midpoint of the scale. The mean importance ratings for the four attributes across sessions indicated that the dispersion of importance was greater in the first session and that it reached its minimum in the post-decision phase. To verify this, the standard deviation was computed for the mean importance for each session. This resulted in standard deviations of 15.50, 9.28, 7.67 and 7.54 for the different occasions. This declining series of numbers in differentiation and consolidation terms may reflect an initial comparatively greater reliance on importance differentiation which is later decreased and used less in consolidation processes. However, this hypothesis would have to be tested in future research.

Interindividual differences in goal conflicts

Subjects perceive the same decision problem in different ways according to the degree to which the problem leads to value or goal conflict. In the group of twenty-one subjects one subgroup (the conflict group) of ten subjects had a decision involving the most or second most important attribute not supporting their chosen alternative. The remaining eleven subjects (the non-conflict group) did not have such a conflict.

The attractiveness advantage of the chosen alternative increased on the two most important alternatives over the decision (from session 2 to 3) in the non-conflict group. However, this trend was not significant and no other relevant significant changes over time were found in the non-conflict group.

The ten subjects of the conflict group indicated a somewhat stronger effect in that there was an increase on the second most important attribute across the decision (sessions 2–3) which was marginally significant ($t = 2.08$, $df = 9$, $p \leq 0.068$). There was also a pattern of slightly increased advantages between the immediate pre-decision and the immediate post-decision period on all attributes (sessions 2–3). This pattern was not significant, but it provides a clue for further analysis.

The subjects in the conflict group had a conflict on the most or second most important attribute not favouring their choice. The conflict group was therefore split into two subgroups. In one subgroup the conflict was on the most important and in the other group on the second most important attribute. Plotting the attractiveness advantage of the chosen alternative across sessions made it clear that it did not matter, for the change over time, whether the conflict was on the most or the second most important attribute. The data in the conflict group were therefore aggregated across (1) 'conflict' attribute, (2) 'other' of two most important attributes, (3) third most important attribute and (4) fourth most important attribute.

The result can be seen in Figure 13.2. It is clear that the initial disadvantage of the chosen alternative before the decision is gradually eliminated. Note that it seems that it is not enough just to reduce the conflict, but it is also necessary to create a sufficient attractiveness difference after the decision. That is, the prior negative advantage of the chosen alternative is changed to an attractiveness advantage (greater than zero). This validates the earlier results of the Svenson and Malmsten (1996) study.

The advantage on the non-conflicting of the two most important attributes *decreases* over time in approximately the same way as the advantage is increased on the conflict attribute. A linear regression analysis for the conflict attribute indicates a significant increasing linear trend

$Y = 5.25X - 13.78$ ($t = 3.074$; $df = 1, 38$; $p \leq 0.05$ for slope).

Correspondingly, the 'other' attribute gave a linear decreasing but not significant trend. This result may indicate a compensatory process in which advantage would be given up on the non-conflicting attribute to compensate for the increase in advantage on the conflict attribute. The net effect of this is a constant difference in overall attractiveness across sessions, as reported earlier. Thus the differentiation and consolidation processes change the *pattern of support* for the chosen alternative, not necessarily its *overall attractiveness*.

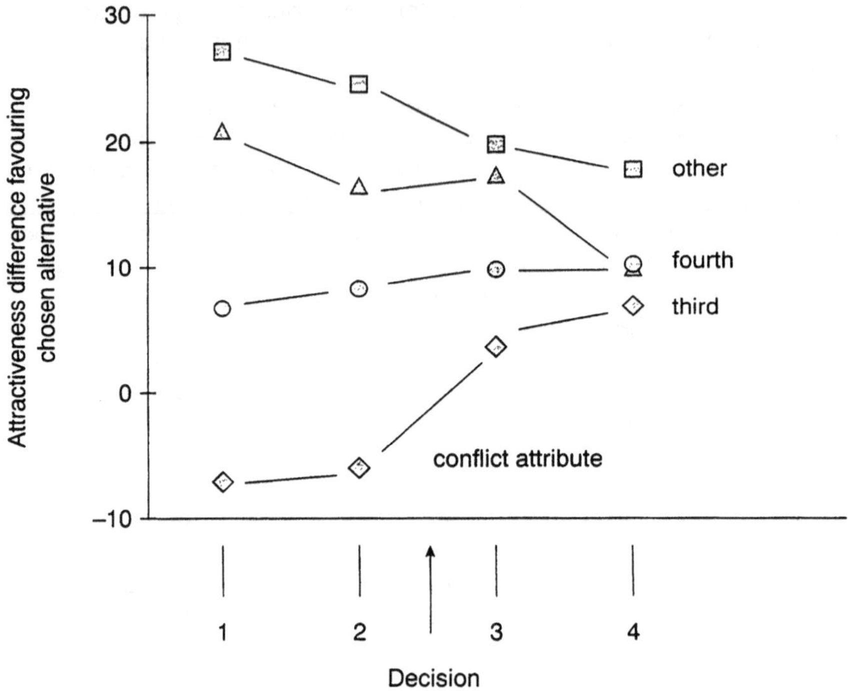

Figure 13.2 Attractiveness advantage for chosen over non-chosen alternative

CONCLUDING REMARKS

The present chapter has illustrated how pre- and post-decision processes follow a pattern of differentiation and consolidation which starts ahead of the final decision and continues beyond that decision. The processing of the information is not unbiased beyond the selection of a preliminary decision alternative but involves systematic restructuring of the subjective representation of the alternatives of the decision problem. In case of value conflicts, the restructuring goes further than just eliminating the conflict, so far that prior disadvantages can be changed to advantages.

The research in the Diff Con framework has also indicated that, in non-involving decisions, less structural differentiation and consolidation will be activated. It has also been shown that the decision maker's knowledge that he or she will later have to justify the decision may serve to prevent structural differentiation and consolidation. Comparatively less research effort has been allocated to studies of how decision rules are used in the differentiation process and even less to the post-decision phase. It is now common knowledge that the differentiation phase includes an initial screening stage, but in the post-decision consolidation phase only structural changes have been studied to the best of the present authors' knowledge. Important future research topics connected to the present study include conflict resolution patterns and the use of decision rules or other processes such as social support as complements and/or as substitutes to structural differentiation and consolidation in human decision making. If we know more about these and other problem areas it will be possible to understand better and hopefully to advise decision makers facing difficult real-life decisions.

ACKNOWLEDGEMENTS

This study was supported by grants from the Swedish Work Environment Fund and the Swedish Council for Research in the Humanities and Social Sciences. The authors want to thank Anne Edland, Nils Malmsten, Anders Johansson, Sanny Shamoun, Bas Verplanken and two anonymous reviewers for valuable comments.

REFERENCES

Beach, L.R. (1990) *Image Theory: Decision Making in Personal and Organizational Contexts*, Chichester: Wiley.

Benson III, L. and Svenson, O. (1992) 'Post-decision consolidation following the debriefing of subjects about experimental manipulations affecting their prior decisions', Lund University, *Psychological Research Bulletin*, 32, no. 3.

Benthorn, L. (1994) 'On post-decision processes', Ph.D. dissertation, Lund University, Sweden.

Festinger, L. (1957) *A Theory of Cognitive Dissonance*, Stanford CA: Stanford University Press.

Festinger, L. (1964) *Conflicts, Decision and Dissonance*, Stanford, CA: Stanford University Press.

Frey, D. (1986) 'Recent research on selective exposure to information', *Advances in Experimental Social Psychology*, vol. 19, New York: Academic Press.

Janis, I.L. and Mann, L. (1977) *Decision Making: A Psychological Analysis of Conflict, Choice and Commitment*, New York: The Free Press.

Kahneman, D. and Tversky, A. (1979) 'Prospect theory: an analysis of decision under risk', *Econometrica*, 47: 263–91.

Larrick, R.P. (1993) 'Motivational factors in decision theories: the role of self-protection', *Psychological Bulletin*, 113: 440–50.

Malmsten, N. (1996) 'On post-decision processes in human decision making', Ph.D. dissertation, Stockholm University.

Montgomery, H. (1983) 'Decision rules and the search for a dominance structure: towards a process model of decision making', in P. Humphreys, O. Svenson and A. Vari (eds) *Analyzing and Aiding Decision Processes*, Amsterdam: North-Holland.

Montgomery, H. and Svenson, O. (1983) 'A think aloud study of dominance structuring in decision processes', in R. Tietz (ed.) *Aspiration Level in Bargaining and Economic Decision Processes*, Berlin: Springer

Payne, J.W., Bettman, J.R. and Johnson, E.J. (1992) 'Behavioral decision research: a constructive processing perspective', *Annual Review of Psychology*, 43: 87–131.

Russo, J.E., Medvec, V. and Meloy, M.G. (1996) 'The distortion of information during decisions', *Organizational Behavior and Human Decision Processes*, 66: 102–10.

Svenson, O. (1979) 'Process descriptions of decision making', *Organizational Behavior and Human Performance*, 23: 86–112.

Svenson, O. (1989) 'Eliciting and analysing verbal protocols in process studies of judgement and decision making', in H. Montgomery and O. Svenson (eds) *Process and Structure in Human Decision Making*, London: Wiley.

Svenson, O. (1990) 'Some propositions for the classification of decision situations', in K. Borcherding, O.I. Larichev and D.M. Messick (eds) *Contemporary Issues in Decision Making*, Amsterdam: Elsevier.

Svenson, O. (1992) 'Differentiation and Consolidation theory of human decision making: a frame of reference for the study of pre- and post-decision processes', *Acta Psychologica*, 80: 143–68.

Svenson, O. (1996) 'Decision making and the search for fundamental psychological regularities: what can be learned from a process perspective?', *Organizational Behavior and Human Decision Processes*, 65: 252–67.

Svenson, O. and Benson III, L. (1993) 'Post-decison consolidation following the debriefing of subjects about experimental manipulations affecting their prior decisions', Lund University: *Psychological Research Bulletin*, 32, no. 3.

Svenson, O. and Benthorn, L. (1992) 'Consolidation processes in decision making: post-decision changes in attractiveness of alternatives', *Journal of Economic Psychology*, 13: 1–13.

Svenson, O. and Malmsten, N. (1996) 'Post-decision over time as a function of gain or loss of an alternative', *Scandinavian Journal of Psychology*, 37: 302–11.

Svenson, O., Ortega Rayo, A., Andersen, M., Sandberg, A. and Svahlin, I. (1994) 'Post-decision consolidation as a function of the instructions to the decision maker and of the decision problem', *Acta Psychologica*, 87: 181–97.

Chapter 14

Post-decisional confidence – can it be trusted?

Dan Zakay

Confidence is a feeling which emerges automatically and which accompanies all of the phases of almost any mental activity. When a goal-directed mental activity is in its planning phase, a prospective feeling of confidence, reflecting confidence in one's ability to accomplish a task successfully, might be felt. Later on, while a task is being performed, an ongoing feeling of confidence in the optimality of one's performance might also be felt. Finally, after performance has terminated, a retrospective feeling of confidence arises. Retrospective feelings of confidence, defined by Peterson and Pitz (1988) as the belief that a given prediction is correct, reflect how confident or non-confident one is regarding the optimality of one's past performance. Feelings of confidence have a strong impact on behaviour, because prospective confidence may determine whether a specific planned task will actually be executed and also which mental strategies will be employed during its execution. Ongoing feelings of confidence may determine whether or not the execution of an ongoing activity will be continued, and, if it is continued, whether any change in strategy will take place. For example, while judgements are being made under conditions of uncertainty, a simple heuristic might be employed. However, if one does not feel confident in this judgement, a shift to a more sophisticated judgement strategy (e.g., algorithmic decomposition) might take place. Retrospective confidence determines the lesson learnt from past experience and the probability of executing a certain activity or employing a certain mental strategy again.

Kruglanski *et al.* (1991) showed that, when the initial level of confidence in a given hypothesis was high, the motivation for acquiring more knowledge in order to test the hypothesis was lower than when the initial confidence was low. In a different context, Zakay and Glickshon (1992) suggested that, while having a reasonable level of confidence in one's knowledge is important for achieving good performance in multiple choice tests, having too high and non-realistic feelings of confidence might lead to the employment of a suboptimal choice strategy. In the latter case, students relying on their initial high level of confidence might choose the first response which comes to mind without checking it carefully.

The inevitable conclusion is that, unless feelings of confidence are accurate in terms of predicting the optimality of future performance or reflecting ongoing and past performance level, feelings of confidence may mislead and bias behaviour. This is confirmed by the common, unfortunate research finding that confidence judgements are unrealistic in the sense that people mostly either overestimate or underestimate the actual level of the optimality of their performance (e.g., Thompson and Mason, 1996).

In the following sections, the inaccuracy of feelings of confidence will be illustrated in various domains of mental tasks, the possible origins and determinants of feelings of confidence will be explored and, finally, an explanation for the lack of reliability of feelings of confidence will be proposed and two empirical tests of this explanation presented.

THE LACK OF SENSITIVITY OF FEELINGS OF CONFIDENCE

Eyewitness testimony

Research on eyewitness testimony has conclusively established that the confidence with which a witness delivers his or her testimony is a strong determinant of whether a jury will be convinced that the eyewitness's testimony is accurate (Cutler *et al.*, 1988). Unfortunately, it seems that the jurors' strong reliance on witness confidence as a measure of accuracy is not justified (Weingardt *et al.*, 1994). Wells and Murray (1984) surveyed thirty-one studies and reported that the average correlation coefficient between accuracy and confidence was only 0.07. Bathwell *et al.* (1987) conducted a meta-analysis on studies in which events are staged so that eyewitness testimony can be tested under controlled conditions. The correlations between confidence and accuracy in these situations was found to reach 0.25. In another meta-analysis (Sporer *et al.*, 1995), similar findings were obtained, although the authors distinguished between witnesses making or not making positive identifications. In the first case, the confidence–accuracy correlation was reliably and consistently higher than in the latter case. Loftus *et al.* (1989) conducted an experiment using the typical three-stage misinformation paradigm (i.e., participants see an event, then read misleading information and finally take a memory test). The authors concluded that participants who are exposed to misleading post-event information are more poorly calibrated and overconfident in their responses than participants who are exposed to neutral information.

Post-decisional confidence (PDC)

In many cases PDC level is not indicative of the optimality of the decision process itself. Wickens *et al.* (1993) found that, as problems required greater dependence upon declarative knowledge, the decisions made were less optimal but were made more rapidly and with greater confidence. Zakay (1985) found that PDC was not sensitive to the optimality of the choice strategy adopted by the decision makers. Nurses were presented with thirty-six choice situations which were so designed that the choice of one alternative would suggest a compensatory decision process, whereas the choice of the other alternative would suggest a non-compensatory process. Results indicated that PDC was higher when a non-compensatory strategy was employed than when the strategy was a compensatory one, although compensatory choices are, by definition, more optimal than non-compensatory choices. The explanation offered by the author was that PDC reflected the amount of conflict experienced while the subject was making the choice, which is higher in the case of a compensatory process than in the case of a non-compensatory one.

Forecasting

Slovic (reported in Russo and Schoemaker, 1989) tested the predictive abilities of eight professional horse-race employees. They were asked to make predictions for numerous races based on past performance charts, with information on each horse and its history. In each case, predictions were based on either 5, 10, 20 or 40 pieces of information per horse. The findings indicated that, whereas confidence increased as a function of the amount of available information, the accuracy of the prediction was not affected by it. Similar findings were found among clinical psychologists who were asked to predict the behaviour of patients with brain damage (Russo and Schoemaker, 1989).

Overconfidence

One of the best examples of the inaccuracy of PDC is the overconfidence phenomenon. Overconfidence (OC) is a widespread phenomenon manifested in a variety of tasks and defined by Slovic *et al.* (1977) as a bias or an 'unwarranted belief in the correctness of one's answer'. Slovic *et al.* found that people were overconfident in assessing the reliability of their memory about facts of general knowledge, a finding which has been repeatedly replicated (e.g., Zakay, 1992). Fischhoff and MacGregor (1982) cite an impressive body of research demonstrating how pervasive overconfidence is in a variety of professional forecasts. Sen and Boe (1991) found that subjects were overconfident when performing a complex problem-solving task, and Solomon *et al.* (1985) found auditors' judgements in a general knowledge task to be significantly overconfident. It seems that OC reflects mainly cognitive processes, because non-significant relationships between scores on a variety of personality measures and the magnitude of OC exhibited by individuals have been documented (Wright and Phillips, 1976).

A puzzling phenomenon of OC is the hard–easy effect (Lichtenstein and Fischhoff, 1977; Keren, 1988; Suantak *et al.*, 1996), which is manifested by an increase in OC magnitude as the difficulty level of the items for which knowledge is to be retrieved increases.

Overconfidence is not confined to naïve people. On the contrary, it has been found among experts, including lawyers (e.g., Loftus and Wagenaar, 1988), medical doctors (Christensen-Szalanski and Busyhead, 1981), clinical psychologists (Oskamp, 1965) and chemical-industry managers (Lichtenstein *et al.*, 1982) in the domain of their own expertise.

WHAT DO FEELINGS OF CONFIDENCE REFLECT? A POSSIBLE EXPLANATION FOR THE LACK OF SENSITIVITY OF CONFIDENCE

We argue that the reason for the lack of sensitivity in feelings of confidence and for their low correlation with performance quality is that feelings of confidence only partly reflect the processes which are responsible for optimal performance. We also claim that feelings of confidence for the large part reflect general factors which already exist prior to the process itself or that emerge after the process has already ended or factors which accompany the process but are irrelevant in assessing its optimality. This argument holds for all types of feelings of confidence, including confidence in memory and in knowledge retrieval or PDC, although in each case unique non-relevant factors might be involved.

In order to demonstrate this argument, we will discuss it with reference to the phenomenon of feeling of knowing (FOK), which is similar in some aspects to feelings of confidence. FOK is the state of believing that a piece of information can be retrieved from memory, even though that information cannot currently be recalled. FOK is a rapid metacognitive process that generally precedes the point at which individuals either retrieve or otherwise determine an answer to a question (Miner and Reder, 1994). Nelson *et al.* (1984) found that there are several determinants of FOK, only some of which support optimal performance later on. Some of these determinants actually create 'noise' which eventually interferes with optimal performance. Koriat (1993) reports that the standard finding regarding FOK is that the predictive validity of FOK judgements is above chance, though far from perfect. Koriat formulated the accessibility model of FOK, according to which the cues for FOK are found in the very information that is activated and accessed during the course of the search-and-retrieval process. He postulated that FOK is a function of the overall amount of retrieved information regardless of its validity in terms of being correct or incorrect in the case of a specific required answer. Since incorrect retrieved information reduces retrieval accuracy it should not contribute to FOK in order to make it a reliable predictor of retrieval accuracy. In reality, however, incorrect retrieved information increases the reported FOK. Allwood and Montgomery (1987) suggest that the phenomenon of FOK be considered a parallel to judgements of confidence in one's knowledge. Following this line of thought and generalising it, we argue that, like the irrelevant contribution of incorrect retrieved information to FOK, many irrelevant (in terms of their relation to actual performance) factors contribute to feelings of confidence, thereby making them a non-reliable index of performance optimality. Some of these irrelevant factors are discussed in the following sections.

Personality traits

Personality traits have been found to have an impact on PDC. Block and Peterson (1955) found a curvilinear relationship between personal balance and adaptiveness and the degree of reported PDC. Individuals with intermediate levels of PDC were found to be more personally balanced and adaptive than those with extreme PDC, either low or high. Individuals possessing a concrete cognitive structure (Sieber and Lanzetta, 1966) as well as dogmatic people (Long and Ziller, 1965) exhibited overconfidence in a situation about which they lacked information.

Amount and quality of available information

Russo and Schoemaker (1989) argue that analysts may feel more confident with more information even if the additional information does not result in increased accuracy at all. This is exactly what was found by Oskamp (1965) regarding clinical judgements. Kahneman and Tversky (1973) have shown that people are most confident in judgement when information is consistent and/or extreme, even though these factors should reduce their confidence. Griffin and Tversky (1992) argue that overconfidence and underconfidence are explained by the hypothesis that people focus on the strength or extremes of the available evidence but pay insufficient regard to the credibility of the source of the evidence.

Perceived expertise

Trafimow and Sniezek (1994) asked introductory psychology students to answer fifty binary multiple-choice questions and to indicate their level of confidence for each question. The first ten questions were either extremely easy or extremely difficult, assuming that high or low perceived expertise would be primed respectively. It was found that those participants who were high in perceived expertise, as identified by the priming procedure, subsequently expressed more confidence than those who were low in perceived expertise, though there were no differences in OC, because performance was also affected by perceived expertise.

Level of internal conflict

The study by Zakay (1985) reported earlier indicates that the level of felt conflict while making a choice might affect PDC. This of course reduces PDC reliability as a measure of choice optimality because strong internal conflict might lead to a better choice than a weak conflict, which might reflect a superficial choice process. The relationship between PDC and level of internal conflict is well documented in the literature. Festinger's (1959) cognitive dissonance theory considers PDC to be a function of the magnitude of post-decisional dissonance reflecting the ratio of consonant to dissonant cognitions attached to each alternative. Adams and Adams (1961) as well as Janis and Mann (1968) also consider PDC to be an expression of the amount of conflict posed by the decision.

Motivational factors

Fischhoff and Beyth Marom (1983) as well as Mayseless and Kruglanski (1987) suggest that the motivational context characterising a specific decision making process may affect the feelings of confidence which are attached to that decision.

Post-decisional factors

We propose that PDC might be affected by heuristics and inferences which occur after a choice has already been made. Zakay and Tsal (1993) propose that factors like the use of a familiar strategy increase feelings of confidence, whereas other factors, such as the feeling of investing a great deal of mental effort in a decision process, decrease the level of confidence. Wagenaar (1988) claims that when people do not know the correct response required in a specific task, they try to infer it. Thus, it is possible that, although a response is incorrect, a respondent will feel very confident in his or her inferential reasoning, a contradiction leading to overconfidence.

To sum up, this review lists various factors which, despite not being relevant predictors of choice optimality or of knowledge-retrieval accuracy, affect feelings of confidence. This state of affairs leads to a lack of sensitivity to the actual level of difficulty of a task requiring knowledge retrieval (Lichtenstein *et al.*, 1982). People, in general, lack the ability to recognise the actual cognitive processes they are employing (Nisbett and Wilson, 1977) and knowledge retrieval and choice processes are no exception. Thus, feelings of confidence are strongly influenced by general and peripheral information, as well as by general considerations (Arkes *et al.*, 1987; Keren, 1987; Trafimow and Sniezek, 1994). In the following section, we demonstrate that one of the most influential determinants of PDC is prospective feelings of confidence which emerge prior to the start of a choice process.

AN EMPIRICAL STUDY OF THE IMPACT OF PROSPECTIVE FEELINGS OF CONFIDENCE ON PDC

Fourteen questions about capital cities throughout the world were designed according to the following format: 'What is the capital of France?: Paris; Rome'. According to a pilot study, seven of the selected questions were easy, with more than 80 per cent correct answers (e.g., France and Paris), while the rest were difficult to answer, with an average of 60 per cent correct answers (e.g., Brazil and Brasilia). Thirty-six high school students, whose studies included global geography, were randomly allocated to two groups. In the control group participants were asked to read fourteen questions, to mark the answer they thought correct and then to state their level of confidence in the correctness of the choice on a scale ranging from 50 to 100 where 50 was defined as chance level and 100 as certainty. It was emphasised to the participants that, if they did not know the answer, they should select the option with a higher level of probability of being correct. The questions were presented in random order of difficulty. Participants in the experimental group were asked, prior to being presented with the questions, to state their general feeling of prospective confidence (GPC) regarding their ability to answer correctly binary questions about capitals around the globe on the same scale as described above. They were then presented with a question (e.g., What is the capital of France?) without seeing the response options and were asked to state their specific prospective confidence (SPC) regarding their prospects of correctly answering the question. Finally, the options were presented, an answer was chosen and a PDC was stated. The same 50–100 scale described above was employed in the cases of SPC and PDC. The following dependent variables were calculated for each respondent: (1) percentage of correct answers in the easy questions (ER); (2) percentage of correct answers in the difficult questions (DR); (3) average PDC in the easy questions (PDE); (4) average PDC in the difficult questions (PDD); (5) overconfidence in the easy questions (OCE); (6) overconfidence in the difficult questions (OCD). Overconfidence (OC) was calculated as the weighted average of the difference between confidence and accuracy across confidence categories, with the number of items in each confidence category serving as the weighting factor. In the experimental group, the following indices were also calculated: (7) average SPC in the easy questions (SPE); (8) average SPC in the difficult questions (SPD) and (9) average GPC.

No significant differences were found between the experimental and control groups in ER, DR, OCE and OCD, indicating that the elicitation of GPC and of SPC did not influence knowledge retrieval and overconfidence levels. A significant difference was found, as expected, between ER and DR across groups, with respective values of 93.92 and 56.56 per cent. The data supported the hard–easy effect: OCE was –11.42 and –13.12 in the control and experimental groups respectively and OCD was 18.83 and 12.98 in the control and experimental groups respectively. In order to demonstrate that PDC was strongly influenced by GPC and SPC, Pearson's correlations between the dependent indices were computed in the experimental group. The correlation coefficients are presented in Table 14.1.

As illustrated in Table 14.1, PDC explains only about 3 per cent of the variance in performance. SPC explains about 80 per cent of the variance in PDC. A multiple regression analysis was conducted with PDC as a dependent measure and GPC, SPC and performance as independent variables. A significant R^2 (0.85) was obtained and the only significant contribution was found to be that of SPC. Performance was not found to have any significant effect. In order to demonstrate further that overconfidence and the hard–easy effect do not necessarily reflect the choice processes, the differences between SPC and performance scores were calculated separately for the easy and difficult questions, yielding prospective overconfidence scores. Analysis of variance revealed a significant hard–easy effect with average prospective overconfidence scores of –28.10 and 6.08 in the easy and difficult questions, respectively.

The findings obtained in this experiment clearly demonstrate that PDC is not a good reflection of the optimality of choice processes and is not correlated with performance. PDC is highly influenced by pre-choice variables, such as general prospective confidence about one's ability to retrieve correct knowledge in a specific domain, but primarily by specific prospective confidence feelings. It is clear that SPC is a pure pre-decision rating

Table 14.1 Pearson's correlation coefficients (n = 18)

	SPC[1]	*PDC*[2]	*Performance (% correct)*
GPC[3]	0.36	0.31	0.05
SPC		0.90	0.28
PDC			0.17

Notes:
1 SPC = specific prospective confidence
2 PDC = post-decisional confidence
3 GPC = general prospective confidence

because at the time of the rating no choice options existed. It should be noted that, although there was a significant decrease in level of PDC from easy to difficult questions, this decrease was not strong enough to compensate for the much larger respective decrease in performance. Whereas the ratio of ER to ED was 1.60, the ratio of PDE to PDD was only 1.11.

AN EMPIRICAL STUDY OF CONFIDENCE IN PROFESSIONAL CHOICES

The following experiment was designed by Zakay and Yaaron (1996) to demonstrate the lack of sensitivity of PDC outside the domain of retrieval of knowledge for general knowledge questions. Twenty-five basketball video films showing NBA games were edited so that in each piece of video 20 seconds of a continuous game was presented and then a player was seen receiving the ball. At this point the picture froze, showing the player holding the ball and all the other players of both teams in their positions. Participants were expert basketball players from three age groups: adults ranging in age from 20 to 30 years, juniors ranging in age from 12 to 13 years and children ranging in age from 7 to 9 years. The adults were professional players in the first Israeli national basketball league. The juniors were players in the first junior Israeli national basketball league and the children were selected by trainers as promising basketball players and had participated regularly in basketball courses. Control groups were matched to the experimental groups in terms of age, education and general lifestyle, but control participants, also being basketball players, were far less expert in the game. Twenty-five video pieces were constructed, each presenting a different game condition. The videos were shown to the participants individually, in a random order, and they were required to decide on the most appropriate move for the player holding the ball (i.e., throwing to the basket, penetrating or delivering the ball to another player whom they were asked to indicate). No time limit was imposed. Three professional high-level trainers analysed each video and decided upon the correct move. Only those videos regarding which the three trainers reached a unanimous choice were presented to the participants. After reaching a decision, each participant was asked to report his feelings of confidence in the correctness of his decision. This was done on a ten-point scale, 1 denoting 'not confident at all' and 10 denoting 'entirely confident'. The proportion of correct decisions (PC) and the average confidence level (PDC) were calculated for each participant. PDC was calculated for all twenty-five decisions as a group and separately for correct and incorrect decisions. Overconfidence scores could not be calculated since it was not possible to discover the exact number of alternatives considered by each participant. The findings are presented in Table 14.2.

Table 14.2 Means of PC and PDC according to expertise and age

	Adults			*Juniors*			*Children*			*Total*		
	PC[1]	*PDC*[2]	*n*[3]	*PC*	*PDC*	*n*	*PC*	*PDC*	*n*	*PC*	*PDC*	*n*
Experts	.80	8.88	17	.80	8.75	15	.55	8.78	13	.72	8.80	45
Non-experts	.68	8.64	16	.67	8.57	15	.25	8.46	14	.54	8.56	45
	.74	8.76	33	.74	8.66	30	.38	8.61	27	.63	8.68	90

Notes:
1 PC = proportion correct
2 PDC = post-decisional confidence
3 n = number of respondents

The following significant results were found for PC scores. As age increased, more correct decisions were made. Additionally, experts of all three age groups made more correct decisions than non-experts. However, the difference between expert and non-expert was larger for children. No significant effects were obtained for age or for expertise for PDC scores, despite the relatively large difference in performance quality. The average levels of PDC across groups were significantly higher for correct than for incorrect decisions (8.88 and 8.26, respectively). However, the decrease in PDC from correct to incorrect decisions was negligible and thus does not reflect the change from correct to incorrect responses.

Another interesting finding was the correlation between the latency times and PDC. These correlations were negative and significant (-0.47) for the juniors and negative and approaching significance (-0.34) for the adults, for both the expert and non-expert groups. This finding indicates that the faster decisions were made, the more confident participants felt. This feeling, however, was not justified since the correlation between latency times and PC was very low and non-significant, especially for the non-experts.

CONCLUDING REMARKS

The evidence reviewed in this chapter suggests that retrospective feelings of confidence in general, and PDC in particular, are based on multi-dimensional sources. Some of these sources are not related to post-decisional factors, and others are pre-decisional factors such as heuristics and inferences, personality traits, and motivational factors. The quality of the individual's background knowledge (May, 1986) and prospective feelings of confidence are also strong determinants of retrospective feelings of confidence. This notion is compatible with Peterson and Pitz's (1988) view that confidence is influenced by salient factors that, people believe, affect the accuracy of their predictions. These factors include the type of strategy used and feelings of comfort while making a decision. Zakay and Tsal (1993) also propose that PDC is a reflection of an ongoing internal cost–benefit interaction between factors which either increase or decrease a decision maker's satisfaction with his or her decision making process. Because of such processes, retrospective feelings of confidence are only moderately correlated with choice optimality or with the accuracy of knowledge retrieval. Unfortunately, feelings of confidence emerge as a result of automatic processes and are therefore difficult to control. Nevertheless, it should not be forgotten that having a feeling of reasonable confidence is necessary from a motivational point of view. When one is not feeling confident, one will most probably feel reluctant to act (Taylor and Brown, 1988). Underconfidence also has its shortcomings because a lack of initiative and ability to be daring are often associated with underconfidence. Therefore the claim that overconfidence should be eliminated is too extreme. Instead, the costs and benefits of both overconfidence and underconfidence should be weighed. Even though Griffin and Tversky (1992) doubt that the benefits of overconfidence outweigh its costs, the problem is more complicated than it appears. Decision makers therefore face the problem not of ignoring feelings of confidence altogether but rather of calibrating them properly. This is a problematic and difficult task. In the context of overconfidence research, most of the so-called debiasing methods aimed at reducing OC have been ineffective (Granhag, 1996; Trafimow and Sniezek, 1994). A possible reason for this is that, in order to calibrate feelings of confidence, all of the various factors which contribute to these feelings must be treated simultaneously, a goal that is not easy to achieve.

Further research should identify all the origins of feelings of confidence and the processes which integrate them. Only if all of the relevant factors, those outlined in this chapter as well as others which will be identified by future research, are taken into account will optimal debiasing methods be developed.

REFERENCES

Adams, J.K. and Adams, P.A. (1961) 'Realism of confidence judgments', *Psychological Review*, 68: 33–45.

Allwood, C.M. and Montgomery, H. (1987) 'Response selection strategies and realism of confidence judgments', *Organizational Behavior and Human Decision Processes*, 39(3): 365–83.

Arkes, J.H., Christensen, C., Lai, C. and Blumer, C. (1987) 'Two methods of reducing overconfidence', *Organizational Behavior and Human Decision Processes*, 39: 133–44.

Bathwell, R.K., Deffenbacher, K.A. and Brigham, J.C. (1987) 'Correlation of eyewitness accuracy and confidence: optimality hypothesis revisited', *Journal of Applied Psychology*, 72(4): 691–5.

Block, J. and Peterson, P. (1955) 'Some personality correlates of confidence, caution and speed in a decision situation', *Journal of Abnormal and Social Psychology*, 51: 34–41.

Christensen-Szalanski, J.J.J. and Busyhead, J.B. (1981) 'Physician's use of probabilistic information in a real clinical setting', *Journal of Experimental Psychology: Human Perception and Performance*, 7: 928–35.

Cutler, B.L., Penrod, S.D. and Sture, T.E. (1988) 'Juror decision making in eyewitness identification cases', *Law and Human Behavior*, 12: 41–55.

Festinger, L.A. (1959) *A Theory of Cognitive Dissonance*, Evanston, IL: Row Peterson.

Fischhoff, B. and Beyth Marom, R. (1983) 'Hypothesis evaluation from a Bayesian perspective', *Psychological Review*, 90(3): 239–60.

Fischhoff, B. and MacGregor, D. (1982) 'Subjective confidence in forecasts', *Journal of Forecasting*, 1: 155–72.

Granhag, P.A. (1996) 'Realism in confidence judgments of semantic and episodic knowledge', Ph.D. dissertation, Göteborg University, Sweden.

Griffin, D. and Tversky, A. (1992) 'The weighing of evidence and the determinants of confidence', *Cognitive Psychology*, 24: 411–535.

Janis, I.L. and Mann, L. (1968) 'A conflict theory approach to attitude change and decision making', in A. Greenwald, T. Bruck and K. Ostram (eds) *Psychological Foundation of Attitudes*, New York: Academic Press.

Kahneman, D. and Tversky, A. (1973) 'On the psychology of prediction', *Psychological Review*, 80: 251–73.

Keren, G. (1987) 'Facing uncertainty in the game of bridge: a calibration study', *Organizational Behavior and Human Decision Processes*, 39: 98–114.

Keren, G. (1988) 'On the ability of monitoring non-veridical perception and uncertain knowledge: some calibration studies', *Acta Psychologica*, 67: 95–119.

Koriat, A. (1993) 'How do we know that we know: the accessibility model of feeling of knowing', *Psychological Review*, 100(4): 609–32.

Kruglanski, A.W., Peri, N. and Zakay, D. (1991) 'Interactive effects of need for closure and initial confidence on social information seeking', *Social Cognition*, 9: 127–48.

Lichtenstein, S. and Fischhoff, B. (1977) 'Do those who know more also know more about how much they know?', *Organizational Behavior and Human Performance*, 20: 159–83.

Lichtenstein, S., Fischhoff, B. and Phillips, L.D. (1982) 'Calibration of probabilities: the state of the art of 1980', in D. Kahneman, P. Slovic and A. Tversky (eds) *Judgment Under Uncertainty: Heuristics and Biases*, Cambridge: Cambridge University Press.

Loftus, E.F., Donders, K., Hoffman, H.G. and Schooler, J.W. (1989) 'Creating new memories that are quickly accessed and confidently held', *Memory and Cognition*, 17: 607–16.

Loftus, E.F. and Wagenaar, W.A. (1988) 'Lawyers' predictions of success', *Jurimetrics Journal*, 437–53.

Long, B.H. and Ziller, R.C. (1965) 'Dogmatism and predecisional information research', *Journal of Applied Psychology*, 49: 376–8.

May, R.S. (1986) 'Overconfidence as a result of incomplete and wrong knowledge', in R.W. Schalz (ed.) *Current Issues in West German Decision Research*, New York: Lang, 13–30.

Mayseless, O. and Kruglanski, A.W. (1987) 'What makes you so sure? Effects of epistemic motivations on judgmental confidence', *Organizational Behavior and Human Decision Processes*, 39: 62–183.

Miner, A.C. and Reder, L.M. (1994) 'A new look at feeling of knowing: its metacognitive role in regulating question answering', in J. Metcalfe and A.P. Shimamura (eds) *Metacognition: Knowing about Knowing*, Cambridge, MA: MIT Press, 48–70.

Nelson, T.O., Gerber, D. and Narens, L. (1984) 'Accuracy of feeling of knowing judgements for predicting perceptual identification and relearning', *Journal of Experimental Psychology: General*, 113: 282–300.

Nisbett, R.E. and Wilson, T.D. (1977) 'Telling more than we can know: verbal reports on mental processes', *Psychological Review*, 84: 231–59.

Oskamp, S. (1965) 'Overconfidence in case-study judgments', *Journal of Consulting Psychology*, 29: 261–5.

Peterson, D.K. and Pitz, G.F. (1988) 'Confidence, uncertainty and use of information', *Journal of Experimental Psychology: Learning, Memory and Cognition*, 85–92.

Russo, J.E. and Schoemaker, J.H. (1989) *Decision Traps*, New York: Simon and Schuster.

Sen, T.S. and Boe, W.J. (1991) 'Confidence and accuracy in judgements using computer displayed information', *Behavior and Information Technology*, 10: 53–64.

Sieber, J.E. and Lanzetta, Y.T. (1966) 'Some determinants of individual differences in predecision information processing behavior', *Journal of Personality and Social Psychology*, 4: 561–71.

Solomon, I., Ariyo, A. and Tomasini, L.A. (1985) 'Contextual effects on the calibration of probabilistic judgments', *Journal of Applied Psychology*, 70: 528–32.

Slovic, P., Fischhoff, B. and Lichtenstein, S. (1977) 'Behavioral Decision theory', *Annual Review of Psychology*, 28: 1–39.

Sporer, S.L., Penrod, S., Read, D. and Cutler, B. (1995) 'Choosing, confidence and accuracy: a meta-analysis of the confidence–accuracy relation in eyewitness studies', *Psychological Bulletin*, 118(3): 315–27.

Suantak, L., Bolger, F. and Ferrell, W.R. (1996) 'The hard–easy effect in subjective probability calibration', *Organizational Behavior and Human Decision Processes*, 67(2): 201–21.

Taylor, S.E. and Brown, J.D. (1988) 'Illusion and well-being: a social psychological perspective on mental health', *Psychological Bulletin*, 103: 193–210.

Thompson, W.B. and Mason, S.E. (1996) 'Instability of individual differences in the association between confidence judgements and memory performance', *Memory and Cognition*, 24(2): 226–34.

Trafimow, D. and Sniezek, J.A. (1994) 'Perceived expertise and its effect on confidence', *Organizational Behavior and Human Decision Processes*, 57: 290–302.

Wagenaar, W.A. (1988) 'Calibration and the effects of knowledge and reconstruction in retrieval from memory', *Cognition*, 28: 277–96.

Weingardt, K.R., Leonesia, R.J. and Loftus, E.F. (1994) 'Viewing eyewitness research from a metacognitive perspective', in J. Metcalfe, and A. Shimamura (eds) *Metacognition: Knowing about Knowing*, Cambridge, MA: MIT Press.

Wells, G.L. and Murray, D.M. (1984) 'Eyewitness confidence', in G.L. Wells and E.F. Loftus (eds.), *Eyewitness Testimony: Psychological Perspectives*, Cambridge: Cambridge University Press.

Wickens, C.D., Stakes, A., Barnett, B. and Hyman, F. (1993) 'The effects of stress on pilot judgement in a MIDIS simulator', in O. Svenson and A.J. Maule (eds) *Time Pressure and Stress in Human Judgment and Decision Making*, New York: Plenum, 271–92.

Wright, G.N. and Phillips, L.D. (1976) *Personality and Probabilistic Thinking: An Experimental Study*, Tech. Ref. 76–3, Uxbridge, England: Brunel Institute of Organizational and Social Studies.

Zakay, D. (1985) 'Post-decisional confidence and conflict experienced in a choice process', *Acta Psychiatrica*, 58: 75–80.

Zakay, D. (1992) 'The influence of computerized feedback on overconfidence in knowledge', *Behavior and Information Technology*, 11(6): 329–33.

Zakay, D. and Glickshon, J. (1992) 'Overconfidence in a multiple-choice test and its relationship with achievement', *The Psychological Record*, 42: 519–24.

Zakay, D. and Tsal, Y. (1993) 'The impact of using forced decision-making strategies on post-decisional confidence', *Journal of Behavioral Decision Making*, 6: 53–68.

Zakay, D. and Yaaron, M. (1996) 'Expertise and duration estimation', Unpublished manuscript, Tel-Aviv University, Israel.

Index

For Product Safety Concerns and Information please contact our EU representative GPSR@taylorandfrancis.com
Taylor & Francis Verlag GmbH, Kaufingerstraße 24, 80331 München, Germany

www.ingramcontent.com/pod-product-compliance
Lightning Source LLC
LaVergne TN
LVHW011121300926
849160LV00008B/462

* 9 7 8 0 4 1 5 5 1 3 5 9 3 *